Thriver Soup

A Feast for Living Consciously During the Cancer Journey

For Nicole,
  May you thrive!
    Injoy,
      Heidi M Bright

Praise for Thriver Soup

"Heidi has something for everyone in *Thriver Soup*: practical tips for coping with the side effects of cancer treatment, notes on healthy living, explorations into how different religious and spiritual traditions can inspire, and most importantly, an invitation to use a life-threatening illness to find renewed meaning and purpose in one's journey."

—Sheryl Cohen, PhD, Psychologist and Director, Temenos

"*Thriver Soup* provides much-needed inspiration that cuts across religious lines for women diagnosed with cancer. So many people in this culture feel, deep down, that they are fundamentally bad and deserving of illness; Heidi's bright spirit radiates Basic Goodness and can be a source of comfort for anyone suffering or challenged. She communicates with an openness and vulnerability that will empower readers to accept and work with their individual situations. Those of us in the helping professions will want to keep a copy of *Thriver Soup* as a reference for people who might be helped by her insights, wisdom, and practical tips."

—Marian Judith Broadus, PhD, Licensed Psychologist, Co-editor,
"Conversations in Psychosynthesis"

"Heidi Bright is one of the bravest women I know. From the moment she received her diagnosis of a rare, aggressive, terminal cancer with an extremely low survival rate, she became determined not to die. She left no stone unturned in her search for anything that would restore her health and vitality. In this invaluable resource, she spares nothing in equipping readers with everything they need to know if they, or loved ones, are on the cancer journey. A cancer diagnosis is not the time to lose hope...it's the time to decide to thrive. That's what Heidi did and she transformed not only her body, but her inner and outer life as well. In this book, she explains in detail how you can do the same. I highly recommend *Thriver Soup*."

—Tara L. Robinson, Publisher, *Whole Living Journal*, and radio host

"*Thriver Soup* helps me see that life is uncertain, fleeting, precious, bursting with opportunity and delight; that the enemy is not death, but fear—fear of living authentically and joyfully, fear of deeply trusting ourselves; that we have at our disposal an incredible array of potent tools for healing and healthy living; that strength comes from connecting with Spirit, connecting with a communion of caring souls, connecting with the intuitive wisdom of our bodies and our spiritual hearts; that acceptance and hard work and taking risks and having fun are harbingers of vibrant health; that we are hardwired to thrive, to love unconditionally, to serve courageously, to bless others abundantly."

—Sam Quick, PhD, Professor Emeritus and Human Development Specialist

" *I* don't think of myself as having a strong willpower, but Heidi has been an inspiration to me in this matter. Through reading her book, she has become my model for a person using utmost willpower to fight for her life, for going the extra mile, for really doing her best. I sincerely respect her and think of her when I need more strength to do what needs to be done. Her ability to blend Western medicine and alternative medicine is really inspiring. I recommend this book for those seeking an original and thoughtful and kind way through the maze of cancer."

—Mim Grace Gieser, yoga instructor and
Certified Emotional Freedom Technique Practitioner

Notifications

Heidi Bright was awarded Ohio Arts Council Artist with Disabilities grants for professional editing in 2012 and for marketing and promotion in 2015.

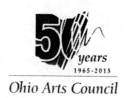

Ohio Arts Council

Thriver Soup

A Feast for Living Consciously During the Cancer Journey

Heidi Bright, MDiv

SUNSTONE
PRESS

SANTA FE

Author's Note

All ideas and information included in this book are intended for informational purposes only, and should not be interpreted as specific medical advice. Neither is any information intended for self-diagnosis or self-treatment. Please consult with a qualified healthcare professional for assistance before making decisions about therapies and/or health conditions.

Sunstone books may be purchased for educational, business, or sales promotional use. For information please write: Special Markets Department, Sunstone Press, P.O. Box 2321, Santa Fe, New Mexico 87504-2321.

Cover Image › Keith and Margaret Klein
Book and cover design › Vicki Ahl
Body typeface › Minion Pro
Display typeface › Vladimir Script
Printed on acid-free paper
∞
eBook 978-1-61139-374-3

Library of Congress Cataloging-in-Publication Data

Bright, Heidi, 1961-
Thriver soup : a feast for living consciously during the cancer journey / by Heidi Bright, MDIv.
  pages cm
  ISBN 978-1-63293-059-0 (softcovers : alk. paper)
  1. Cancer--Treatment--Popular works. 2. Cancer--Psychological aspects--Popular works. 3. Self-care, Health. 4. Mental healing. I. Title.
  RC270.8.B75 2015
  616.99'4--dc23

                          2015006210

WWW.SUNSTONEPRESS.COM
SUNSTONE PRESS / POST OFFICE BOX 2321 / SANTA FE, NM 87504-2321 /USA
(505) 988-4418 / ORDERS ONLY (800) 243-5644 / FAX (505) 988-1025

Contents

C. Mapping the Emotions — 183
Introduction to Mapping the Emotions: Linking Heart and Body

D. Mending the Mind — 235
Introduction to Mending the Mind: Entering Peace Like an Arrow

E. It Takes a Village — 277
Introduction to It Takes a Village: Sharing the Moment...Sharing Life

F. Soaring with Spirit — 295
Introduction to Soaring with Spirit: Wrestling with the Divine

9. GPS: Guides Providing and Sustaining — 330
Introduction to GPS: Guides Providing and Sustaining, Even a Donkey

Glossary — 355
Sources — 358
Other Resources — 376

Acknowledgments

*J*ust as it takes a village to survive cancer, it takes a group of people to birth a book. With deep gratitude, I would like to acknowledge all of the people who helped me with idea formation, editing, and writing the manuscript and its proposal. These individuals also offered a variety of other forms of assistance and support during the time I was dealing with cancer. They are listed in alphabetical order. My apologies to anyone my chemo brain failed to record or recall: Tami Boehmer, Roselie A. Bright, ScD, Trish Bright, Judith Broadus, PhD, Bonnie Crawford, MSW, Laura Dailey, MSW, Clark Echols, MDiv, Janine Hagan, Wendy Henry, Vince Lasorso, Mark Lewandoski, PhD, Judy Merritt, PhD, Kathy Nace, Kathryn Martin Ossege, Maria Paglialungo, Judy Peace, Sam Quick, PhD, Barb Spidel Smith, and Ruthy Trussler. Providing further editing support were Patricia Garry, Kathleen O'Neill, Theresa P. Maue, PhD, and Sheila Mudd Baker, MSOL.

I feel special appreciation for my friend Mim Grace Gieser and my psychotherapist Sheryl Cohen, PhD, both of whom read and provided valuable feedback on the entire manuscript. And my thanks to the Ohio Arts Council for fully funding a grant that enabled me to obtain some professional editing of the manuscript and proposal by Rebecca Woods, MDiv. I am grateful to Tara L. Robinson who wrote a letter of support when I applied for the grant.

I am thankful Anyaa McAndrew, MA, put me in touch with Linda Star Wolf, DMin, PhD; and that Star Wolf believed in me and my manuscript.

I will attempt to list all those who helped me during this terrible time in my life, and to whom I feel gratitude.

My then-husband took me to nearly every chemotherapy session and surgery for sixteen months and proposed a life-saving choice of surgery before more chemotherapy. He stepped in to do a lot of caregiving during this time even while working long hours at his engineering job.

My father, Charles D. Bright, PhD, provided generous assistance and helped fulfill my long-time desire to eat at the top of the Space Needle.

My step-mother, June Bright, brought my dad to Cincinnati for a visit, during which she took me to and from chemotherapy.

My sister Roselie called upon all her friends and colleagues to help her find and connect with the best uterine sarcoma oncologists in the country. She met three of these oncologists with me, taking notes and providing valuable insights, questions, suggestions, and assertiveness with the oncologists. She secured housing and transportation for us and my brother Jim for some of the time we were in Houston. She also gave me smiley-face buttons to wear, a quilt, and some wigs, and made a silly hat for me. Roselie and her husband Mark provided my then-husband and me with housing through his friend Cindy in Manhattan, NY, and with transportation during our visit to the Memorial Sloan-Kettering Cancer Center. After I settled on an oncologist in Ohio, Roselie attended my visits over the phone. Roselie helped me and the rest of our family understand my particular sarcoma by translating my medical records and technical cancer literature into terms we could all understand.

Roselie and I are also grateful for two of her resources who helped her assist me: Current and former employees of the National Cancer Institute for finding the best uterine sarcoma oncologists in the country; and the librarian at the MD Anderson Cancer Center patient library in Houston, who helped Roselie quickly identify and copy the most recent relevant lay- and medical-level literature at no cost.

My brother Jim Bright met with Roselie and me at MD Anderson. He offered insights into how we should approach the physicians. His assertiveness ensured I got the straight answers I needed. He provided transportation assistance and secured housing for Roselie and me with his friends David Prasse, MSEE, and Ellen Prasse, MS, in Houston. Jim, his wife Janet Bright, MS, and their two children, James and Mindy, offered their hospitality and generously gave thoughtful gifts throughout my treatments.

My brother Charlie Bright, MSME, and his wife Sheila Bright, RN, helped out greatly with our kids and sent thoughtful, enjoyable gifts.

My brother Walter Bright and his wife Trish Bright gave me a Vitamix high-speed blender. They extended their hospitality to my then-husband and me before our Alaskan cruise and helped fulfill my long-time desire to eat at the top of the Space Needle. They continued to send gifts to delight and entertain me. Their daughter Grace painted a black panther that was imprinted on a tote I used during each chemotherapy treatment.

Maria Paglialungo, an energy intuitive, supported and assisted me before and during my two years of treatment, offering numerous valuable and life-altering insights and wisdom along the way.

Brecka Burton-Platt gave me several intuitive healing touch sessions and blessed me with gifts of wisdom, insight, time, and tea.

Laura Dailey drove me to and from many appointments, offered kind hospitality, and gave gifts of time, a listening ear, and beauty.

Mim Grace Gieser taught me how to do the Emotional Freedom Technique and offered her generous hospitality.

Tracy Lilly and her children, Avery and Austin, graciously opened their home to Roselie and me; our connection was that Tracy's sister worked with Roselie.

Cathy Robbins picked me up from medical procedures, even driving two hours one way to bring me home. She created a helping community on the Lotsa Helping Hands website. She also crocheted a beautiful shawl that kept me warm during CT scans, along with some woolly warm socks.

Connie and Vince Lasorso, co-owners of Whatever Works Wellness Center and White Willow School of Tai Chi, continually offered energy work, life-altering wise counsel, and thoughtful gifts. Vince, a tai chi master, taught me Level 1 of tai chi as well.

Paula Overstreet drove more than two hours to take me to surgery, and provided constant encouragement throughout my process.

Trudy Deutsch assisted with many neighborly chores, helped my kids, brought over several meals, and gave thoughtful gifts.

John Hill taught me a healing chi gong practice and the Bengston image-cycling technique.

Debbie Dougan, RN, and Cynthia Wells helped with wound and house care after my second lung surgery.

Kathryn Martin Ossege set me up on a CaringBridge blog site and gave me my most dog-eared book, *Waking the Warrior Goddess*, by Christine Horner, MD.

Charley Sky wrote a lovely column for a local magazine, asking the community to support me with prayer, visualizations, and affirmations.

Many people helped with watching our sons and/or providing transportation for them at various times, as well as other gifts of support, including Rebecca and Dan Woods, Morissa Ladinsky, MD, and Loveland soccer coaches Michael and Jim.

Shannon and Galen Mills gave me several needed rides.

Amma, the hugging saint, specifically prayed for me and ensured that I would receive holy and blessed ashes to use during my treatments.

I feel deep gratitude for my health care team, including Larry Copeland, MD; James Pavelka, MD; Patrick Ross, MD; Sheryl Cohen, PhD; Hari Sharma, MD; Edward Lim, MD; Victoria Mosso, RN; Michael J. Panyko, DC; Lani J. Lee, LAc; Linda Havenar; and the chemotherapy nurses at Ohio State University's Gynecologic Oncology center in Hilliard, Ohio, and St. Elizabeth Cancer Care Center in Edgewood, Kentucky.

For the myriad of other thoughtful, loving gifts and support that helped me through this journey, I wish to thank the following (in alphabetical order by first name or word): Anne McQuinn, Barb Mount, Becky and Doug Jones, Marybeth and Helmut Wolf, Charoula Dontopoulos, Cynthia Wells, Denise Fuqua, Diane Faul, Dona Sarno, MA, Eric Ornella, DDS, MSD, Fran Matteson, MS, Fay Gano, Gary Matthews, Geoff Hodges, MSEE, Gillian Mayer, Heather Duncan, Hillary Pecsok, Jean Koppes, Jill Becker, Joanne Ziolkowski, MBA, Jorjann Chezem, Judi Winall, MDiv, Judy Leamy, RN, LSN, Karen Wagner, Kathy Nace, Kay Smay, Kelley Hall, Lesley Jackson, Li Bradshaw, PhD, Lois Clement, MA, Loretta Novince, PhD, Louis Valentine, DC, Loveland's Boy Scout Troop 888, Marilyn Moore Hudson, MSCE, Marlys Book and Chris Book, MAE, Mark Zeiner, Marnie Poirier, Mary Lu Lageman, MS, Mary Manera, MA, Mica Renes, ND, Michael and Sarah Davis, Morgan Dragonwillow, Nancy Lawlor, MA, Norma Gracia Munive-Prime, Norma Wirt, Northeast Community Challenge Coalition, Pat and Jim Brugger, Philip G. Helburn, MA, Erik Madsen, Renate Madsen, MA, Sharon Howison, Steve Edwards, Susan Smith-Sargent, Teri Dettone, Valerie DeMathews, and the women of Galveston United Methodist Church.

I also wish to thank all those thousands of individuals who supported me through prayers, phone calls, emails, and my CaringBridge blog.

Thank you, from the bottom of my heart, for helping to save my life and for making this book possible.

Reference Acknowledgments

Scripture quotations marked (NIV) are taken from the Holy Bible, New International Version, NIV. Copyright © 1973, 1978, 1984, 2011 by Biblica, Inc. Used by permission of Zondervan. All rights reserved worldwide. www.zondervan.com The "NIV" and "New International Version" are trademarks registered in the United States Patent and Trademark Office by Biblica, Inc.

Scripture quotations are taken from the Complete Jewish Bible, copyright 1998 by David H. Stern. Published by Jewish New Testament Publications, Inc. www.messianicjewish.net/jntp. Distributed by Messianic Jewish Resources Int'l. www.messianicjewish.net. All rights reserved. Used by permission.

Scripture quotations are taken from *God Talks with Arjuna: The Bhagavad Gita*, by Paramahansa Yogananda, copyright 1995, 1999. Published by Self-Realization Fellowship, Los Angeles, California. Used by permission.

Scripture quotations are taken from the New American Standard Bible, Copyright © 1960, 1962, 1963, 1968, 1971, 1972, 1973, 1975, 1977, 1995 by The Lockman Foundation. Used by permission. (www.Lockman.org)

NET Bible scripture quoted by permission. Quotations designated (NET) are from the NET Bible® copyright ©1996-2006 by Biblical Studies Press, L.L.C. http://netbible.com All rights reserved.

Quotes from the Qur'an, unless otherwise noted, are from a translation by Yusuf Ali in The Holy Qur-an, published in Lahore, Pakistan, in 1934. The text was copied with permission from www.sacred-texts.com/isl/yaq/index.htm and retrieved April 25, 2014.

Introduction

Beloved, I pray that in all respects you may prosper and be in good health, just as your soul prospers.
—3 John 2, Christian Bible, New American Standard Bible

I thought I had been sentenced to die. Instead, I had been invited to live joyfully so my soul could prosper.

In March 2009 I awoke from a dream in which an ogre stole the contents of a large, beautifully carved egg. To me, this indicated some aspect of my feminine nature had been abducted. The dream answered my question—yes, I would commit to a nine-month gestation with a circle of women. We would assist each other with birthing the Divine feminine within ourselves and bringing that consciousness into the world. Psychotherapist Anyaa McAndrew would lead us through this "priestess process."

At the same time, my family doctor ordered an ultrasound for a hard mass in my lower abdomen. The diagnosis: benign uterine fibroids. The chances of there being cancer were slim, especially since I was so healthy. I saw no need to continue testing; I chose to work with the fibroid through nutritional supplements and tai chi exercises until I reached menopause, a time when benign uterine fibroids generally disappear.

During a meeting with the women's circle in June, one of the participants, Judy Merritt, suggested I read *Bluebeard,* a French folktale in which a man kills his successive wives. Judy, a psychologist, intuited that my uterus had a story to tell and provided me with an important metaphor.

During the first week of July, I used my imagination to pretend I was entering Bluebeard's castle. What did the murderer have to do with me, if anything?

The fierce answer came: Bluebeard lopped off my left arm and carved out all my reproductive parts below my ribs, stuffed them into a bag and threw them into his frozen dungeon. Later, a healthy inner masculine figure arrived and took me to a hospital. He returned to Bluebeard's castle with a pistol—a sufficiently potent masculine weapon—to rescue my sack of feminine body parts and return them to me. All was restored.

The imaginary experience soon manifested in physical reality. Within two weeks I lay under the surgeon's knife. Out came my cancer-filled cervix, uterus, fallopian tubes, ovaries, and six inches of small intestine.

Bluebeard had accomplished his evil deed.

Scans exposed a cancerous spot on my lung. The highly undifferentiated endometrial sarcoma had metastasized and I was flung headlong into the fight of—and for—my life.

My heroine's journey to survive stage IV of an incredibly rare and highly aggressive cancer took me deep into my soul and far away to specialized physicians. I chose to use both conventional methods and complementary healing modalities—a choice that most likely saved my life. A village of lovely people supported and prayed for me every step of the way.

One of them was my friend and energy intuitive, Maria Paglialungo. During the winter of 2011 she told me about her experiment making soup from scratch. At first it tasted pretty good. So she added something else. And something else. And something else. By the time she finished adding, the smorgasbord soup tasted awful.

Just as Maria learned that her way of preparing such a meal didn't work too well, cancer patients who dabble in a wide variety of treatments might find limited benefit. A smorgasbord approach might even be dangerous. Instead, I think a recipe-style template might work better, providing a strategy for reaching the goal of healing or even a cure. I have seen this approach to cooking in magazines. A certain type of food will be suggested, such as vegetable soup. The author will present a few categories for the basic ingredients: stock bases, herbs, vegetables, and fats. Select one or more items from each list and you'll probably have a meal. Throw everything in and you might produce an unsavory mess.

When applied to surviving cancer, there are major treatment categories to seriously consider: conventional treatments of surgery, chemotherapy, and radiation, along with complementary options for healing the body, emotions, mind, and spirit.

As others urged me to do, I now also highly recommend staying with the conventional recommendations of a Western oncologist who specializes in the type of cancer you have. I believe this is particularly true if your doctor has set the cancer beyond stage I. My sister, Roselie Bright, proved an invaluable encourager and supporter of my conventional medical treatments, working tirelessly to find and help me get appointments with the best uterine sarcoma oncologists in the United States. She, my brother Jim Bright, and my then-husband pressed for answers during my medical appointments and provided useful advice—and recall—while I still reeled from the shock.

I also wanted guidance for selecting complementary healing methods. Vince and Connie Lasorso, co-owners of Whatever Works Wellness Center, possessed decades of experience with cancer patients and provided exquisite insights. They encouraged me to approach the illness 100 percent from each of the following non-medical areas: nutrition, body care, emotional healing, mental attitudes, spiritual exercises, and social relations.

For those living with a stage IV diagnosis, I now believe this whole-person approach is key for any chance of reaching a physical cure and for psychological and spiritual healing. In my desperation for a cure, I approached the cancer from every category. I tried out almost every healing modality I mention in this book. Some worked for me; some didn't. I needed to sift and settle upon the treatments I found most beneficial for my particular body and circumstances. I am sure I saved myself much suffering by following a variety of practices; I also became a better human being. Eventually I found a Thriver Soup mix that worked best for me.

So, too, I believe a cancer patient could benefit from reviewing the various ideas presented here, and then selecting those that one feels are most comfortable and manageable. Be cautious about your choices before spending a lot of money. Reading "Recognizing Scams: Buyer Beware" in the "Mending the Mind" section could be a useful first step.

Ultimately, I believe we, as spiritual beings who entered into human form, came here to learn certain things. We are given a span of time in which to glean precious gifts for our souls. To a large extent, I think we have free will to choose to learn or not learn; to live or not live. I have two friends whose souls, I believe, accomplished their purposes, and both passed after months of struggling with cancer because it was their time to go. Neither was cured. In my opinion, even though both accomplished their purposes in their lives, one was healed and one was not. One experienced wisdom and acceptance, while one faded away. When I think of Treya Wilber, in the book *Grace and Grit: Spirituality and Healing in the Life and Death of Treya Killam Wilber*, I see a woman who was healed at the deepest levels, and who probably even experienced enlightenment, yet cancer still claimed her life. In my opinion, her soul had accomplished its purpose and it was time for it to move on.

I know a couple of other woman who probably could have lived far longer than they did. In my opinion, they experienced too much fear to do what was needed to survive, to make the paradigm shift required to live beyond the diagnosis. One had access to the knowledge that could have saved her life; the other did not have the guidance that could have taken her along a better path. Neither was to blame; neither was wrong. They simply did the best they were able to do with where they were at.

I understand the terrible and tremendous challenges I had to meet to save my life and fulfill at least one aspect of my soul's overall purpose. As far as I am concerned, the woman I had been, who was diagnosed with cancer in 2009, died. I am a new creation, and I continue evolving. If I had not made some terrifying yet crucial decisions, I am certain I would have died. I believe I am still alive for one or both of these reasons: I have more to learn, and I have more to give.

In my final analysis, the end results are not up to us; they are up to the Divine. I'm not convinced that everyone who works toward a physical cure long enough, or well enough, or who tries it all, can live longer. I think Treya did her absolute best to live, making changes in every aspect of her life, yet she passed anyway. It is my opinion that we are cured in Divine time, for Divine reasons, or we move on to the next life.

We can, however, positively affect our experiences along the way. While I gleaned much from trying out various ideas and treatment options, I learned that healing and curing are not always found in specific techniques or in trying everything. Rather, they probably require an internal shift that involves a transformation of one's physical, emotional, mental, spiritual, and/or social being.

For me, the changes took about eighteen months to solidify and I accepted that I had to greatly reduce stress in my life if I wanted to live. For you, the shift might involve something entirely different. And that is why I wrote this book—to ease your journey and possibly provide a key ingredient for your health and healing. Many of these entries were written while my experience was still fresh and raw, and reflect my own confusion. I am letting them be as they are, because those thoughts might be similar to your thoughts, and might provide you with more acceptance of your own sense of powerlessness and lack of understanding. Life is full of mystery, and you might land in a different place from where I landed. And that is perfectly fine; each of us must find our own ways and access our own inner wisdom and experiences of peace.

If you are newly diagnosed, I would suggest starting with a look at Heidi's Top Ten Quick-Start Tips. For more guidance along the way, you will find suggestions for how to select ingredients for your Thriver Soup recipe in the introductions to the conventional and complementary sections. Skim the entry headings to find whatever appears most relevant or useful to you. Select ingredients that resonate with you and make your own Thriver Soup.

To bring a spiritual dimension into the journey, each *Thriver Soup* entry begins with a relevant portion of sacred scripture or an ancient text from the world's great wisdom traditions. Humanity's variety of religions has brought meaning and purpose within different cultures and personal experiences. I believe the Divine speaks to people where they are at and in ways that offer individual guidance and meaning. I see value in all wisdom traditions and believe all can be of assistance, even to people of different faiths. Because of the multiplicity of traditions and names given to the Source of All, I have selected the more generic words Divine and Spirit as reference points. As you read, substitute whatever term feels most comfortable to you.

Each entry continues with a personal story concerning the cancer journey. A practical tip rounds out each reading, providing a suggestion for applying the concept. Many are offered for fun; others might provide you with insights for your own journey. Taste the *Thriver Soup* ingredients that appear appetizing to you and create your own feast.

A glossary in the back explains a variety of terms used within the book. For example, I use the term "ankhologist" instead of oncologist, because the Egyptian ankh is the symbol for life. My nephew, James Bright, provided this insight. Connie referred to chemotherapy as chemosabe, a Native American term for trusted friend, and an important companion for those who choose that route of care.

It is my prayer that all who read this book will prosper, be richly blessed, and will experience good health in every aspect of life.

Thriver Soup Ingredient:

It might be useful to keep a blank journal on hand to write about how different ideas in *Thriver Soup* work or don't work for you. I have found inspiring, gorgeous, and delightful blank books in bookstores. The nicer the cover, the more you might be drawn to fill the pages with your heart's offerings.

Heidi's Top Ten Quick-start Tips

1. Get at least one other opinion or pathology report following the initial diagnosis. Pathology is more of an art than a science, and the reports will help determine your treatment plan.

2. Select an experienced physician who understands the ramifications of your particular diagnosis, has the most experience with treatment options for your personal situation, and has good ideas for dealing with the side effects of surgery, chemotherapy, or radiation.

3. Find someone who will assist you with researching your options and organizing basic support, such as scheduling others to help you get rides, obtain nutritious meals, and receive assistance with other practical needs.

4. Search for a support community in your area. Many research studies show that women who feel highly supported survive longer than those who experience low levels of assistance. The international Cancer Support Community offers more than fifty U.S. locations, 100 satellite locations, and online aid. See the entry "Cancer Support Community" in the Complementary Care section, "It Takes a Village." This organization provides a good starting point as they might have access to more information in your area. Also ask your physician for referrals to support groups in your community.

5. Start taking proteolytic, or pancreatic, enzymes, which help the body digest protein. Find out why in the entry "Proteolytic Enzymes: The Bigger Picker Upper" in the section "Let Food be Your Medicine."

6. Add curcumin to your day, because it is the leading anti-cancer spice, inhibiting the illness in at least ten different ways. "Curcumin: Go for the Gold" provides more details in the section "Let Food be Your Medicine."

7. Work at eliminating processed foods and sugar from your diet. Processed foods lack the vitality you need during treatment and recovery, and cancer thrives on sugar. Shop the perimeter of your grocery store and avoid the aisles. Review the entry "Treat Yourself Right" in the section "Let Food be Your Medicine" for ideas on how to let go of the sugar. Unless you have a specific medical condition that prevents you from eating dark leafy greens, include plenty of these nutritional powerhouses daily. See "Dark Leafy Greens: Emerald City" in the section "Let Food be Your Medicine."

8. Reduce sources of stress as much as possible. When the body is under stress, it dumps sugar into the bloodstream. This makes cancer cells happy. For more information, read the entry "Stress Trek" in the section "Minding the Body."

9. If you have a sarcoma, the best treatment is surgery. Take a look at the "Softening Surgery" section.

10. Start a mindfulness meditation practice. Australian psychiatrist Ainslie Meares reportedly found that meditation inhibited the growth of tumors in ten percent of the cases he studied. That's better than most chemotherapy-induced remission rates. For ideas, scan the entry "Mindfulness Meditation" in the "Soaring with Spirit" section.

I.

Conventional Methods

Introduction to Conventional Methods: Whatever Works

Were I to be felled and cut in pieces, were I to be grounded in a mill; were I to be burned in a fire,
and blended with its ashes, I should still not be able to express Thy worth;
how great shall I call Thy Name?
—"Sri Raag, Mahala 1," Sri Guru Granth Sahib

Cut into pieces, ground in a chemotherapy mill, burned in a radiation fire. Those are our choices with current conventional cancer treatment. They work, to some degree, even though they might seem counter-intuitive. Did I really want to go that route?

At the start of my cancer journey, I had a long talk with Vince and Connie Lasorso at Whatever Works Wellness Center. For decades they have offered complementary treatment methods and emotional support to cancer patients. They told me the story of a woman who worked in the local holistic community and got cancer. She rejected all conventional treatments and focused on a variety of alternative healing practices. She ended up dying of cancer, acknowledging at the end that if she had received conventional medical care in the beginning, she probably would have survived. That story struck a note with me and I decided to follow what my doctors recommended. Oncologists, after all, have far more experience than a solitary patient.

Later, during a visit to see the Hindu hugging saint Amma, I asked her what to do. She said follow what the doctors recommended.

The simple fact that the metastasis from my uterus to my lungs had advanced from one nodule in July 2009 to four nodules within six weeks, despite enormous amounts of energetic prayer, meditation, visualization, affirmations, energy work, and dietary modifications, indicated that holistic healing by itself, and faith alone, probably were not going to get me through this crisis. The highly aggressive, fast-growing sarcoma cells were not to be leisurely trifled with. I needed to take full responsibility for my future by taking advantage of everything available to me; I needed conventional medical intervention. If nothing else, traditional care would buy the time I needed for complementary healing methods to exert their own influence.

Connie called the treatments "chemosabe," a play on the Potawatomi (a Native American language) word *kemosabe*, which means "faithful friend." My nephew James Bright, who at the time was fascinated by the ancient Egyptians, coined the phrase "ankh-ologist" (rather than oncologist) because the Egyptian ankh is the symbol for life. I later came to realize the word "che*mother*apy" contains the word "mother." So I looked up "che." It is the name for traditional Vietnamese puddings, dessert soups, or sweet drinks. And APY refers to annual percentage yield.

So chemotherapy can be viewed as a sweet, nourishing mother with an annual percentage yield. For me, any positive spin on chemo, no matter how silly, was helpful.

This is not to say holistic methods were ineffective; to the contrary, Vince noted how slowly the cancer had spread in my body, compared to what could have happened. The doctors I saw after surgery all expressed surprise at how few nodules showed up in my lungs, considering how much the sarcoma cells had spread throughout my abdomen. They had expected my lungs to be filled with tumors.

About the time I decided to heartily pursue every avenue of healing open to me, someone sent me an email confirming my choice: "[I]n many cases it takes faith AND serious medical work to be healed. And in some cases even that might not be enough."

Cancer is deadly serious. I urge you to do whatever it takes to survive. Make your choices based on what you believe is best for you, your body, and your future. In this way, any treatment you choose will have the best possible effectiveness it can produce. Know that the Spirit is with you every step of the way—even during the pain of being cut into pieces, the grinding of chemotherapy, and the burning of radiation. Whatever side effects you experience, view them as labor pains because you are in a birth canal. When you emerge, whether on this side of the veil of tears or the other, you will be a new creation.

Thriver Soup Ingredient:

If you select conventional medicine, do some research for yourself about what your physician proposes for your treatment plan. See other doctors as well to find the one whom you believe can provide the best possible care. I ended up selecting an ankhologist two hours from home because I felt confident he knew the most about my particular form of cancer. Be persistent; if you lack the energy, find someone who can be persistent for you.

A. Cushioning Chemotherapy

Introduction to Cushioning Chemotherapy: Chemosabe, Trusted Friend

> *Wounds from a friend can be trusted.*
> —Proverbs 27:6a, Christian Bible, NIV

To help me feel that chemotherapy really was chemosabe (from *kemosabe*, a Native American word for "faithful friend")—my trusted friend—even though its mission was to kill, I worked with my psychotherapist to create visualizations to assist me through treatment.

During my first round, my body entertained the chemo agents Gemzar and Taxol. I saw Gemzar as pinkish red gems that my guides, friends, and family shot at the sarcoma nodules. Docetaxel became silvery beams of light.

My next set of treatments involved doxorubicin and cisplatin. "Doxo" in Greek means to honor, as in the Christian doxology, "Praise God from whom all blessings flow...." This drug provided an opportunity for me to honor my desire for life. The next part of the name is "rubi," which looks similar to the word ruby. When I thought of this drip working on my nodules, I saw it as ruby-colored harpoons that all of us were injecting into the rebel cells. Cisplatin contains platinum, so I visualized this infusion as platinum-colored harpoons. When I arrived for my treatments, I told the receptionist I was getting a platinum ring with a ruby on top.

My psychotherapist created a visualization tape for me to use during each infusion process. I sent her a description of what each drug did and she used those as the basis for each visualization. She played off the "stealth" ability of doxorubicin to sneak past the defensive systems of sarcoma cells and deliver magic bullets inside the cancerous membranes and to prevent DNA from dividing. Cisplatin worked by handcuffing the base of each DNA double helix so the strands could not split apart and replicate.

Reframing chemotherapy as a faithful friend whose wounds can heal, as a tool which the Divine can use to rid your body of evil, and as a way to honor your drive toward life, might help the drugs work more effectively.

Thriver Soup Ingredient:

Play with the names and actions of your chemotherapy agents. See if you can come up with imaginative uses for the names and visuals to accompany them while you are in treatment.

～～～

Heidi's Top Five Chemotherapy Quick-start Tips

1. Find out the major side effects for the chemotherapy drugs you will be receiving. Then research how to prevent or reduce them. This section of *Thriver Soup* offers a host of tips I

found helpful. A lot of unnecessary pain can be prevented if you are able to plan ahead and follow some simple steps.

2. Start out taking the other medications your oncologist suggests. Back off slowly, and only after talking to your doctor. I was able to reduce the Benadryl injections to one-fourth the typical dose, and cut back on the steroids and anti-nausea medicine as I was able.

3. To help prevent neuropathy, ask about taking vitamin B6 with a vitamin B complex and r-lipoic acid. Discuss the pros and cons of glutamine powder. If you start these nutrients ahead of time, it might save you some nerve damage. Take a peek at "Neuropathy: Tingle Town."

4. To help slow issues that develop on the hands and feet, try icing them during chemotherapy and occasionally during the following day or two. This prevents blood flow to the extremities, and can reduce hand-foot syndrome. Again, discuss first with your oncologist, as there might be a risk of cancer spreading to your extremities, in which case you won't want to reduce the chemotherapy in those areas. For more information, see "Socks Discrimination."

5. To remove the chemo taste from your mouth, try the oil pull. For instructions, read "Chemo Mouth: Anointing with Oil" in this section.

~~~

Finding Chemo

A song of ascents: If I raise my eyes to the hills, from where will my help come? My help comes from ADONAI, the maker of heaven and earth.

—Psalm 121:1-2, Complete Jewish Bible

From where would my help come? I was newly diagnosed, lying in a hospital bed after nine hours of surgery, in shock, all drugged up and exhausted, and needed to start chemotherapy. How could I even begin to find the right doctor for an extremely rare, highly undifferentiated endometrial sarcoma?

My family, friends, and I looked to heaven in prayer.

The first ankhologist I saw was unable to locate much in the way of treatment information.

At about the same time, great help came from my sister Roselie Bright, who tirelessly assisted me with finding an ankhologist who might have experience with the orphan sarcoma. She contacted the American Cancer Society along with acquaintances she knew in the field. She also found the Sarcoma Alliance with lists of doctors who treated sarcomas.

Within a matter of days she created a list of physicians and wrote them emails seeking assistance and appointments. Everyone seemed quite helpful. Soon Roselie and I were off to visit two specialists at MD Anderson Cancer Center in Houston (with assistance from my brother Jim Bright) and the world's most well-known researcher in a similar type of sarcoma at Memorial

Sloan-Kettering Cancer Center in Manhattan, New York (with assistance from my then-husband and Mark Lewandoski).

During the meetings, I found myself unable to focus, which meant I was incapable of understanding the doctors or of finding the best treatment options. I desperately needed my sister's help because of her knowledge of medicine. I also needed the assertiveness of my supporters to push the ankhologists for honest answers.

All three specialists seemed to agree on a protocol quite different from the one proposed by the first ankhologist I saw. Unfortunately, they wanted me to come to their offices for treatments. While they welcomed additional opinions, they would not participate in joint management because then no one would be responsible—which would not be good for me, the patient.

That would have meant either moving to those locations or flying there every few weeks. Neither was a good option, especially because I had a preteen living at home.

Roselie suggested I see one of the leading members of the Sarcoma Alliance, Dr. Larry Copeland. Known to the chemotherapy staff at the Ohio State University as The Great Oz, because he always seemed to have a plan, Dr. Copeland had almost a decade of experience at MD Anderson; was president of the Society of Gynecologic Oncologists during 2006–2007; and was Chief of Staff of the James Cancer Hospital during 1995–1997.

We met him and felt he had not only suggested the best treatment options—similar to those suggested by the other physicians—he also was only a two-hour drive from our house. We felt confident I was in the best hands getting the right chemotherapy.

When it came time to try a third regimen, we agreed the best course of action was to surgically remove the existing nodules and have them cultured and tested for responsiveness to a handful of other chemosabe agents, most likely ifosfamide combined with one other drug.

Ifosfamide required hospital stays of three to five days every three weeks for a lifetime limit of six stays. I wanted to move my treatments to Cincinnati, and Dr. Copeland willingly selected an ankhologist for me and worked with Dr. James Pavelka on a consultation basis. I had the benefit of both Dr. Copeland's vast experience and Dr. Pavelka's proximity, knowledge, and flexibility.

I received a list of the potential drugs and combinations and meditated on the possibilities. I came to a conclusion and did not mention it to the ankhologists until after they received the results of the chemo FX assay of my nodule cells. (Be aware this expensive procedure, and others, might not be covered by your insurance.) Both doctors agreed on using paclitaxel with the ifosfamide, which was the same answer I had received during meditation.

If I had followed the original ankhologist's recommendations, I might have died within a year or two. Instead, my sister exhaustively gathered information and we reflected on my options. Then I accessed my inner wisdom by contacting the Spirit during meditation. Through intuition, I received the information I needed to make my decision, and I followed through on my desire.

As it turned out, the drugs I received prolonged my life enough for surgery and complementary aid to extend my existence beyond chemo. Assistance arrived from the hinterlands, like the proverbial cavalry, through many, many people. And I looked to the hills for help—hills that can be considered a feminine feature of a landscape, representing the motherly aspects of the Divine. The help came from the Creator of heaven and earth in creative ways.

Thriver Soup Ingredient:

If your cancer is fairly common and the chemotherapy choices fairly straightforward, it's probably a good idea to follow protocol. Otherwise, ask people for assistance with doing research to find out what's been done with other patients who have the same or similar diagnosis and how they responded to treatment.

Go see the specialists, wherever they are located. Ask the ankhologists' office for organizations that provide assistance with travel if that's what is necessary to get the help you need. There are programs available that can provide transportation and even housing while you investigate your options (see the Resources section at the end of *Thriver Soup*). Ask your friends if they might know people living in the cities you are visiting who might open their homes to you.

When you see the ankhologists, ask for treatment plans, including dosages of chemotherapy drugs and the numbers and frequencies of cycles. Be assertive—ask, push for honest answers, and ask some more. Your life is at stake. If you can't be assertive, ask someone to be your advocate during the meeting. When my sister could not attend meetings, she participated by conference call.

Your life is in your hands. If you don't feel right about your final choices, perhaps you can explore other options. The more confident you feel in your choice of treatment, the more effective your treatment probably will be.

〜〜〜

Bonfire of the Veinities

For this reason I remind you to fan into flame the gift of God, which is in you through the laying on of my hands.

—2 Timothy 1:6, Christian Bible, NIV

Plenty of hands were laid on me, filling my veins with fire for healing, during two years of chemotherapy treatment. The chemo injected into my arms was a gift from the Divine that burned its way through my body. For two years I allowed my hands and forearms to be used as pincushions. Each time I had a new regimen, I expected to be done with chemotherapy. Yet I ended up on the IV pole for three different types of combined treatments.

Had I known what lay down the road for me, I would have opted to have peripherally inserted central catheter lines in my upper arms or a port placed in my chest.

My ignorance was not bliss. Two days following my second infusion of gemcitabine and docetaxel, I took a heavy bag of trash out to the garage, then started cooking. My right forearm felt odd, so I pulled back my sleeve.

I gasped.

The infusion vein bulged a good quarter inch out of my arm. Shaking, I raised my arm above my head and called the ankhology station. The chemosabe nurse wanted me to take more drugs, use warm compresses, and keep my arm elevated. Instead of drugs, I took anti-inflammatory supplements, but followed her other instructions. Gradually the vein settled down, though it stayed purple and red.

Before the next infusion, my Kodak nurse, Vicky, suggested putting a warm compress on my other arm for fifteen minutes before infusion to prevent the same issue in the next blood vessel.

The warm compress helped open up the vein and reduced the burning sensation when the gemcitabine made its entrance. The nurses also started diluting the gemcitabine with saline. A fair trade—more chair time for less burning.

Friends Judy and Rusty suggested I use arnica homeopathic ointment on my forearms to assist with healing between treatments. It helped, yet at times I succumbed to using the topical cream given to me by the nurses. It relieved the itching, yet the redness and mild swelling persisted for days. I also began icing my arms following chemo and gently stroking them from my hands to my elbows.

At one point I had a red, bruised vein all along my forearm.

By the end of sixteen such treatments, a swollen rash stretched four inches long and one and one-half inches wide.

Red and purple patches on my forearms persisted for a good year following the gemcitabine and docetaxel treatments. Vince Lasorso reminded me that these stripes on my arms were not unlike the stripes Jesus bore for humanity—so, in a small way, I was imitating Christ.

My veins, understandably enough, began to hide. Whoever was the lucky winner of my forearms for each blood draw or drip patted numerous locations to find a spot that would dare to rise again.

About a year into infusions, a nurse accessed a small volunteer on my hand and used a slow drip, yet the drugs leaked out onto my hand. She ended up pulling the IV and, with the help of another nurse, scoured for another possibility.

My Kodak nurse had ideas for opening up and exposing the veins for subsequent infusions: Squeeze two squishy fist-sized balls with my hands, as long as I can tolerate it, at least three to four times daily. Lift three- to five-pound weights as often as I can to exercise my biceps, triceps, and chest. I decided to try these out, since I was done with the burning chemos and on to other types. I lost the fear of exploding veins and exercised, yet my blood vessels still hid.

It took a long time for my veins to heal. Bruising left one forearm purple and then brown for years. Whenever I had to get another puncture, I asked for the best phlebotomists on duty and told them they won the lucky prize for most challenging patient. I wanted only the best to lay their hands on my forearms so that I could receive a gift from the Divine—an easy stick for better care of my whole body.

Thriver Soup Ingredient:

If you frequently have your forearms and hands punctured, ask your doctor if you can use some light weights to do hand exercises. Exercise will help the veins heal between sticks. If the weights are too much, simply follow these suggestions without the weights. Don't force anything; be kind and gentle, respectful of your body, yet give your blood vessels a little something to stimulate blood flow.

Sit in a chair and grasp the weights in your hands. Hang your hands over your knees, facing downward. Lift your hands up and down a few times.

Turn your hands to face each other, still hanging over your knees. Move your weights back and forth a few times.

Keep your hands in front of your knees and turn your palms up. Move the weights up and down.

Do this at least once a day and gradually increase your number of repetitions to strengthen the muscles and improve circulation.

~~~

Antihistamines: Flying the Friendly Chemotherapy Skies

Unattracted to the sensory world, the yogi experiences the ever new joy inherent in the Self. Engaged in divine union of the soul with Spirit, he attains bliss indestructible.
—*God Talks with Arjuna: The Bhagavad Gita*, 5.21

I found my bliss in the chemotherapy infusion room.

Unfortunately, it was no yogic ecstasy attained by union with the Divine. This bliss was entirely too destructible.

During my first infusion session, the nurse found a receptive vein in my arm and started pumping in saline. She then pushed fifty milligrams of diphenhydramine right into my bloodstream.

Woo-hoo! Woo-zee baby. The room spun. My speech slowed and slurred. I asked the nurse: "Please bring me my hair."

This temporary heavenly state proved to be the highlight of my two years in Club Chemo.

I got high on the diphenhydramine because it was injected directly into my vein. The medication, which blocks the effects of histamine in the body, is used to counteract any allergic reactions to the chemo drugs.

To help with chemo, I used my WholiSound Serenity Box, dabbed holy water on my body, placed guru Paramahansa Yogananda's healing rose petals on my chest, and placed pictures of my Spirit guides on the intravenous bags, their visages facing the fluids.

Around me lounged many women who napped during infusion, probably because of the diphenhydramine. I, however, wanted as few drugs as possible, so for subsequent treatments I found I could reduce the diphenhydramine injection to twelve and one-half milligrams since my body accepted the chemotherapy as the life-extending friend it proved to become. I also wanted to stay awake to perform my ice torture—keeping my mouth, fingers and toes cold to reduce side effects at those locations.

I had received a taste of the yogic joy that occurs after years of meditative practice. My high lasted less than an hour. A mystic can exist in a perpetual state of bliss. Rather than rely on any temporary, fleeting experience, I wanted to live long enough to get closer to union with the Divine. Chemotherapy became one of the disciplines I used to deepen my spiritual awareness.

Thriver Soup Ingredient:

Collect small images of any angels or spiritual guides you call upon for assistance. When you go to chemotherapy, tape the images together vertically and hang them so they face your infusion bags. Ask your guides to send divine healing light into the fluids so the molecules carry that energy into your bloodstream to help cure your body.

$$\approx\approx\approx$$

Chemo Die-off Phase: O Burn That Burns to Heal

But for the burning of their souls and the sighing of their hearts, they would be drowned in the midst of their tears, and but for the flood of their tears they would be burnt up by the fire of their hearts and the heat of their souls. Methinks, they are like the angels which Thou hast created of snow and of fire. Wilt Thou, despite such vehement longing, O my God, debar them from Thy presence, or drive them away, notwithstanding such fervor, from the door of Thy mercy?
—Bahá'u'lláh, *Unlocking the Gate of the Heart*

Bahá'u'lláh (1817–1892), founder of the Bahá'í Faith, knew intense suffering and the fire of Divine energy in his bones.

My whole body knew well the internal burn of devouring flames, and it wasn't the fire of my heart or the heat of my soul. It was the chemotherapy die-off phase. After the drug infusion fulfilled its purpose and I emerged from the nausea stage, the fire of destruction incinerated my cells and they began to die off. The drugs hadn't discriminated. They were equal-opportunity destroyers of any fast-growing cells in the body.

During this stage, I developed an odd fatigue—not the usual tiredness that a nap could cure. No, this was unremitting and could last for days. A dull, dark, prickling ache gnawed at every cell. I usually didn't bother getting out of bed. I spent listless hours staring at nothing, thinking nothing. When I felt good enough, I roused myself to watch nap-inspiring family videos. If I managed to gather more energy, I listened to visualizations and Emotional Freedom Technique recordings, inducing more naps. Sometimes I managed to get vertical long enough to creep into the kitchen and warm up chicken broth with brown rice. I felt like I was living in a dark cave with no escape.

During this phase, other issues cropped up. My eyes watered excessively. My mouth tasted nasty. The veins on my arms burned. My stool scorched my bottom. Sometimes my hands chapped. I felt like I was burning from the inside-out—which probably was close to the truth. I put drops into my eyes, rubbed arnica homeopathic ointment on the infusion area, and drank up to a tablespoon of baking soda in water to prevent the burning stool. I frequently used my WholiSound Serenity Box to reduce pain and inflammation.

A couple of times at night I experienced a fever, a pounding heart, and uncontrollable shaking combined with gasping breaths. I could not even muster the energy to pull up another blanket. I felt incapable of relaxing or breathing deeply. This continued for about three hours before subsiding.

I talked with another woman about this phase of chemo. She said she stays busy so she doesn't feel it. I don't know how she did it. And staying busy was the last thing I needed. My friend Maria Paglialungo kept reminding me to stay in my body during this process rather than escaping into busyness, movies, or thinking. Sitting with the ache helped me stay connected to my body, an important skill I had to learn the hard way. As I felt my muscles, I usually noticed a lot of tension. When I managed to relax, I often napped.

On the plus side, I found it humorous and pleasant that even when repeatedly interrupted, I could still cat nap six or seven times during a span of two hours. I could even nap during a car trip. This—for a woman who frequently experienced insomnia all her life and never slept in cars or planes. Green tea helped when I needed a bit of extra energy.

One time at the end of the die-off phase I dreamt that I had a nice stack of $100 bills. Money in dreams usually indicates energy. Sure enough, my energy surged back up the next morning. How nice to feel a little more normal again.

I learned to let the chemo scorch away all corruption so I could progress toward the possibility of a cure. I allowed my smoldering body to burn away as much of the unwanted invasion as possible, yet attempted to keep my mind stayed on my remembrance of the Divine. I wanted the door of mercy opened...

Thriver Soup Ingredient:

During the chemo die-off phase, use the time to feel the inside of your body. What are your muscles doing? What are you experiencing? Where are you feeling it? Stay connected to your sense of soul and Spirit, and allow the drugs to burn up all that is not needed within you.

During this time you also might consider meditating upon this poem by Christian mystic St. John of the Cross (1549–1591):

> O burn that burns to heal!
> O more than pleasant wound!
> And O soft hand, O touch most delicate,
> That dost new life reveal,
> That dost in grace abound,
> And, slaying, dost from death to life translate!

~~~

Chemo Stool: Think Outside Your Buns

Pride goes before destruction, a haughty spirit before a fall.

—Proverbs 16:18, Christian Bible, NIV

The medical establishment has left me humiliated so many times that I no longer feel concern about my dignity. Practicality wins over pride. Getting through the day matters the most.

And so it's time to deal with the messiest issue. Chemotherapy can kill cells throughout the digestive system. Two unpleasant outcomes can drop down: constipation and diarrhea.

Your ankhologist should have information for dealing with these issues, yet I found the materials incomplete.

The chemosabe drug docetaxel produced black diarrhea that burned its way out—enough for me to dab on diaper rash cream after each deposit. Following the first treatment, I discovered that drinking two teaspoons of baking soda in two to three cups of water before bed took out the sting. I drank it on an empty stomach because it caused a lot of burping. I read that long-term use might soften bones, so I used it only as needed.

Later my digestive system flipped to the opposite extreme—constipation. Peaches, pears, plums, and prunes can assist with constipation, as can exercise and water, yet I found I needed more help.

My doctor suggested Milk of Magnesia. I found it a little helpful because it contains magnesium, which can assist with softening stool.

I didn't use fennel or senna leaves, yet they can help if your doctor thinks it's a good idea. Fennel seeds relax the muscles in the digestive tract. You can soak two to four teaspoons of fennel seeds overnight, then steep for ten to twenty minutes in one cup of hot water. Strain and drink one to three times each day. Senna leaves mixed with ginger, peppermint, or cardamom (to decrease flatulence) in a cup of warm water can be drunk at night to relieve constipation.

Recalling how harmless alfalfa tablets helped with both constipation and acid reflux when I was pregnant, I bought a bottle. At the time I was on the chemo drugs paclitaxel and ifosfamide, which caused acid reflux and constipation, so I had the perfect solution for my body. My ankhologist reassured me that alfalfa would not interfere with the action of the chemo agents. I started with one pill a day and quickly learned three tablets at each meal fixed the problem. When I didn't use the alfalfa tablets enough, I clogged toilets. Once I clogged two on the same day. Pride? It got flushed down the drain.

Thriver Soup Ingredient:

My arms were dramatically weakened by chemotherapy, especially because my forearms were used for pincushions and then I had a line placed in my upper arm. When I was alone and clogged a toilet, I could not use a plunger with even remote effectiveness. Big (ah-hem) problem.

In such a situation, I suggest flushing periodically while on the toilet so only small amounts need to go down at once. If that doesn't work, plan to have a throw-away plastic container (like a large yogurt tub) with a lid or a plastic bag and a kitchen tool, like a long-handled spoon or tongs, next to the toilet. Use as needed.

≈≈≈

Chemo Mouth: Anointing with Oil

Is anyone among you sick? Let them call the elders of the church to pray over them and anoint them with oil in the name of the Lord. And the prayer offered in faith will make the sick person well; the Lord will raise them up.

—James 5:14-15a, Christian Bible, NIV

Anointing with oil was practiced in ancient times as a means of consecrating someone for a holy purpose, bringing Divine influence to bear upon a person or situation. It also provided a means of spiritual healing to effect physical cures. Soon after the diagnosis, I discovered that anointing the inside of my mouth with oil could help me heal my taste buds.

When starting my infusions, I recalled how my mother complained, during her chemo-therapy treatments, that everything tasted metallic. She could only tolerate eating lemon drops after chemo. Fortunately, I had learned from two friends about a procedure called an oil pull and wanted to see if it could prevent any nasty chemotherapy taste in my mouth.

My theory worked. Even through eight treatments with the platinum-based drug cisplatin, my mouth never tasted metallic and my taste buds worked perfectly. I waited each chemosabe cycle until the drugs had run their course, on day four or five after treatment, before doing the oil pull, and would continue daily through the morning of the next infusion.

I stopped the oil pull once for about a month and the taste in my mouth gradually worsened. It grew especially unpleasant during the die-off period, which lasted about three days. Brushing didn't do a thing, and filtered water tasted unpleasant. I took to drinking mostly herbal and decaf teas. I couldn't wait to start the oil pull again.

Only the oil pull worked to keep my taste buds happy. It was like anointing my mouth with oil as a prayer to keep my taste buds clean and to aid in my healing.

Thriver Soup Ingredient:

First thing each morning after the chemotherapy die-off days are completed, and before anything else (except water) goes into your mouth, do the oil pull to get rid of chemo mouth.

What you will need for the oil pull:

A plastic throw-away tub with a lid

Raw, organic sunflower or sesame oil

1 tablespoon measuring spoon

¼ teaspoon measuring spoon

Baking soda

Cup of water

Measure out one tablespoon of oil, place the oil in your mouth, and swish it around for three to four minutes. Spit the used oil into the tub and rinse your mouth with water. Repeat two more times. Then measure out ¼ teaspoon of baking soda and stir it into a quarter cup of water. Swish in your mouth and spit it out. Rinse with water.

Some people brush their teeth and use a tongue scraper after the final rinse.

Continue daily until the morning of your next infusion.

~~~

Hair Today

I also want the women to dress modestly, with decency and propriety, adorning themselves, not with elaborate hairstyles or gold or pearls or expensive clothes, but with good deeds, appropriate for women who profess to worship God.

—1 Timothy 2:9-10, Christian Bible, NIV

During the first century AD, women left their tresses long and created elaborate hairstyles for when they left their hovels. I had long locks, yet after my first hospital stay I knew I needed to get it cut for all the lying around I'd be doing.

A month after my first surgery, my sister-in-law Janet Bright took my sister Roselie Bright and me to her hair dresser for a cut and style. The stylist showed me a picture of the hairdo she thought would go best with my face. It was the last type I would ordinarily have chosen. Well, I thought, it's time for the new Heidi, and heck, it probably won't last more than a month anyway, so go for it!

Everyone seemed to like it.

And the cut stayed. Even though my hair thinned, I still had plenty. Two other women I met who were on docetaxel lost their hair within two weeks. I decided every day with my own hair was a good hair day.

I read that people on "the red devil" chemotherapy drug Adriamycin were practically guaranteed to lose their hair. Then someone did a study with vitamin E supplements and found that sixty-nine percent of the patients taking the vitamin kept their hair. I had been taking 400 international units of the vitamin E for several months prior to chemo. During my second and third treatments, my ankhologist was surprised I still had enough hair to look decent.

I began taking vitamin E again four days after each treatment and stopping it three days before the next infusion.

My hair got noticeably sparse and I lost some eyebrows and eyelashes. By the sixteenth treatment, my eyelashes are quite sparse, giving my face an odd appearance. I had read that raw apple cider vinegar was good for hair growth, so occasionally I sprayed my scalp with it and left it on for about an hour before washing it. I appeared to have lots of short hair growing on my scalp, especially up front where it had been sparse.

These tufts made my style appear strange, so I got another haircut. I was on doxorubicin, a kinder cousin of the red devil, and again I kept the vast majority of my hair.

In preparation for my final chemo I got a third haircut because I knew I would be in and out of hospital beds for four months. During my initial surgery in 2009, with a nine-day hospital stay, I never got my long hair combed. It took my neighbor about an hour to untangle the rat's nest I'd developed. I wanted to avoid such a mess again, because I didn't expect to lose my hair this time.

Oh, well...third time was the charm. Hair today, gone tomorrow. The only elaborate hairstyle I was going to sport was a wig. Yuck.

Thriver Soup Ingredient:

Talk to your ankhologist before taking vitamin E, which is an antioxidant.

$\sim\sim\sim$

Hair Loss: Fallout

Are not two sparrows sold for a penny? Yet not one of them will fall to the ground outside your Father's care. And even the very hairs of your head are all numbered. So don't be afraid; you are worth more than many sparrows.

—Matthew 10:29-31, Christian Bible, NIV

All the hairs on my head might have been numbered, but despite my worth in Divine eyes, that number dropped dramatically during my third type of chemotherapy.

I had been told I would lose my hair with the first two types of chemotherapy. My hair thinned, yet I still had plenty. Unfortunately, the third type of chemotherapy proved too much for my hair follicles. Sixteen days after the first paclitaxel treatment, my scalp became tender. The nurse said it was the pain of dying hair follicles. Drat.

Two days later I was shedding more than a sheltie in summer. I wore a scarf to catch it so I wouldn't have to tie a broom to my backside. I still looked like I had a normal head of hair.

By day nineteen, the wind yanked out my hair like a teenage girl in a catfight. I held my scalp while outside to reduce the sharp pin-pricks I felt.

Four days later, I owned a couple of quite noticeable bald spots on the back of my head, and the hair in front of my ears was gone. I used a pet hair roller to clean off my pillow, clothes, and even the bathroom sink. I got a clump of hair from my comb about every hour. My boys' eyes grew large when they saw how easily the hair departed my head.

Twenty-seven days after my first paclitaxel treatment—thirteen days after the second infusion—I celebrated that chemosabe was working, because most of my hair was gone. No more "any day with hair is a good hair day." I had no plans, however, to clean the rest off because even a little hair felt better than none.

My sister noted of all the chemotherapy effects, this was the easiest to cope with. I also found it the most blatant. I got plenty of stares, especially from young women. It was like waving a flag that says, "Hey, guess what! I'm in cancer treatment!"

After my third type of chemo, I became fascinated by my scalp. The hair right over the crown of my head was still intact, even though I was supposed to lose it first. A bald ring surrounded the tuft, and then I had another ring of hair. Maybe my halo fell onto my scalp?

I had been doing Reiki energy healing on myself nearly every day for four months. The way I understand Reiki, Divine energy enters the body through the crown chakra at the top of the head, then goes where most needed in the body. Apparently this energy was sufficiently strong so I could keep the hair covering my crown healthy enough to temporarily survive paclitaxel.

Finally, just shy of two months after receiving my first paclitaxel drip, I shaved my head.

A month later I was down to two lashes on my right eye and a half dozen on my left. I still had some eyebrow hair, which was nice.

Three and one-half months into treatment, I had none of the original eyelashes, yet I had a few nubs growing on my right eyelid. I still had eyebrows.

The Divine knows the number of hairs on our heads, including our eyebrows and eyelashes. None falls to the ground without the Spirit taking account. That is how valuable we are, how deeply we are loved. Believe in that love, feel that love, know that love, even if you feel ugly and unlovable without hair.

Thriver Soup Ingredient:

If you know your hair probably will fall out, purchase a pet hair roller. It makes cleanup a snap.

~~~

Hair Pieces: Turbanator

It is for this reason that a woman ought to have authority over her own head, because of the angels.
—1 Corinthians 11:10, Christian Bible, NIV

"It's a miracle!" I told the chemotherapy nurses. "The angels are watching over my head. Taxol has the opposite effect on me. I grew long braids overnight!"

I wore my Willie braids (fake dark brown braids hanging from a red bandana folded like a headband) to my appointment. They called me Pocahontas.

This brought to my mind 1 Corinthians 11:3-16 in the Christian Bible, in which the Apostle Paul writes about head coverings for Christians at church in the ancient city of Corinth. A male (who might go bald) is not to wear a head covering during worship because his head symbolizes or reflects Christ. A woman (who generally doesn't go bald) is to keep her head covered during worship because her head reflects the glory of humanity. She is to cover up her hair so she also can reflect the glory of God.

I especially like verse ten: a woman should have authority or power on her head—like a queen's crown—because of the angels. My remaining hair formed a tuft on my seventh chakra, the center of the crown on my head. I learned this spot symbolized Divine power working in my life in both a metaphorical and a tangible, physical way.

Soon I didn't even have enough hair to get away with the Pocahontas look. I switched to a turban supplied by the local Cancer Family Care office. As Turbanator, my re-mission was to baldly go where this woman had never gone before. Turbans and scarves and wigs, oh my!

I had to get my driver's license renewed while starting to wear the turban, since my hair was falling out in gobs. That meant three years as Turbanator, at least on my license.

Cancer Family Care also provided one free wig, and a family member sent me two more. I wore one of them while chaperoning a school field trip. As I'd heard, the wig was hot and itchy. While I'd always wanted poufy hair (mine was fine as silk and hardly kept a curl), the wig felt so not-me that I decided I didn't like the abundant-hair look.

Since I only wore the wig for one outing, I was glad I didn't get into the habit of wearing one around the house. A friend in Club Chemo baked cookies one day, and singed the top front of her wig while leaning into the oven. I have heard this is not uncommon.

I imagined painting my scalp with henna after shaving, until I heard that it would only last three weeks because of all the oils on the head. So, I didn't bother. I had kept so much stubble anyway, it would have looked strange.

I preferred wearing cotton and silk scarves over my scalp. They were more comfortable than a wig, and worked because I was not employed in an office setting. I found a neutral-colored headband covered with glittery beads that I could wear with each scarf I owned. I folded the scarf into a triangle, put the long edge on my forehead, placed the headband on top of the scarf around my head, and then tucked the pointed ends of the scarf into the headband at the back of my head. The bling held the scarf securely in place.

The American Cancer Society offered an occasional program called Look Good, Feel Better. Teachers demonstrated how to use makeup, including how to apply eyelashes and draw eyebrows. They also demonstrated how to wear scarves and how to turn an old, large T-shirt into a turban. Each participant received a bag of cosmetics. Together we earth angels dressed up our faces and placed our new queenly crowns on our heads, reflecting the glory of the Divine while the heavenly angels watched over us.

Thriver Soup Ingredient:

Have fun with your new style. Roselie Bright, my sister, knit a silly cap, which I wore to laughter yoga. Or find some Willie braids. Or surprise your partner with an inexpensive Halloween wig—perhaps a rainbow-colored clown wig (and get a matching bulbous red nose) or a long blond wig. Not everyone gets an opportunity like this to play around with a bald scalp.

~~~

Baldilocks

Your beauty should not come from outward adornment, such as elaborate hairstyles and the wearing of gold jewelry or fine clothes. Rather, it should be that of your inner self, the unfading beauty of a gentle and quiet spirit, which is of great worth in God's sight.

—1 Peter 3:3-4, Christian Bible, NIV

After nearly two years on chemotherapy, I finally accepted that I would become Baldilocks. I shaved my scalp. No elaborate hairstyles for me. While adjusting to my new look, my younger son began rubbing the stubble on my head. I was surprised how much there was—almost all on top.

Gradually I got used to seeing myself bald. I was reminded of Ilia, a character in Paramount's "Star Trek: The Motion Picture." The actress shaved her head, yet still had plenty of eyebrows and eyelashes, lacking the "I'm bald from chemo" look.

Baldness evokes an egghead air, especially when one wears glasses. I could always pretend that too much brain power blew out all my hair.

My brother shaves his head every day and feels quite comfortable without hair. I suggested we get our picture taken together if I became bald, yet by the time he arrived in town I had stubble all over my scalp.

A friend of mine who lives near the Arctic Circle lost her hair to chemotherapy in the dead of winter. Brrr! Her head felt cold all the time. When I shaved my head, the summer heat arrived. I felt grateful for the warmth at night, keeping my head from freezing. However, I didn't like the way my ears stuck to my scalp when I laid on my pillow. Long after my hair grew back, someone suggested dusting cornstarch behind the ears to prevent the sticking.

I envied people with hair just as I felt jealous of overweight people when I weighed 108 pounds. I also noticed how attached my ego was to my hair. Since the spiritual life generally involves growing beyond the limited self (or ego) and moving into the larger Self (Spirit), I discovered plenty of room for inner growth, never mind hair growth.

And so I challenged my ego, pushing the limits of my comfort levels. For my first foray into baldom, I warned my two teenagers I was going wigless around the house. My thirteen-year-old had a hard time adjusting to it. Initially, he gave me several hugs and repeatedly came up to touch my scalp.

I grew bolder, deciding to stay cool while driving around in the summer heat. I figured most people wouldn't notice I was a bald female. It wasn't long, though, before one of my neighbors and her daughter stopping at a nearby intersection, recognized me, and waved. Oops! My face reddened a bit. I survived.

It was time for my inner Self, the unfading beauty of a gentle and quiet spirit, to shine forth without obstruction. It was worth far more than the most beautiful coiffure in the world.

Thriver Soup Ingredient:

To help my hair regrow, my friend Morgan Dragonwillow suggested rubbing peppermint essential oil onto my scalp. I rubbed it on twice daily. It made my scalp tingle, so I guess it increases blood flow to the hair follicles. I suspect it dried out my scalp, because the skin grew dry, itchy, and flaky. So I cut back to one application daily and greased up later in the day with raw jojoba oil. Worked like a charm.

∽∽∽

Hair Regrowth: Fuzzy Wuzzy

White hair is a crown of honor obtained by righteous living.
—Proverbs 16:31, Complete Jewish Bible

I went on chemotherapy to prolong my life. My crown of honor, however, appeared early in my span of years. While sporting a shaved head and still receiving my sixth hair-removing paclitaxel treatment, I found a circlet of white fuzz all over my scalp. It felt so soft and pleasant, I called myself a peach and frequently stroked it.

Within two weeks I could feel the breeze move my fuzz. I smiled.

It grew about a quarter of an inch the first month. My thirteen-year-old enjoyed rubbing it.

Stubble appeared where my eyebrows had been, and I grew mini eyelashes. Many people told me their hair came in curly, so I thought I might get lucky. My dad felt fortunate after he lost all his hair to pneumonia. When my mom's final hair grew back, it was reddish and curly. So why not me? Vince Lasorso suggested I visualize myself with the kind of hair I wanted.

Well, I didn't put energy into that. Maybe I should have. My hair came in limp, sparse, and brown. How boring. Still, it was my hair, and I felt grateful for it.

It took another four months for the skin sores to finally disappear from my scalp. At about the same time, I looked like I'd been given a crew cut, so I finally shed the scarves and came out of the hair closet. The stubble had grown barely long enough to lie down instead of stick straight up. I could not tell what color it was since it was so short and sparse. I suspected it might be grey mixed with dark brown, or maybe some dark brown with blondish highlights. Whatever it was, I loved it—it felt much better than no hair at all. And in my opinion, far better than a hoary head.

It took another month for me to actually need to run a comb through it after a shower. I still was unsure of the color—it appeared dark brown, yet seemed to have blond and grey highlights. It also remained fairly sparse. No luscious waves or cute curls. Shirley Temple, you still steal my show.

Another month went by before I ran into a woman who had done some hair dying. She looked at my hair and said it was brown with blond and grey highlights. According to the Livestrong website, grey hair can be returned to its natural color through nutrition. It specifically mentions vitamin B12, which I hadn't been taking regularly. It came as no great surprise to me that a biggie in preventing grey hair was folic acid, which comes from dark green leafies. I get those daily in my Vitamix blender, so that might be why I didn't have a full head of grey like many chemotherapy patients whose hair returns. I commented about this on my CaringBridge blog. Someone questioned those comments about the cause of grey hair. She probably was right—for some, maybe it's genetic and no amount of good nutrition can alter it. And the website mentioned taking PABA, but I didn't know what that is so I didn't mention it on my blog.

Another cancer survivor once said she was told her hair would come in different after going bald from chemotherapy. "No one ever said it would come in gray," she joked.

I should count my blessings—almost no gray hairs. And she could count hers—the gray head in ancient times represented a life well-lived, since most people never quite got that far along. At some point I plan to have my crown of honor. In the meantime, I can pretend to be younger than I am.

Thriver Soup Ingredient:

You can help stimulate hair growth by dabbing raw organic apple cider vinegar where you want your hair to grow. I suggest waiting until you have no sores on your scalp, though, as the vinegar might burn the open skin.

~~~

Chemo Side Effects: How Can You Spell "Relief"?

Then Mary stood up and greeted all of them and said to her brethren, "Do not mourn or grieve or be irresolute, for his grace will be with you all and will defend you. Let us rather praise his greatness, for he prepared us and made us into men." When Mary said this, their hearts changed for the better, and they began to discuss the words of the [Savior].

—The Gospel of Mary

Mary Magdalene, for whom the apocryphal "Gospel of Mary" is named, encouraged her Christian brothers to praise the greatness of the Divine rather than mourn and grieve. She wanted them to shift their focus from the negative to the positive, and they did—their hearts "changed for the better" and they began discussing the words of the Christ. In this translation, the editors wrote, "he prepared us and made us into men." In another translation, by Willis Barnstone and Marvin Meyer in *The Gnostic Bible*, the ancient fragment reads "He...made us truly human." In their version, Mary seemed to delight in becoming truly human, truly who she was created to be.

My own humanity was dredged up during every chemotherapy die-off phase. I still had to live in this human body, this flesh so prone to breakdown. Yet breakdown can lead to breakthrough.

The effectiveness of chemosabe could be directly proportional to the intensity of the side effects it produces. Since these drugs are designed to kill fast-growing cells, if the patient experiences no secondary results, the drugs might not be working. I often heard—and experienced myself—that after a period of treatments, the side effects subside, indicating the drugs' effectiveness on cancer cells has diminished and it's time to switch to another treatment plan. Generally the ankhologists have an idea how many treatments will work, yet each person responds in her or his own way and time.

Several perpetual side effects seemed to span most of my chemo time. My hands inflated. My lower legs stayed swollen. My skin dried out despite copious amounts of raw flax oil. My gums bled. My tongue gradually grew a fur coat. My eyelids flushed pink and puffy. My clothes smelled bad by the end of the day.

I also had some occasional side effects. One day I felt chest pressure and had an irregular heartbeat. After some internal debate—I didn't want more medical intervention—I called the ankhology station. My trepidation had only worsened the symptoms. The chemo nurse reassured me that my issues probably stemmed from dehydration. What a relief. It made sense—I had been much more focused on eating healthy food than on drinking enough water. Sure enough, I drank a bunch and the symptoms magically disappeared.

Hearing can be adversely affected by the drug cisplatin, so I did a little research and learned that r-lipoic acid could prevent or lessen hearing loss. I got a supply and took it daily. My ears did start ringing, and yet my hearing remained fine. I have since learned that potatoes provide a rich source of this helpful nutrient.

Not every side effect felt uncomfortable. One actually proved a boon for me. While some women found that odors made them nauseous, I relished my dramatically improved sense of smell. I discovered I could sniff things out better than my then-husband, which was no small accomplishment.

Whatever the side effects are, we can always look beyond our tears and grief to the breakthrough that comes after the breakdown. Be firm in your resolve to live. Allow yourself to feel Divine grace protecting you. And accept your humanness as the gift it is.

Thriver Soup Ingredient:

My psychotherapist suggested that I visualize what I want physically as I move through chemotherapy. Depending on the side effects you experience, perhaps you can imagine the opposite for yourself: soft skin, the enjoyment of your favorite food unencumbered by chemotherapy-doused taste buds, or sweet-smelling clothes.

~~~

Chemo-induced Hand Sores: Cool Hands, Luke

[W]hen you walk through fire, you will not be scorched—the flame will not burn you. For I am

ADONAI, your God, the Holy One of Isra'el, your Savior—I have given Egypt as your ransom, Ethiopia and S'va for you. Because I regard you as valued and honored, and because I love you. For you I will give people, nations in exchange for your life. Don't be afraid, for I am with you.

—Isaiah 43:2b-5b, Complete Jewish Bible

We are dearly beloved of the Spirit, and are encouraged by the writers of the Jewish Bible not to be afraid.

Easy for the prophets to say. They haven't been on chemotherapy for end-stage cancer. Many patients know well the fire that erupts in one's bones, induced by drugs designed to target and kill fast-growing cells in the body.

Some drugs produce what's called hand-foot syndrome—dryness, redness, swelling, even blistering. Some people lose their nails. The intensity of symptoms depends on several factors, including the type of drug and the dose.

The first chemo combo I received—paclitaxel and gemcitabine—was known for causing nail loss. I decided I preferred the ice torture. I packed a cooler with ice cubes, pint-sized plastic tubs, and two hand towels. Before succumbing to the infusion, I placed a hand towel at each hip while my then-husband filled the tubs with ice and water and set them on the towels. Then I allowed an arm to be hooked up. During the infusion hours, I dipped my fingers in and out of the ice water to keep them cold. This reduced circulation in my fingers so less chemo would invade those capillaries.

My fingernails remained fairly normal through sixteen treatments, though I had to keep them short to prevent them from ripping. I talked to another woman receiving the same drugs. She wasn't doing the ice torture, and she quickly developed brown spots on her fingernails. I don't know if she ever lost her nails.

The next two drugs I received, doxorubicin and cisplatin, were notorious for hand-foot syndrome. Some women reported severe blistering on their extremities. Uh, no thanks. I marched into a drugstore and bought ice wraps for my wrists and ankles. The night before seeing my ankhologist, I would pop them into the freezer. The next day they stayed cold for several hours during infusion.

Starting the following morning, I wrapped myself in blankets and soaked my hands and feet in ice water for twenty minutes, three times each day. I did this daily during the first three post-chemo days.

My hands and feet still got dried out, red, rough, and swollen, despite my liberal intake of omega-three fatty acids. The skin on my hands peeled, even between my fingers. I tried many creams and lotions, yet a beeswax lotion bar worked wonders—on par with lanolin (a fat extracted from sheep's wool) without the strong smell. It provided much soothing comfort every day.

One ankhologist suggested nicotine patches to prevent these sores, but I never felt that was necessary.

The fire of chemotherapy doesn't need to burn terribly; there are options to diminish the pain. Even in the midst of the burning flames, it might help to recall that we are honored and loved by the Divine. We are asked to let go of fears because the Spirit is with us and dwells within the cells of our bodies—even during chemotherapy.

Thriver Soup Ingredient:

I tried several creams to reduce the chapping on my hands and feet. The best I found were made of beeswax and/or lanolin, both natural products. If your skin gets dry and you decide to use cream, check the ingredients on products and stick with those that avoid alcohol and names of chemicals. I obtained my beeswax lotion bars from Mark Zeiner, a local beekeeper. If you opt for lanolin, there are tubes made for breastfeeding mothers that work especially well, though pure lanolin is thick, slow to absorb, and I don't care for the smell.

∾∾∾

Foot Sores: Socks Discrimination

He brought me up from the roaring pit, up from the muddy ooze, and set my feet on a rock, making my footing firm. He put a new song in my mouth, a song of praise to our God. Many will look on in awe and put their trust in ADONAI.

—Psalm 40:2-3, Complete Jewish Bible

I needed a lift out of the thick mire of water retention and help getting my steps reestablished. The edema was a side effect of the chemotherapy drugs. My feet were swelling and my socks started leaving creases around my ankles. I tried using ice packs during infusions, keeping my feet elevated, and soaking with ice water (also known as the ice torture) for three days following each infusion.

My feet kept expanding. I bought larger, looser socks, yet they, too, soon shackled my ankles.

My friend Kathy Nace suggested I try socks for diabetics because she found them soft and stretchy.

I bought four pairs and they worked perfectly. I used them throughout the rest of my treatments, completely wearing them out.

The socks also assisted with growing toenail issues. My nails softened and were easily torn, and even a little pressure on them—such as from blankets while in bed—hurt. The smaller nails turned dark brown during the first two types of treatments, then developed crusty white coatings during the final type of chemosabe.

Just after I started on the drip, a fellow cancer patient told me that hydrogen peroxide was helpful for preserving the nails and nail beds. I put some in a spray bottle and sprayed my toes, sometimes several times during the day. This helped the nails return to a more normal color and stay neatly inside their beds.

My nails also thickened and rose up about half-way along their beds. This made wearing dress shoes painful, so I stayed with walking shoes. This growth also prevented me from cutting the nails with trimmers. I went to a drugstore and asked for their roughest nail file. With some steady sawing, I managed to keep the nails in check enough to wear walking shoes. I jokingly threatened my then-husband to finally paint my nails, since they looked pretty disgusting.

With the ice torture, hydrogen peroxide spray, diabetic socks, and a hefty nail file, my nails and feet kept sturdy. I had a firm standpoint throughout treatment, a gift from my friends and the Divine.

Thriver Soup Ingredient:

Purchase a spray bottle and a bottle of hydrogen peroxide. Spray your toes in the shower or tub after you are clean, or put a towel on the floor before spritzing. Do this at least once a day and allow the fluid to sit for a few minutes to maximize the benefits.

～～～

Bee Products: Sweet Healing Gifts

And thy Lord taught the Bee To build its cells in hills, On trees, and in (men's) habitations; Then to eat of all The produce (of the earth), And find with skill the spacious Paths of its Lord: there issues From within their bodies A drink of varying colours, Wherein is healing for men: Verily in this is a Sign For those who give thought.

—Qur'an 16:68-69

Bees are so important that the Qur'an encourages people to reflect on the healing qualities of their honey, their "drink," which comes from within their bodies. A honeybee uses a long, tube-like tongue to suck nectar out of flowers. She stores the nectar in her second, or honey, stomach, which can hold almost seventy milligrams of nectar. She must visit between 100 and 1,500 flowers to fill her storage tank. When full, the honey stomach weighs almost as much as the bee.

Back at the hive, a worker bee sucks the nectar out of the honeybee's stomach and chews it for about half an hour. The bee's enzymes break down the sugars, making the honey more digestible and less vulnerable to bacterial attack. Then the honey is spread throughout the honeycombs until it is eaten.

Honey has been used since ancient times as part of traditional medicine. It works as an antibacterial, antioxidant, antitumor, anti-inflammatory, and antiviral agent, probably because of its flavonoids.

These flavonoids are available only in raw honey. This might be why Ayurveda, the ancient Asian Indian medical system, teaches that honey should be consumed raw—to take advantage of all its healing properties. Heating can destroy these qualities, leaving only a sweetener.

In my search for natural products following the diagnosis, I was aware of the healing qualities of bee products, including their honey, so I contacted a local beekeeper, Mark Zeiner. To help me out, he provided raw honey. I loved his lip balm, hand lotion bars, and soap made from beeswax prepared with other natural, fragrance-free ingredients.

I used the lip balm and soap daily. His lotion bar worked wonders when chemotherapy ravaged my hands.

In the future, even bee venom might help some cancer patients. When a bee stings something, it pumps in a toxin called melittin. Because melittin ruins membranes around individual cells, researchers at the Washington University School of Medicine have been experimenting with placing this substance into tiny particles they call nanobees. Nanobees are designed to destroy cancer tumors.

The honeybee's myriad gifts for healing are sweet indeed.

Thriver Soup Ingredient:

Contact a local beekeeping organization for the names of members who might have bee products to sell. One way to find local organization is via the Back Yard Beekeepers Association. They list clubs by state at www.beeculture.com/content/whoswho/.

~~~

Mouth Sores: Melt in Your Mouthwash

He also saw in her pores all the sentient beings who had been liberated by her from the calamities of unfavorable circumstances, evils, and miserable conditions.
                    —"The Flower Ornament Scripture," *Avatamsaka Sutra*

Sudhana, a youth depicted as an acolyte in Buddhist, Taoist, and folk stories; has gazed into the night sky and seen the goddess Vasanti, known as the lady of springtime. In the pores of her skin—the night sky—he saw all of the beings whom she had freed and turned into stars.

As a patient of the evil disease cancer, I wasn't among those whom she had liberated. I longed to be set free from my miserable condition, which included painful sores in the pores of my mouth, brought on by the calamity of chemotherapy.

During my second type of chemosabe treatment—with doxorubicin and cisplatin—my mouth hurt so much I lost twenty-five pounds in eight months.

At first I thought that by simply sucking on ice during the infusions I wouldn't have to give up the citric acid (namely my organic raw apple cider vinegar) or spicy foods. After all, ice had worked well for my fingers and feet while I was on paclitaxel and Cisplatin for eight months.

The sores appeared innocently enough. Mildly bothersome. No big deal. I swished with baking soda and salt water, as recommended by the chemo nurses, did the Emotional Freedom Technique and used the WholiSound Serenity Box to reduce pain and inflammation. I figured I could keep taking my apple cider vinegar each morning.

Big mistake.

The sores intensified. I shifted to a diet of mush so I could avoid chewing and sucking. Then I backed down to gentle drinks. Even sucking through a straw that emptied into the back of my mouth proved painful. I avoided talking.

I slurred to Connie Lasorso about the sores. "Great!" she said. "The chemosabe is working."

Okay, maybe I can keep tolerating this, I thought.

A few hours later—on Friday night, of course, long after the chemo filling station had closed for the weekend—I slurred to a pediatrician friend, desperate for some relief. She suggested mixing one part over-the-counter liquid antacid with one part children's liquid diphenhydramine, then swishing.

I raced to a nearby store, bought the two products, mixed them in my car, swished for five minutes, and spat. Ahhhh.... Relief! I could sleep, even if it was upright in my cushy chair so I could avoid pressing my painfully tender cheeks and lips into my teeth.

On Saturday I swished periodically. The sweet relief lasted about two hours. When numb enough, I could consume the cottage cheese/flax oil mix, green vegetable sludge—er, liquid sunshine, and plenty of coconut ice cream.

Saturday night I realized the mixture was making the mouth sores worse. So back to baking soda and salt, Emotional Freedom Technique tapping, and the sound pad. And plenty of pain.

What a long weekend. Finally, Monday crept around the corner. I slurred to a chemo nurse, who sent in a prescription for magic mouthwash. Real relief! I found it numbed my mouth for one to four hours. I advanced to soft foods.

She also suggested taking the amino acid lysine. I used lysine daily for a year. I don't think it did much for me.

Rather than swish my whole mouth with the wash, I switched to drowning a cotton swab in the medicine, then painting it onto the sore spots. This kept the rest of my mouth from going numb so I could still taste my food. Sometimes I ended up dribbling, yet felt grateful I could get the food down.

This miserable condition eventually subsided and I found liberation from mouth sores. Maybe not the total liberation of enlightenment with the Divine Feminine, yet the freedom to eat and speak again felt pretty darn good.

Thriver Soup Ingredient:

If you are receiving a type of chemotherapy known for mouth sores, I suggest asking for a prescription for magic mouthwash before leaving your first infusion. David Simon, MD, suggests gargling with a non-alcoholic herbal mouthwash that might contain or can be created from sage, goldenseal, slippery elm, licorice, or raspberry leaf (steep two tablespoons in one cup boiling water and allow it to cool). Also follow all advice about avoiding salt, spicy food, and citric acid, at least until after finishing the die-off phase. I found I had to avoid consuming those foods altogether during the months of harsh drug treatments. I remember well the deep satisfaction of my first taste of mustard after months without anything the slightest bit spicy.

~~~

Dry Eyes: My Eyes Will See the Glory

[M]y face is red from crying, and on my eyelids is a death-dark shadow. Yet my hands are free from violence, and my prayer is pure.... With friends like these as intercessors, my eyes pour out tears to God

—Job 16:16-17, 20, Complete Jewish Bible

Job, a character in the Hebrew Bible, has suffered terribly even though he has lived a righteous life. His friends try to guide him, but they only make him feel worse. And so his tears pour out to God.

I didn't need terrible suffering or unhelpful friends to cry copious tears. My eyes could drip onto a floor without a flicker of emotion. I would be walking around, not feeling anything in particular, when tears would start coursing down my face. It got so bad I went to see an optometrist. Laura Fiorenza, OD, said my problem wasn't excessive tearing; it actually was dry eyes. My lower eyelids, which normally excrete fat to help keep the water on the cornea from evaporating, were not producing much fat. Docetaxel was drying them out.

She suggested I use a hot compress on my eyelids once every day for three minutes, then press hard on the lower lids with an upward motion to encourage the ducts to excrete fat.

I did this every day right after my shower, when hot water already flowed out of my faucet.

She suggested at night I put a cream with a high mineral oil content into my eyes before going to sleep. During the day I could use eye drops also containing mineral oil.

The first time I used the drops, my eyes suddenly felt normal again—I hadn't realized how abnormal they had been feeling during the previous year.

While the shadow of death upon my eyelids came from both the cancer and chemotherapy, my face also shriveled from weeping about my condition. Job would have understood my pain and my tears, and might even have cried along with me. And yet, despite his terrible suffering, he wrote that his prayers were pure. He remained faithful despite every disaster that could be thrown his way. May I be able to do the same.

Thriver Soup Ingredient:

While on chemotherapy, I had trouble with my eyes clouding up from excessive fluids as my body worked at releasing toxins. I went to see my optometrist for a new prescription, and she urged me to wait until six months after ending chemotherapy before updating my prescription lenses. This is the amount of time it takes for the eyes to adjust to a new normal.

~~~

Booster Shots: Bringing Good Things to Life

Upon the corpse hung from a stake they directed the fear of the rays of fire, Sixty times the food of life, sixty times the water of life, they sprinkled upon it, Inanna arose.
—Inanna's Descent to the Nether World

According to ancient Sumerian mythology, the goddess Inanna descended into the netherworld, where her sister Ereshkigal reigned as queen. Ereshkigal promptly killed Inanna and put her corpse on a meat hook. When Inanna did not return to the surface, Inanna's messenger Ninshubur stormed heaven on her behalf. Enki, Inanna's maternal grandfather, responded by creating beings to go into the underworld to raise Inanna from the dead. After these beings sprinkled the food and water of life on Inanna's corpse, the goddess is resurrected.

For me, this myth resonated deeply during chemotherapy. Ereshkigal acted like chemotherapy in the body, killing off her own kind. During a chemotherapy treatment, the first cells to die include white blood cells because they grow quickly, just like cancer cells. Their numbers usually drop precipitously. Like chemo, Ereshkigal energy can cause patients, like Inanna, to languish, corpse-like, with low blood counts.

Keeping white blood cell counts high enough to stay on one's chemosabe treatment schedule can prove quite the challenge. Ankhologists routinely prescribe shots to boost white blood cell production between treatments. They are like Inanna's maternal grandfather, Enki. This man showed his wisdom and healing powers by providing a means for Inanna to return to life. Enki supplied two creatures to sprinkle the food of life and the water of life on the corpse. Their gifts brought new vitality into Inanna's veins, and she rose as if from the dead.

I was determined to stay on my chemo schedule to ensure its maximum effectiveness. And I didn't want any more drugs than necessary. After sixteen months on the drip, however, I bowed to necessity and accepted a shot of the food and water of life: granulocyte colony-stimulating factor, injected to increase my beleaguered white blood cell count.

I didn't want to take this drug any more than absolutely necessary. Its most common side effect is aching in one's bones, muscles, and joints. The night following the shot, my bones ached and my stomach queezed. Knowing these were normal side effects helped me cope. Thirst also kept me awake, and I must have drunk a quart during the night.

It was a good time to absorb Psalm 42:10 of the Christian Bible, NIV: "my bones suffer mortal agony." The night after my shot, I had some idea what agony in the bones felt like.

In the Bible's psalms, David cried out in his soul's anguish, just as any chemo patient might weep: "O Lord, how long? I am weary from my sighing; every night I sully my bed; I wet my couch with my tears." After all, as David reasoned, how can we praise the Divine if our voices lie silent in a grave?

The shot worked a miracle. For me, it was worth the pain. My white blood cell count shot up to 10.0, six points above the minimum acceptable range. During the following treatment, my mid-cycle count still remained 3.7, a high number for me (yet still below normal range, which begins at four). The count stayed high enough for the next drip. My inner Inanna had risen from the dead.

Thriver Soup Ingredient:

 If you are taking a white-blood-cell-stimulating drug and your body hurts, seek to support what your body is trying to do—help you survive. Sit or lie down and relax as much as you can. If you have the energy, try some slow, deep breathing. As you breathe in, imagine the oxygen bringing healing white light into the marrow of your bones. Gently let the breath go out, then inhale again, drawing in more healing light. Ask the Spirit to saturate, strengthen, balance, and heal your bone marrow.

<p style="text-align:center">~~~</p>

Heterogenius Cells

I have called upon thee, for thou wilt hear me, O God: incline thine ear unto me, and hear my speech. Shew thy marvellous lovingkindness, O thou that savest by thy right hand them which put their trust in thee from those that rise up against them. Keep me as the apple of the eye, hide me under the shadow of thy wings, From the wicked that oppress me, from my deadly enemies, who compass me about.

—Psalm 17:6-9, King James Bible

Wicked rebel cells had robbed me of my health, and my own cells had risen up against me, becoming my deadly enemy. I called upon the Divine for protection. It arrived via mortals using petri dishes.

 In my struggle to survive, I learned I could get a laboratory test to see if a sampling of my tumor cells had receptors for the hormones progesterone or estrogen.

 Results showed the cells lacked these receptors. This meant the progestin Megace, which the ankhologist could have prescribed, would probably have had little or no effect on my condition. Why take something you don't need, especially if one of the side effects is rapid weight gain? I felt so relieved that I had asked to have the cells tested.

 I then asked my doctor if I could take bio-identical hormone replacement therapy. He reminded me that tumors tend to be made up of heterogeneous cell populations, so there might have been some tumor cells with hormone receptors. He strongly recommended I stay away from all things estrogen, probably for the rest of my life.

 This explained what I found to be a strange phenomenon: When a tumor appears to respond to chemotherapy by shrinking, and then suddenly explodes in size, this rapid growth is caused by cells in the tumor that are different from those responding to the chemo. Phillip Sharp, a Nobel Prize-winning molecular biologist, calls the complexity of cancer cells "stunning."

 This confirmed my desire to continue with my healing practices, from the faith-based to the bizarre. As Vince Lasorso said, whatever works—I'd probably try it. I had everything to gain. I learned to rely more on my intuition to help me understand what did and did not work for my body. My growing ability to live in my body provided a huge boost in my confidence with this practice.

Vince reminded me to think globally while acting locally. Don't think about taking out each individual cell with the chemotherapy, he explained. This puts focus on the small stuff, and gives it more power.

Rather, focus on transforming your entire self. Use the grace of life already embodied in every cell to transform your whole body, making it healthy. I later realized this is a feminine way of healing, a concept that grew in importance for me.

Remember to take refuge in the Spirit, seeking protection from the foes residing within your own body. See yourself wrapped in heavenly wings, and feel cherished like the apple of Spirit's eye. Experience the wonder of Divine love that now makes so many treatments available to patients. Ask for healing light to fill, surround, and assail the rebel cells and transform your entire body.

Thriver Soup Ingredient:

Keep asking questions. Find out if samples of your cells can be tested for hormone receptors or responsiveness to other agents. Check with your medical insurance company to find out if any special procedures you want are covered.

Hope: To Have and Have Not

For in this hope we were saved. But hope that is seen is no hope at all. Who hopes for what they already have? But if we hope for what we do not yet have, we wait for it patiently.
　　　　　　　　　　　　　　　　　　—Romans 8:24-25, Christian Bible, NIV

Hope can survive doubt and despair. And we can always hope despite what is seen.

Following my final chemotherapy, I had a PET/CAT scan. Two days later I went to the hospital's medical records department to pick up my scan report. I read it as I walked toward the elevator. I read it again, and again, the paper slightly shaking.

Oh nooooo! Another nodule.

I scheduled my second lung resection.

During my post-operative check-up, I asked about the pathology report. She said the half-inch nodule from the July 23 scan had grown to two and one-half inches when it was removed August 31.

I understood better what the doctors meant when they said a type of cancer is aggressive. That growth, even with all I was doing...

The nurse, who had more than three decades of experience in that department and seen thousands of cancer patients, urged me to do more chemotherapy just to try to control the growth of anything else that might be lurking. It took a while for her to convince me. It was chemo or get ready for Hospice in a few months.

The next day I talked with my ankhologist. He reminded me that we had already tried everything known to work on uterine sarcomas. No other chemo agents had shown any measureable effectiveness, so there was no point in doing more chemo. Since he gets paid to give chemo, it was clear I had no more approved drug options.

He added that there was a new trial drug for soft-tissue sarcomas going on in Louisville, Kentucky, that had shown some measureable effect on leiomyosarcomas. I qualified in every way except they required measurable evidence of disease.

I used to think it was awful that people lived on chemo for five to ten years. At this point, however, I moved into jealousy. Tears flowed. Then I remembered to spend some time focusing on the sensations inside my body. The urge to jump out of my skin peaked, yet I stayed put, riding the waves.

By sitting with my hopelessness for a while, truly feeling and experiencing it, I miraculously moved into acceptance.

Amazingly, two months later I had a clean scan. Hope survived doubt and despair, moving me beyond what I could see.

Thriver Soup Ingredient:

No matter what you are told, everything is curable. To believe anything less is an insult to the Creator. One caveat: We do not know the mind of the Divine, and it might not be for our highest and best good to continue living this particular life. So hold onto hope, and demand a cure, if that is what you want. Miracles happen every day.

∽∽∽

Tax-o-Tears

Those who sow in tears will reap with cries of joy.

—Psalm 126:5, Complete Jewish Bible

My first ankhologist, Dr. Larry Copeland, learned from one of his patients that the chemotherapy drug docetaxel (Taxotere) tends to induce scar tissue that can completely close up a patient's lacriminal tear ducts.

We quickly scheduled outpatient surgery to thread thin, clear, two-inch silicon stents through each side of my face. These tubes would keep my ducts open, as the lacriminal ducts were threatening to permanently scar closed.

As I sat in the waiting area, I felt tremors in my lungs and watched my rapid, shallow breathing. In the pre-operation room I dressed in a gown and was hooked to a monitor. A nurse provided saline through an IV and acquiesced to my request that she hang a sign that faced the bag: "Easy, successful surgery, positive outcome."

The ophthalmologist decided to use sedation with local anesthesia rather than put me to sleep because I already was loaded up with chemotherapy drugs. Even though I was supposed to be in twilight sleep, I felt fully awake.

The surgery was painful, possibly because my tear ducts had already started closing up. The sedative didn't seem to do much for me. In recovery I let the tension go by allowing my body to shake, which frightened the nurses until I explained what I was doing.

At home again, my then-husband brought me two bags of frozen peas so I could drape them over my eyes. They worked great for about twenty minutes. His friend Helmut asked why we didn't use bags of corn. "Because I'd eat it," I said.

One of my swollen eyes had turned black, and by the next day I had swelling, bruises, and blood coming out my nose, all of which was normal. I used the pea bags as much as seemed reasonable to reduce the swelling and help the bruises fade.

Each day my eyes and nose felt better, although ten days after surgery my eyes still felt like they had hard contacts in them.

One month later, the docetaxel was causing excessive tearing, so my ankhologist's suggestion proved wise.

The stents appeared as tiny clear holes on the inside corners of my eyes—not noticeable to the casual observer. I was warned that the tubes could be pulled out if I rubbed my eyes. Sure enough, two months after surgery I rubbed my eyes and pulled one of the stents out about one-third of an inch. It felt fairly uncomfortable. I dreaded a visit to the surgeon the next day to have the stent moved back into place. Within a few minutes, I made a mental connection between pulling out the stent and not wanting to look at an old emotional issue with which I had been wrestling. About half an hour later my eye felt more comfortable, so I looked in the mirror. The stent had returned to its original position. I released a sigh of relief.

I didn't mind my eyes being excessively tearful. For one thing, I still needed to work on letting go of sadness. I had gone forth weeping, sowing many tears, and returned joyful that my tear ducts were saved.

For another, these tears might have been a channel for the docetaxel toxins to exit my body. I cried out seeds of poison to make room for sheaves of health. Cry on!

Thriver Soup Ingredient:

If you are involved with docetaxel, talk to your ankhologist about seeing an ophthalmologist to determine if you could benefit from having stents placed in your lacrimal ducts. If so, discuss timing for the surgery as it relates to your chemotherapy schedule, so you can take as much advantage of sedation and anesthesia as possible.

~~~

Taxanes: Hecate's Slips of Yew

Whom she [Hecate] will, she greatly aids and advances....

—ll. 404-452, *The Theogony of Hesiod*

According to ancient Greek mythology, the maiden goddess Persephone was abducted into the underworld by its king, Hades. Persephone's mother, the goddess Demeter, was beside herself with grief. She consulted with the virgin goddess Hecate on how to retrieve her daughter. Hecate suggested to Demeter that she talk to the sun god for assistance. After Demeter successfully negotiated her daughter's release from the underworld—for a season—Hecate became Persephone's companion for each journey to and from the kingdom of Hades. This gave Hecate experience with moving back and forth through the gateway between the realm of life and the world of shadows and death.

Subsequently, the funeral trees alder, poplar, and yew were associated with Hecate. Yew trees are known for their longevity; one of the oldest known examples lived at least 1,200 years. During ancient Greek ceremonies, Hecate's attendants honored the goddess by placing yew wreaths around the necks of sacrificial black bulls before the animals were slaughtered. Her potions contained "slips of yew," and the bough's seeds were extremely poisonous. Yew boughs, considered especially sacred to Hecate, were burned on funeral pyres because they symbolized death as only a transition to immortality.

The Greek word for yew, *toxos*, is similar to *toxicon*, their word for poison. Today, the scientific name for yew is *taxus*, and it provides Hecate's power to poison as the source for the chemotherapy taxanes such as paclitaxel (made from the bark of the Pacific yew tree). Paclitaxel is known for its ability to disrupt the action of proteins inside cellular structures so cancer cells can neither function nor reproduce.

I took paclitaxel even after two clean scans. How was I supposed to visualize paclitaxel debilitating cancer cells when there might not be any left in my body? Mica Renes, a naturopath, suggested I simply focus on the light and love that lives in each of my cells and within me. And just in case there were a few cells floating around in my bloodstream, they were "the dumb, confused ones that forgot to be part of the whole, and were thus sensitive to chemo," she wrote.

I also asked Judy Winall, who helped lead the Cincinnati Bruno Gröning Circle of Friends group, how to meditate when I had chemosabe in my body, assuming the cancer was gone. She suggested meditating on the drugs being effective as needed, with minimal side effects. That would be more of a verbal practice than a visualization exercise.

And I could call on the power of the goddess Hecate to greatly aid and advance my quest for health—watching her drip the poison from her cauldron into my veins and guide it to any cancer cells so they would shrink into oblivion.

Thriver Soup Ingredient:

If you take any of the taxanes, such as paclitaxel or docetaxel, you can call on the energy behind the goddess figure Hecate to poison the cancer cells by disrupting their protein functions. Perhaps you could see her poison as toga-clad ancient Greek peacekeepers swarming around, handcuffing, and hobbling all members of the rebel cells so they no longer can function.

~~~

Ifosfamide: Spa Chemosabe

I bless the Lord who has guided me; my conscience (lit. *kidneys*) *admonishes me at night.*
—Psalm 16:7, *The Book of Psalms*

According to the ancient Hebrews, the kidneys were the seat of one's conscience and emotions. My kidneys were going to take a beating from the chemotherapy drug ifosfamide, and I felt pretty scared, knowing I risked stupor and coma. If caught early, these potential side effects were treatable. To ensure the nurses could keep a close watch on me, I would receive this type of chemosabe for three days in a row in the hospital every three weeks. I would receive six treatments, the maximum lifetime dosage. Because ifosfamide affected the kidneys, my treatment included mesna to help keep them rowing. I also received the chemo drug paclitaxel.

To prepare, I talked to my ankhologist about which hospital was the better place to go for treatment. Once I settled on the hospital, I called the dietetic department to ensure I would receive the kind of food I wanted, when I wanted it.

With a little research, I learned that parsley, nettles, cranberries, and dried juniper berries could support the health of my kidneys during this treatment regimen, so I added them to my diet. I attempted to drink plenty of water. My psychotherapist created a visualization on cassette tape for when I was back under the bag. Not knowing how I would feel during my treatments, I brought home movies to view during my first session.

On day one I received eight hours of paclitaxel infusion, then mesna, then ifosfamide, then mesna four hours later, then mesna another four hours afterward. The mesna/ifosfamide/mesna/mesna routine repeated on days two and three.

After the second infusion of mesna on day three, I took home my final mesna treatment. It came in a needleless syringe. My ankhologist for this chemo, Dr. James Pavelka, heard from other patients that the bitter liquid was tolerable in pomegranate juice. I found a half cup of juice worked well—bitter yet not horrid.

After a couple of treatments, I decided my chemosabe sessions were spa treatments—someone else cooked and cleaned; I feasted on fresh produce, lean meat, and even brown rice; and I could do my nails (by spraying them with hydrogen peroxide to lessen the effects of chemotherapy on them). I brought different projects along to pass the time, such as painting my horse figurines and clay angels. On one stay I spent my three days writing more than 100 thank-you cards.

As treatment progressed, I found my fingers had more difficulty controlling a pen. Since neuropathy was a major known side effect, I wasn't surprised. And the neuropathy continued for years after treatment ceased.

With a cheerful attitude, however, I was able to turn this hospital time into a pleasure. This stance eased the burden of the continuous drips and lightened the yoke of my spa stays.

Thriver Soup Ingredient:

If you know you will be receiving chemotherapy in a hospital, call the dietitians ahead of time and ask for their assistance in planning appropriate meals for you. If you are going to have extended hospital stays, perhaps you could plan on taking a fun, easy project to do. Or, gather movies you've been wanting to watch but haven't yet. I took my laptop and used it for watching movies when I was too tired to paint or write. Most of all, do what you can to make the experience as fun as possible.

~~~

PIC Line: Seven of Nine

[F]or We Are nearer to him Than (his) jugular vein.

—Qur'an 50:16b

The Divine is closer to me than my own jugular—and it is through my veins that I received the gift of life extension through chemotherapy.

I never wanted a port placed in my chest for chemotherapy infusions. I chose, instead, to have my arms pierced for blood draws and treatments. For the final chemo, I chose to have a peripherally inserted central catheter (PICC or PIC line) placed under my upper left arm.

The tube insertion is relatively easy. Local anesthesia is given, ultrasound is used to find a vein, and then the tubes are inserted. Two tubes come out of the arm, run through a stabilizer and end in colored caps.

PIC lines can stay in the arm a maximum of three months; any more time brings a higher risk of infection. When the dressing is changed weekly, the lines are flushed. Blood can be drawn and infusions can be given. The dressing and beads need to be kept dry, so no showers or baths are permitted during this time.

I chose to leave my PIC line in for three treatments, have it removed, and reinserted when starting the fourth of six infusions.

After my first PIC line was inserted, the surgeon asked me when my initial surgery had been. "Seven of oh-nine," I answered—and realized I was virtually repeating the name of the human—turned Borg—turned human character from the "Star Trek: Voyager" television series, Seven of Nine. As Borg, she had been covered with tubes; now I had two tubes coming out of my arm.

When a PIC line is removed, you hold your breath as the nurse pulls. It's easy and painless. Then you have to lie flat for thirty minutes to prevent the formation of blood clots. No lifting with the arm is allowed for two days afterward so the wound can heal.

If you have a PIC line, remember that the Divine is with you—closer than your own jugular.

Thriver Soup Ingredient:

Some people enjoy the ease and comfort of getting a port in their chests for chemotherapy. I didn't want the scar. The PIC line can be a good option if you aren't getting a lot of chemotherapy for a long period of time. These lines are good for about three months, and the actual procedure can generally be done a few times.

~~~

Neuropathy: Tingle Town

Then I would feel consoled; so that even in the face of unending pain, I would be able to rejoice; for I have not denied the words of the Holy One.

—Job 6:10, Complete Jewish Bible

Unending pain can be caused by chemotherapy-induced peripheral neuropathy (CIPN). The nerves in your hands, forearms, feet, and lower legs will probably get damaged if you are on chemotherapy long enough. For me, it felt like I was constantly hitting my funny bone, primarily in my forearms and hands. Sometimes my forearms and hands felt numb, and became painful enough to prevent sleep. Writing by hand in my journal became difficult. On one chemo regimen I entered a phase of dropping things, even though I still could feel with my fingers.

The chemosabe nurse gave me instructions for taking large quantities of glutamine powder and vitamin B6. I learned that the B6 would be more easily absorbed if I took it with a vitamin B complex.

My CIPN continued long after I got off the drip. It felt especially painful in the morning. If it becomes severe enough, seek out the assistance of a chronic pain management specialist. Over a period of many months following chemotherapy, my neuropathy gradually eased, yet it still persists years later. I take consolation in knowing I am beloved of the Spirit, no matter what conditions my body faces.

Thriver Soup Ingredient:

Before you start chemotherapy, ask your ankhologist if the proposed treatment drugs are known to cause CIPN. I took taxanes and platinum-based drugs, both of which induce CIPN. If so, ask about taking vitamin B6 with a vitamin B complex and r-lipoic acid. Discuss the pros and cons of glutamine powder. If you start these nutrients ahead of time, it might save you some nerve damage.

Also ask for symptoms to watch for so you can be alert if CIPN develops. Let your health care team know so you can discuss more options.

≈ ≈ ≈

Visualizations: Imagination at Work

Inanna says to Ninshubur: "O (thou who art) my constant support, My messenger of favorable words, My carrier of supporting words, I am now descending to the nether world. When I shall have come to the nether world, Fill heaven with complaints for me...."

—The Descent of Inanna

I came to love the story of Inanna, queen of heaven and earth and the goddess of love for the ancient Sumerians. Her myth was my story as well. Through cancer, I descended into a hellish realm and, like Inanna, did not know if I would be able to return to the land of the living. I needed help from an inner source to fight by my side as I walked through the world of shadows.

The proverbial cavalry arrived in the form of my own imagination. Some people found benefit from visualizing the video game character Pac-Man eating cancer cells; one woman visualized a white killer rabbit.

During my first type of treatment, I visualized all of my friends and family as an army dressed in black, all carrying pouches around our waists. Inside the pouches were long spears—ruby red spears for the gemcitabine chemotherapy molecules and silver for the docetaxel molecules. We walked on the surface of a sarcoma nodule, each of us thrusting a ruby and a silver spear into each black sarcoma cell. Then my animal guides, a black panther and a snake, pushed the dying sarcoma cells into a black coffin-shaped trough for Glinda (the good witch of the North from the movie "The Wizard of Oz") and Jesus to carry into the white light of the Holy Spirit for permanent disposal.

After several months, I realized I could see the chemosabe attacking the shell-like cells that surrounded the tumor. When I attempted to take an intuitive look at the nodule, I could still see the outer shell that needed to be dismantled and removed.

Later, I visualized tearing down and removing the nodule walls. Afterward, I talked with Vince Lasorso about my realizing I could see all of us on the inside of the nodule attacking the cancer cells with our spears. He said because that image came up organically for me, it most likely indicated that the nodule was ready to break up and was dying. In the beginning, he said, cancer patients typically view the chemo attacks only on the outside of tumors because this method feels safer. To feel brave enough to enter the nodule, risking the spread of the cells, indicates by itself that the nodule wasn't spreading—it was breaking up and dying.

On my final scan with this regimen, two of the original nodules had died. Unfortunately, one was regrowing. Like Inanna, I was still wandering around in the underworld. But I wasn't yet ready to ask someone to set up a lament for me at the ruins of my life. If I needed to spend more time in the dark realms, I would hunt for a new approach.

Thriver Soup Ingredient:

Ask your ankhologist or chemotherapy nurses how your particular drugs work on cancer cells. Use that as a basis for creating a visualization that feeds your mind and soul in a positive way.

～～～

White Cell Counts: Great White Hope

We have created man from an extract of clay; then we made him a clot in a sure depository; then we created the clot congealed blood, and we created the congealed blood a morsel; then we created the morsel bone, and we clothed the bone with flesh; then we produced it another creation; and blessed be God, the best of creators.

—Qur'an 23:12-14, Palmer edition

According to the Qur'an, we humans are made from a clot of blood. Monitoring that life-sustaining liquid is a key component of managing chemotherapy. If white blood cell counts dip too low, the body runs the risk of infection. Chemosabe was only given when my blood levels rose high enough to sustain another chemical onslaught.

Several people contributed to my ability to maintain high-enough counts. For forty-two treatments during a two-year span, I only needed one shot to increase my white blood cell levels.

Vince Lasorso provided me with a relaxation CD designed to increase the production of white blood cells. "Bone Marrow Healing" involved feeling each of my bones, from my toes to the crown of my head, lighting up and becoming strengthened, balanced, and healed.

Emotional Freedom Techniques taught to me by Mim Grace Gieser and practiced regularly contributed to my ability to stave off the shots.

With a little snooping around on the internet, I found acupressure points I could press for the thymus gland (which contributes to white blood cell production) and to increase immunity.

I learned carrots and mushrooms help the body produce more white blood cells. This explains the emphasis on carrot juicing among health practitioners. Beta-carotene, which makes carrots orange, apparently protects the thymus gland. Maitake mushrooms are helpful as well.

Keeping my levels high without additional drugs proved challenging, even with all this assistance. White blood cells are designed to fearlessly move toward danger. Mine certainly did, as reflected in their high death toll. A minimum count usually required for treatment (along with other factors, such as platelet counts) often was 3.5. Once my mid-cycle count dipped to 1.6. The chemosabe nurse warned me not to lick the sidewalk or eat the soles of my shoes.

Toward the end of my treatments, my brave white blood cells got even better at playing limbo, reaching a new low—0.9. That's zero-point-nine.

Fortunately, my white counts rallied so I always managed to gain acceptance into Club Chemo. The Creator—whom the Qur'an says made me from a clot of blood, formed flesh from it and then marrow of bones—infused me with enough life for my thymus gland and bone marrow to rally with sufficient white blood cells.

Thriver Soup Ingredient:

My chiropractor, M. Jay Panyko, suggested visualizing white blood cells emerging from my thymus gland like popcorn. Or you can try the image of a blizzard emerging from your bones. Play with various images until you find what works for you.

～～～

Fatigue: You Snooze, You Cruise

Haven't you known, haven't you heard that the everlasting God, ADONAI, the Creator of the ends of the earth, does not grow tired or weary? His understanding cannot be fathomed. He invigorates the exhausted, he gives strength to the powerless. Young men may grow tired and weary, even the fittest may stumble and fall; but those who hope in ADONAI will renew their strength, they will soar aloft as with eagles' wings; when they are running they won't grow weary, when they are walking they won't get tired.

—Isaiah 40:28-31, Complete Jewish Bible

If the Divine is supposed to invigorate the exhausted and give strength to the powerless, where was this energy? Fatigue is a major complaint resulting from chemotherapy treatment. I had a friend so worn out by chemo that she stopped taking it. She passed away in a matter of months.

I forged ahead, taking exquisite care of my body and soul, determined to do all the chemo available to me. I wanted to live a full life.

As if to spite my healthy diet and disciplined self-care, my energy levels began dropping, even during the better week before the next infusion. I had a hard time getting motivated to do much of anything besides lie around and watch videos.

As the months wore into years, energy intuitive Maria Paglialungo reported the gradual decline of my *chi* or *qi*, otherwise known as my life-force energy. The drugs were persistently draining the life out of me.

It wasn't until six months after my final chemo infusion that the length of time before I wanted a nap stretched into twelve hours. That became awkward because in sixteen hours I wanted to be sleeping for the night. I decided the best way to place myself in a position to renew my strength and have a power surge was to do the sitting technique taught by Bruno Gröning. With a timer set for fifteen minutes, I sat upright, palms up on my lap, and asked to be filled with Divine healing energy. Then I simply noticed what was happening in my body during those minutes. As I waited upon the Spirit, my strength rose and my weariness abated.

I'm not running. Walking, yes; and even soaring—yes, with the Spirit in those quiet moments of respite.

Thriver Soup Ingredient:

Relax. Take your time with everything. Rest when your body wants to rest. Your "job" right now is to get well, and resting gives your body a chance to recover its equilibrium.

A little Indian valerian can help calm restlessness. David Simon, MD, suggests placing an ounce of dried ground roots and underground stems into a silk pillow and placing it where you can breathe in the aroma at night. If you don't have a silk pillow, a cotton sock tied off at the end can probably work just as nicely.

~~~

Chemo Brain: A No-brainer

And when they came to Jordan, they cut down wood. But as one was felling a beam, the axe head fell into the water: and he cried, and said, Alas, master! for it was borrowed. And the man of God said, Where fell it? And he shewed him the place. And he cut down a stick, and cast it in thither; and the iron did swim. Therefore said he, Take it up to thee. And he put out his hand, and took it.
<div align="right">—2 Kings 6:4b-7, King James Bible</div>

One of the prophets in Elisha's company was cutting down a tree when his borrowed axe head fell into the river. The group learned from Elisha that they could ask for assistance with anything that distressed them—nothing was too inconsequential, not even a borrowed tool.

I found this true as well, even with chemo brain.

It didn't take long for this mental fog to manifest. Two months after starting chemotherapy, I found that once or twice a day I struggled to find a word, and experienced brief lapses in short-term memory. Coming from a family of intellectuals, this was not a little distressing.

During the third month I began forgetting words, losing track of what I was saying, and putting things in wrong places. I went back to the eye doctor for my post-surgical follow-up and complained about excessive itching, tearing, and redness in my left eye. He plucked a few eyelashes and, bingo, the itching stopped. Was chemo brain really so bad that I couldn't have figured that out on my own?

Ah, it only got worse.

By December I knew I needed to take my time when talking, and everything I needed to remember had to be written down. I found if I needed to get something from another room, I had to say out loud what it was or I would get into the other room and have no clue why I was standing there.

Eight months into chemo I frequently forgot the names of common household objects or rooms.

The following year I could hardly bring myself to read. I would pick up a book and just stare at the words, hardly able to absorb their meaning. Reading had become a struggle and I didn't want to put forth the effort unless it was necessary. What a huge disappointment for a voracious bibliophile.

And then there were the conversations. I could hardly string three thoughts together. Everything I talked about had to be simplified. Now I knew what "no-brainer" really meant.

My friend Laura Dailey wrote, "The brainiac part of you probably despises that. At least you have an excuse now for putting a book in the freezer and ice cream on the bookshelf! Every magazine you reread can seem new!"

Fortunately I knew this fog would pass. Both the chemotherapy nurse and my doctor said most of the murkiness would resolve a few months after chemosabe ended, even though I had been on the drugs for years. Usually it's gone within a year. I found it persisting.

In the meantime, I made it a habit to ask for help, even with the small things in life. Assistance usually showed up, like the axe blade that reappeared for the prophets.

Thriver Soup Ingredient:

Ask the Divine for assistance while you cope with chemo brain. Then, as my friend Charley Sky suggested to me, whenever you do remember something, say "Thank you" out loud to the Spirit or to your mind. This reinforces recall.

≈≈≈

Corticosteroids: I'm Melting, Melting...

What is fragile is easy to dissolve; What is minute is easy to disperse. Act when there is yet nothing to do. Govern when there is yet no disorder.

—Tao Te Ching, 64

Through my chemotherapy experiences, I learned how easily joints and bones can dissolve. About four months after finishing two years of chemotherapy, a nurse measured my height. I was half an inch shorter than I normally measured. I thought it odd but didn't question her—I figured she was rounding down.

Soon thereafter, one of my brothers said he found out steroids lead to deterioration in the musculoskeletal system, causing people to shrink.

Oh, crap. I had been on Decadron, a corticosteroid, for forty-two chemotherapy sessions.

Soon thereafter I took my kids to the doctor and measured my height for myself. I hadn't lost half an inch. I have lost a full inch of height.

My gut clenched. I felt like the Wicked Witch of the West from the movie "The Wizard of Oz" when Dorothy poured water on her: "I'm melting, melting..." In my ignorance, I had not dealt with my shrinking cartilage before the problem emerged.

I went online to search the National Institutes of Health website. It reports that Decadron can decrease bone formation and increase bone resorption. It may lead to the development of osteoporosis at any age.

There wasn't anything I could do except try to keep my bones and joints as healthy as possible. I needed to put forth greater effort in preventing osteoporosis, dealing with the possibility before it could emerge. That meant frequent weight-bearing exercise and a diet rich in bone-building nutrients.

Unfortunately, it was too late to save my hips. They had been in bad shape before starting chemotherapy, yet I am fairly certain the Decadron cleaned out the remaining cartilage. I had to undergo two total hip replacements the following year.

Fortunately, the orthopedic surgeon said my bones looked healthy. It was my joints that had suffered from the steroids. Perhaps my bones hadn't melted too much. There still was time to put my musculoskeletal system back in order.

Thriver Soup Ingredient:

Talk with your ankhologist about avoiding steroids as much as possible. See if you can opt for another medication to deal with the nausea, vomiting, and potential allergic reactions, at least part of the time. If you do accept the corticosteroids, ask your ankhologist what you, specifically, can do to reduce bone and cartilage loss.

~~~

Finishing Chemo: Good to the Last Drip

Say to the fainthearted, "Be strong and unafraid! Here is your God; he will come with vengeance; with God's retribution he will come and save you." Then the eyes of the blind will be opened, and the ears of the deaf will be unstopped; then the lame man will leap like a deer, and the mute person's tongue will sing. For in the desert, springs will burst forth, streams of water in the 'Aravah; the sandy mirage will become a pool, the thirsty ground springs of water. The haunts where jackals lie down will become a marsh filled with reeds and papyrus. A highway will be there, a way, called the Way of Holiness. The unclean will not pass over it, but it will be for those whom he guides[;] fools will not stray along it. No lion or other beast of prey will be there, traveling on it. They will not be found there, but the redeemed will go there. Those ransomed by ADONAI will return and come with singing to Tziyon, on their heads will be everlasting joy. They will acquire gladness and joy, while sorrow and sighing will flee.

—Isaiah 35:4-10, Complete Jewish Bible

Be strong, and do not fear, because at some point Divine recompense will come and chemotherapy will end. One way or another, I believe the wasteland of everyone's life will end and each of us will experience gladness and joy—even if it is in the great beyond.

During one of my final chemotherapy treatments in the hospital, I watched the movie "Champions." It's a true story about British jockey Bob Champion who was training to ride in the Grand National steeplechase horse race. He learned he had metastatic testicular cancer and went through chemo. During this time his horse injured a tendon and was confined to his stall for six months. Everything appeared to be falling apart. After several treatments, Bob "lay groaning and kept pleading, 'Please let me die, Frank (Bob's friend, Frank Pullen). Tell them to leave me alone.'" (This was in the days before Zofran, a fabulous anti-nausea medicine I took.)

Bob told the nurse to remove the drip. She did, and suggested he walk around the hospital. Bob ended up in the children's cancer ward. In the movie, one of the kids asked him if he was going to live or die. Bob was startled into choosing to live, and later wrote that the incident was an important life lesson. He admitted he had been whining and thinking only about himself, while downstairs were "poor little kids" going through the same difficulties without complaining. He experienced a turning point in his life. "If they could take the treatment," he reasoned, "so could I."

He completed all the chemo and was cured. (He was told ahead of time if he did that course of treatment he could put cancer behind him—testicular cancer is one of three types of cancer that have known cures). Amazingly, two years later he and his horse won the Grand National, he got married, and the following year had a son.

I had two friends with metastatic cancer. Both had chemotherapy and stopped before finishing their treatments. Both turned to alternative healing modalities. Both passed away in less than a year.

Chemosabe can keep people alive for many years. Two friends of mine had sisters kept alive for ten years with regular infusions. One of them rode horses until she passed.

Bob Champion chose to endure into the cure. For many people, this is possible, and they will be redeemed. They stayed strong and eventually achieved gladness and joy. They gave me the courage to continue.

Thriver Soup Ingredient:

If you are thinking about quitting chemotherapy, talk at length with your ankhologist. How have others with a similar situation survived, both with and without continued infusions? What other options did they choose, and how did they fare? What else can be done to support and assist you if you decide to continue with chemo? Gather all the information you possibly can. Think carefully through your options. Pray and ask for Divine guidance.

～～～

Ending Chemo: Take a Licking and Keep on Ticking

The Menat of Hathor, Mistress of Kusae, that She may show you favor, that She may prolong your life, that She may overthrow your enemy.

—Rock tomb of Meir

Hathor, the Egyptian goddess of love, often was depicted as a cow, and also was known as the eye of the sun. I needed the loving nature of the Divine feminine to show me favor, to overthrow my enemy, to help me replenish my body after chemotherapy came to an end, and to prolong my life.

The end can come in more than one way. Maybe it's a clean scan, or the ankhologists run out of drugs known to be effective, or the cancer has spread too far.

After my first round of treatments, I expected to be done with chemo and have a clean scan. Yet my abdomen still tightened when I thought about the aftermath of treatment. What would happen next? How long would I have clean scans? How could I protect myself with alternative treatments?

Someone else who had recently finished treatment and was in remission wisely commented, "I do believe that these feelings and doubts...are a typical part of the cancer journey. I also think it is quite typical that they come at the end of chemotherapy.... What happens when the chemo is over? The protection is gone. That can make one feel very insecure, of course!" She expressed in words what had been growing like a bubble in my mind.

"What long-time effects will the chemo have? Will I get metastases? When shall I go back to work? Was my heart damaged? When will my brain function normally again?" she wrote. "I noticed that I didn't stress so much with exercising any more. There was no more chemo I had to prepare for; I could just sit at home and relax on the sofa. That was when I noticed how big the pressure had been to come through the chemo time as well as possible."

She wisely noticed that this post-drip insecurity makes us easy prey for others who make money by selling products or services to ease our jitters. "I am not immune to them, I noticed. It is so difficult to see what can be useful information and what is pseudo-scientific junk or just bad ideology."

For me, the end came when the doctors ran out of conventional chemotherapy drugs known to have any effectiveness. Yet I still had one option—the best option of all. I could let go of my need to control by doing something. Instead, I could simply receive from the Spirit of Love who might show favor, who might prolong my life, and who might overthrow the enemy and heal me. I rested in the warmth of the Divine Mother, imagining her enfolding me in her maternal care.

Thriver Soup Ingredient:

If you have finished chemotherapy, be cautious about claims regarding alternative therapies. This is a time when you probably are more vulnerable than usual, and there are plenty of mistaken ideas lurking on the internet. Discuss with your ankhologist any ideas you might encounter. Search online for reviews of products. Sometimes you might have to dig through several pages of online links for useful information. Once I had to read through ten pages of internet search results before I found a scientist's website that told the truth about a certain product. I was glad then that I had not thrown away thousands of dollars on a scam.

B. Softening Surgery

Introduction to Softening Surgery: Scarred—>Scared—>Sacred

Surely he has borne our griefs, and carried our sorrows: yet we did esteem him stricken, smitten of God, and afflicted. But he was wounded for our transgressions, he was bruised for our iniquities: the chastisement of our peace was on him; and with his stripes we are healed.
—Isaiah 53:4-5, American King James Version, Christian Bible

*P*erhaps getting scarred up—being stricken, afflicted, pierced, crushed, and wounded—is one way of doing a form of devotion to the Divine reminiscent of what Thomas à Kempis, a late Medieval Catholic monk, called imitating Christ. If the Divine has borne my pain and suffering, the Spirit has been one busy dude. I own more battle scars than most soldiers ever get.

Evidence of a horizontal C-section already creased my abdomen. The hysterectomy added a long vertical blemish with a little s-curve around my navel. I call it my Superwoman tattoo. Maybe in another life I was Scarbelly, meanest pirate on the Caribbean, branded with an anchor-shaped disfigurement covering my entire abdomen.

Later I had nodules removed from my lungs, adding five more slits. What kind of a nickname would cover seven dents scattered over a woman's torso?

Marion Woodman, widely known Jungian analyst, endured a two-year trauma with a uterine carcinoma. I was in great company. She recorded her experiences in *Bone: Dying into Life*. Being a word lover myself, I read with fascination her connection among the words scarred->scared->sacred. She included a picture of ceremonial scarring done on the abdomens of women in Nigeria—a ritual oblation. She wrote that perhaps her surgery was the sacrifice of her feminine organs as a preparation for her next step in her inner development. Her round belly, like the navel of her world, would be cut and scarred to make room for more spiritual development.

Cancer can leave a multitude of scars. If Woodman is right, those blemishes became a sacrifice of more than my feminine organs in preparation for the next chapter in my spiritual textbook.

Scars are the trophies of a life well lived, according to my dad, a World War II veteran. Men are proud of theirs—so why shouldn't women be? These wounds testify to the many ways I have fought to survive, am living my life well, and am continuing that process. The seven scars on my torso represent a number of perfection and completion. The creases themselves are made of stronger, more resilient material than neighboring normal skin, just as the scars to my soul have given it strength and power beyond my expectations. By my wounds the Spirit has healed me on many levels. I am at peace with them.

Thriver Soup Ingredient:

If you have a scar, transform it into something sacred. Connie Lasorso told me about a woman who had the image of a phoenix placed on her chest after a mastectomy. What lovely symbolism, and what wonderful acceptance of her new body, rather than torturing it with the painful surgeries required to regain a breast.

~·~·~

Heidi's Top Five Surgery Quick-start Tips

1. If you are able and have enough advanced notice, try exercising the muscles around the area where you will have surgery. Most likely, when the surgeon makes his first slice, your body will experience less shock; you might reduce the risk of complications; you probably will feel better after surgery; and recovery could progress more rapidly.

2. When surgery is being scheduled, talk with your doctor about what supplements need to be halted, and when, so your body is in optimal condition for the stress of the knife. Find a list in "Pre-operative Testing: Fit for a Queen" in this section.

3. Consider asking for tramadol for pain management after surgery, rather than morphine or other opiates. Opiates tend to suppress the immune system, which is the last thing a cancer patient needs. Tramadol, on the other hand, has shown some indication that it might improve immune functioning. Tramadol can cause more nausea, while morphine can lead to constipation.

4. Consider getting a copy of the Monroe Institute's "Hemi-Sync Surgical Support CD Series." Listen to the first CD with headphones as much as possible, and follow the other instructions provided. It helped me get out of the hospital a day early with most of my surgeries. Learn more in "Preparing for My First Lung Surgery: Eve's Rib," located in this section.

5. The day before surgery take a dropperful of the liquid homeopathic remedy arnica four times by mouth. The day of surgery, rub a drop of the arnica fluid in the crease behind the bottom of each ear every two hours. Continue until you can consume solids again, then restart the pellets. Read more in "Preparing for My First Lung Surgery: Eve's Rib," located in this section.

~·~·~

Hysterectomy: The Road Will Never be the Same Again

The afflicted, the questers for wisdom, the cravers for power here and in the hereafter, and the wise— these, O Arjuna, are the four kinds of righteous men who pursue Me.
                    —*God Talks with Arjuna: The Bhagavad Gita*, 7.16

My pursuit of the Holy suddenly twisted me around a terrifying bend on the road of life, slapped me onto a hospital gurney, and landed me in a pre-operative suite. I was prepped, wheeled into surgery, transferred to the operating table, and put to sleep. The surgical team removed my cancerous uterus, cervix, fallopian tubes, ovaries, and about six inches of my small intestine. They washed my abdomen until there was no more visible cancer. My lymph nodes were declared clear.

I felt horrible in post-surgical recovery. I don't remember being told I had cancer. When I finally came to in my hospital room, I simply knew.

Recovery was hell. By day three, I was hallucinating. In the hospital. It wasn't from the opiates. That day, five people in white coats, including a social worker, traipsed into my room holding clipboards. How was my stay? they asked.

I told them I hadn't slept more than a handful of minutes since coming out of surgery, and was experiencing hallucinations. After that I was finally given some space and started getting one- and one-half-hour naps. What a relief.

Gorgeous bouquets poured in, and my room looked and smelled like a floral shop. Marybeth Wolf wrote, "Flowers remind me of God in His glory, because they are so delicate, strong, and beautiful all at the same time."

The blossoms lifted my spirits, which I needed. A few days later I learned the sarcoma cells had invaded my bloodstream. A CAT scan of my chest showed a one-centimeter spot on my left lung's lower lobe.

I had fallen among the afflicted. I reacted by craving the Divine more ferociously.

Thriver Soup Ingredient:

When I had my hysterectomy, I expected my abdomen to eventually flatten.

No such luck.

When I got home more than a week after surgery, I measured it. Thirty-five inches. The nurse told me to expect the swelling to continue for a couple of months, not unlike the after-effects of giving birth.

And no, my abdomen—even after being so thoroughly cleaned out—never did flatten. No washboard tummy for me. It's a good thing I never wanted one. I decided bridling such expectations and focusing on the Spirit instead was a better use of my limited energy.

Stomach Tube: Elephant Woman

Varenya said, "In the world of birth and death many difficulties arise, and they are very hard to endure. Remover of obstacles, kindly show me the path to liberation now."

—"Ganesha Gita," from *Ganesha Purana*

In the world of those near death, many difficulties arise that are hard to endure. I woke up from my first surgery with a tube arising from my stomach and exiting through my nose; a plastic remover of obstacles in the belly. The tube irritated my throat, making swallowing and speech painful. The hose, light as it was, weighed down my head. I had to use my hands to lift my face so I could look up. I didn't have much strength, so I mostly let my head hang. My forearms swelled up from an IV gone bad. I felt not only like the cartoon character Popeye, with huge forearms, but also like an elephant woman with a long trunk. My condition reminded me of Ganesh, the Hindu god with the head of a pachyderm. This god of wisdom and learning is the remover of obstacles. Whoa, did I have obstacles.

The movie "The Elephant Man," released in 1980, also came to mind. The story follows the life of Joseph Merrick, who had a rare disorder called Proteus syndrome. The overgrowth of his skin and bones disfigured his body terribly. During the movie, Merrick cried out, "I am a human being." Moaning on the hospital bed, with gauze bandages covering my belly, needles pumping fluids into my forearms, and a tube hanging perpetually out my snout, I frequently felt the urge to repeat his words.

In one deeply moving scene, Merrick quoted the Bible's Psalm 23, "The Lord is My Shepherd." Wallowing in my misery, I recalled the Christian King James version of the psalm from memory—I hadn't thought about it in twenty-five years—and said it several times, absorbing comfort from its message: "The LORD is my shepherd; I shall not want. He maketh me to lie down in green pastures: he leadeth me beside the still waters. He restoreth my soul: he leadeth me in the paths of righteousness for his name's sake. Yea, though I walk through the valley of the shadow of death, I will fear no evil: for thou art with me; thy rod and thy staff they comfort me."

Slowly I emerged from the shadow of immediate death, impatiently awaiting the removal of my elephantine appendage. The tube had to stay in my stomach until my bowels woke up. That typically takes three to ten days. My intestines started to move on day five, so the doctors were willing to pull—yet I felt afraid I still wouldn't keep anything down. I refused their offer, because waiting seemed more tolerable than the possibility of getting the tube removed and then re-inserted. On the morning of the sixth day I felt confident enough to allow a nurse to pull the plastic pipe.

Oh, what a relief. One difficult endurance test completed.

Liberated from the obstacle of a stomach tube, I started on a clear liquid diet. The next morning I ate white rice. I had no idea plain white rice could taste so good...

Thriver Soup Ingredient:

If you are in the hospital with a tube through your nose and down to your stomach, remember Ganesh; your trunk is removing obstacles from your belly so your bowels have a chance to recover and you can receive some measure of liberation. Even while walking that Valley of the Shadow of Death, remember the Spirit is with you, able to provide comfort in whatever form you can receive it.

$$\sim\!\sim\!\sim$$

Bag Lady

Come to me, all you who are weary and burdened, and I will give you rest. Take my yoke upon you and learn from me, for I am gentle and humble in heart, and you will find rest for your souls. For my yoke is easy and my burden is light.

—Matthew 11:28-30, Christian Bible, NIV

Overnight I became a bag lady, weary and burdened.

Throughout my nine-day hospital stay after my 2009 hysterectomy, I remained perpetually chained to intravenous bags. Fluids, blood, iron, potassium, drugs, drugs, and more drugs. I still shudder inside when I hear squeaky IV pole wheels.

Thirty-six hours after my first lung resection, I was told to take three walks during each day. Okay, I was chained to an IV pole, a temporary bladder bag, and two 12x12 hard plastic trunks for my lung fluids. Take a walk? While yoked to all those accessories? When I was shaky at best?

They did provide a walker and someone to pull the pole for me. How symbolic. Trundling around, dragging all this luggage with me, I received support from the walker and extra assistance while I needed all my baggage. Gradually, after I did my exercises, and when I was ready, portions of paraphernalia were removed. They no longer served any useful purpose and were disposed of by those helping me. Finally, the hour arrived when I could joyfully stride upright, accessory-free, through the hospital corridors.

The Spirit helps carry our burdens while we need them—and removes them when we truly are ready. Nothing is forced—there's simply a gradual progression from one level to another, each previous stage creating a stairway for the next, each new platform bringing a greater sense of freedom...until we are unyoked and free to live the lives the Divine created us to live.

Thriver Soup Ingredient:

If you are tied to IV bags or other luggage, begin to see them as metaphors for your spiritual walk. Whether they represent baggage you will eventually shed, or assistants on your closer walk to the pearly gates of heaven, encourage yourself to find the joy, rest, and gratitude in the circumstances you are given.

Paying Someone to Knife You

Whoever is soft and yielding is a disciple of life.

—Tao Te Ching, 76

By being receptive to my body's responses during a consultation with my ankhologist and by choosing to yield to the knife, I was able to ascend a step closer to a healthy life.

My opportunity presented itself after the second set of chemotherapy treatments proved to no longer be effective; one of the nodules was growing again.

My then-husband and I sat in my ankhologist's office, sinking deeper into our chairs. The doctor suggested two other drugs to pair with ifosfamide, and didn't have a good feel for which would be more effective. He'd only known less than half a dozen people in thirty years who got rid of their nodules with such a regimen.

Then my former husband sat up. What about surgically removing the nodules and testing them for the best chemo drug to combine with ifosfamide?

A rush of positive energy washed up my body. Yes, that felt so right. Especially because there were only two nodules to remove.

We agreed on the surgery, then testing of the cells, then a final type of drip.

By being receptive to the rise of positive energy in my body at the suggestion of surgery, and by yielding to the process we selected, I acted as a student of life, moving closer to better health. The surgery left me with clean scans for seven months—a long time with the diagnosis I'd been given.

Thriver Soup Ingredient:

If you are heading for surgery, my friend Kathryn Martin Ossege suggests the following: Visualize collecting all the traumas and illnesses held everywhere in your body and moving them into the body part being removed by surgery. Then approach your surgery as a ceremony to remove all that negative energy.

~~~

Pre-operative Testing: Fit for a Queen

And the LORD God formed man of the dust of the ground, and breathed into his nostrils the breath of life; and man became a living soul.
—Genesis 2:7, King James Bible

I wanted my dirty lungs cleared so I could remain a living soul, receiving into my body the breath of the Spirit.

Before having a planned surgery, doctors will want to ensure your body can manage the operation. So for my lung resections, I had preoperative assessments performed. The day-long process started with placing a wristband on my arm (a bracelet for the day). My neck was measured (for a necklace?), an instrument was put on my finger (a ring?), they asked me to sign an electronic signature pad called Topaz, and they set me down on a golden throne.

I'm royalty.

Blood was drawn and anesthesiologists questioned me.

The stress test was a little fun for me. I was not allowed to ingest water or food two hours before the appointment. Then the nurse injected an intravenous isotope. While waiting, I sipped ice water. Then I walked on a treadmill until my heart rate climbed into their target range.

The least pleasant test was for breathing capacity. I sat in a Plexiglas box with a tube and nose clips and performed numerous breathing exercises. These included exhaling over and over until I felt I had nothing left to expire. I can still hear the technician: "Keep going, keep going, keep going..." Nothing painful, yet uncomfortable and certainly unenjoyable.

It turned out I had mild asthma (inflammation of the lung's airways), yet nothing of any real concern.

I passed all the pre-op tests both times. My body must be brilliant.

My chest was ready for the blade—a procedure that would clear my lungs of rebel cells so I could freely breathe in the soul of life supplied by the Divine.

Thriver Soup Ingredient:

If you want to have your tumor tested after surgical removal, ask your surgeon to collect all tumor tissue. Check with your insurance company to find out what is and is not covered, and gather cost estimates so you can prepare.

When surgery is being scheduled, talk with your doctor about what supplements need to be halted, and when, so your body is in optimal condition for the stress of the knife. Anything with anticoagulant properties needs to be avoided for a week before surgery. These include chamomile, melatonin, inositol, passionflower, skullcap, hops, valerian, GABA, and 5-HTP. Ginseng can interfere with anesthesia. Also avoid fish oil, garlic, vitamins C and E, ginger, and gingko because they thin the blood.

In addition, consider asking for tramadol for pain management after surgery, rather than morphine or other opiates. Opiates tend to suppress the immune system, which is the last thing a cancer patient needs. Tramadol, on the other hand, has shown some indication that it might improve immune functioning. Tramadol can cause more nausea, while morphine can lead to constipation.

～～～

Preparing for My First Lung Surgery: Eve's Rib

The Lord God said, "It is not good for the man to be alone. I will make a companion for him who corresponds to him." The Lord God formed out of the ground every living animal of the field and every bird of the air. He brought them to the man to see what he would name them, and whatever the man called each living creature, that was its name. So the man named all the animals, the birds of the air, and the living creatures of the field, but for Adam no companion who corresponded to him was found. So the Lord God caused the man to fall into a deep sleep, and while he was asleep, he took part of the man's side and closed up the place with flesh. Then the Lord God made a woman from the part he had taken out of the man, and he brought her to the man.

—Genesis 2:18-22, Christian Bible, NET

Just as Adam was alone before his surgery, I wanted some time alone before mine. I felt I needed to rest, get centered, pray, meditate, and simply be. I chose to spend nine days at Grailville, a nearby women's spiritual conference center. I moved in during early January, so I had the huge, old Victorian House of Joy all to myself. I soaked up the silence in my little nesting area to prepare for the coming physical trauma.

Since I'd heard exercising before surgery improves recovery and reduces complications, I exercised with more discipline, even during my retreat, for the weeks before my lung surgery. I worked my muscles gently twice each day to maximize any benefits I might accrue. I focused on strengthening my torso, especially my chest area.

My psychotherapist loaned me her copy of the Monroe Institute's "Hemi-Sync Surgical Support CD Series." I listened to them without putting on headphones. I didn't really see any value in the program. I talked about it with my therapist, who told me one of her clients got out of the hospital a day early after using it. Then I talked to Vince Lasorso. He had introduced the series to my therapist. His wife, Connie, had studied the series at a local hospital and found the patients fared better. The producers say they use sound frequencies to alter one's brainwaves so both sides of the brain work in coherence. Audible suggestions are embedded in the CD. So I decided to use headphones at least once a day to listen to the pre-surgical CD.

The day before surgery I followed the recommendation provided by my Ayurvedic physician, Hari Sharma, MD. He suggested taking a dropperful of the liquid homeopathic remedy arnica four times by mouth.

The day of surgery I could not take anything by mouth. Following Dr. Sharma's suggestion, I rubbed a drop of the arnica fluid into the crease behind the bottom of each ear every two hours.

I sat in the waiting area feeling my fear, primarily in my lungs. I watched my shallow, rapid breathing. Later, as I sat on the cot and met all the surgical attendants, I allowed myself to shake out the tension. I was rolled into the operating room, shifted onto a table and disappeared into oblivion. Like Adam, I was placed in a deep sleep for part of my chest to be removed.

Perhaps all of these preparations did the trick; who knows. However, I got to go home after about two days (I was supposed to stay three to five days); I was off the pain medications in 3.5 days (I was expected to be on them for two to three weeks); and I recuperated quickly. Like Adam, I had been put to sleep, my flesh closed up, and I recovered beautifully.

Thriver Soup Ingredient:

If you have time and are able, try preparing for surgery with meditation, prayer, time alone, exercise, and relaxation techniques. Perhaps even try liquid arnica behind the bottom of your ears every two hours during the day of surgery, and afterward if you are unable to consume liquids.

If you can't find arnica in liquid form, purchase the pellets. Place five pellets into a small, dark, glass container with a tight-fitting lid and add two fluid ounces of purified water. Shake ten times. When you are ready to use the arnica liquid, shake twice before opening the bottle.

~~~

A Second Lung Surgery: Short Cuts

O Descendant of Bharata (Arjuna), take shelter in Him with all the eagerness of thy heart. By His grace thou shalt obtain the utmost peace and the Eternal Shelter.

—God Talks with Arjuna: The Bhagavad Gita, 18.62

It was time again to seek the Eternal Shelter because I lacked peace. Even while on my final chemotherapy, a new nodule silently grew. It showed up on a PET/CT scan three weeks after the last treatment.

My ankhologist explained that the half-inch tumor sat in the hilum, a depression where the bronchi, pulmonary veins, and pulmonary arteries entered my lung—right next to my heart. There was no space on the scan between the tumor and a major pulmonary vein. He doubted whether a surgeon could completely remove the nodule.

I immediately made an appointment with Dr. Patrick Ross, who performed my first lung surgery. He seemed confident he could get the nodule out. It might be a resection, yet if the pulmonary vein was too diseased, or more disease was found in other parts of the lower left lobe, the lobe would be removed.

Recovery would take five to seven days in the hospital and four to six weeks at home. Even with a lobectomy, recovery would depend on the incisions, not on the extent of lung removal. He said I would not notice a missing lower lobe, and wouldn't appear sunken-in from the missing tissue. That knowledge encouraged me.

From the time of my scan to the surgical date, five weeks passed, yet I felt so grateful that it was even possible for the surgeon to remove the nodule.

Unlike for my first thoracic surgery, I did not focus on exercising and strengthening my core muscles or my arms and hands before arriving at the hospital.

I paid the price.

It took the intake nurses five tries before they could find a useful IV vein into my forearms or hands. That was painful.

While awaiting anesthesia, I did not shake like I did for the first surgery. This time I felt more confident in the surgeon and the procedure.

I brought ear buds so I could listen to my intra-operative "Hemi-Sync Surgical Support" CD (created by the Monroe Institute) throughout the long hours in the operating room. Fortunately, a nurse remembered to switch to my "Recovery" audio file while I was in recovery.

I noticed a huge difference in my ability to wake up when asked. For the first lung surgery, without this CD, I had tremendous difficulty responding to the nurse; this time I opened my eyes and nodded right away. Perhaps this had to do with the CD I used; perhaps it was due to my having only three incisions on one side this time, instead of two on each side of my chest. Whatever the reason, I felt glad about my rapid recovery.

While trying to move around on the hospital bed, I probably pulled muscles in my back and abdomen. These caused more pain than the three small incisions. I recall being better able to move around after the double-lung resection because my muscles had been stronger and didn't knot up as much from tension and pain.

I was supposed to be in the hospital at least three days. I headed home in less than two.

By focusing on the Spirit, I received peace before the surgery that lasted well beyond the hospital.

Thriver Soup Ingredient:

If you are able and have enough advanced notice, try exercising the muscles around the area where you will have surgery. Your body will most likely experience less shock; you might reduce the risk of complications; you probably will feel better after surgery; and recovery could progress more rapidly.

~~~

Recovery: Master the Possibilities

Cast all your anxiety on him because he cares for you…. And the God of all grace, who called you to his eternal glory in Christ, after you have suffered a little while, will himself restore you and make you strong, firm and steadfast.

—1 Peter 5:7, 10, Christian Bible, NIV

Sometimes in life, we suffer for a little while. Or a long time. Sometimes we can come out on the other end restored. Good preparation can possibly improve our outcomes.

What a huge difference planning ahead can make in recovery time. It not only cut down on my anxiety, it reduced my post-surgical suffering. I learned the hard way.

While in recovery after my initial hysterectomy, my whole body felt entirely wiped out. I heard people talking but don't remember anything that was said.

After my first lung resection, while in recovery it took all my strength to respond in only the tiniest way to the nurse who prodded me. First the struggle to open my eyes. Then to nod. Then to talk. Then to move my hands, then arms.

I felt utterly beat up, even though I experienced no pain. I let my Monroe Institute "Hemi-Sync Surgical Support: Recovery" CD play hour after hour while I slid in and out of consciousness.

When the nursing staff tried to get me into the horrible stiff chair, I could barely stay upright. I kept dozing.

Yet every hour I could feel a slight improvement in my condition.

I was given a breathing apparatus called an Inspiron—ten times I would slowly breathe in to raise the foam pad, and did this every hour. The nurses also urged me to practice coughing each hour to prevent pneumonia. Imagine coughing when you have tubes sticking out of your lungs, not to mention stitches. The Kodak nurse Vicky suggested I hold a pillow against my chest and wrap my arms around the pillow before coughing. It helped. It also helped me to grab my thighs when I was sitting or lying down to ease the difficulty of getting up.

The nurses pushed me to take a walk, so finally I mustered enough energy for a brief walker walk.

The next day I could do more after each nap. By day two I was free of tubes and walking the halls. I quickly shed all pain pills.

The oral pain medicine, oxycodone, made me nauseous, and I threw up twice on the day after surgery. It also dried out my mouth. I asked to be switched to another medication. They provided hydrocodone, which worked better for my body.

My second lung resection went far easier, partly because I was only having one side cut. This time I took ear buds that inserted neatly into my ears so they would not interfere with how the surgeon wanted to move my body during the operation. I placed fresh batteries in the player so there were no loose cords to deal with. As a result, my surgeon allowed me to listen to the "Intra-Op" CD throughout my time in the operating room. Also this time, a nurse had the presence of mind to remember to switch to the "Recovery" CD once surgery was over. I believe these two elements greatly accelerated my healing process.

For one thing, when the nurse asked me to wake up after surgery, I did so quite easily.

Second, while recuperating, the anesthesiologist asked me why I was taking so little pain medication. I didn't need it.

Once home, I put my large exercise ball on a chair and curled my chest over it. That brought some relief to my back muscles which had been strained in awkward ways.

Bowel movements were slow to resume, and usually were rock hard from the pain medications. I found the stool softener helpful, along with milk of magnesia and alfalfa tablets.

I suffered a little while, and then the Divine restored my strength and steadfastness.

Thriver Soup Ingredient:

Find audio files that will assist you with preparing for surgery, the surgery itself, and recovery. I find subliminal CDs and those using brainwave synchronization most useful.

C. Conventional Companions

Introduction to Conventional Companions: Open to Options

Ask and it will be given to you; seek and you will find; knock and the door will be opened to you.
For everyone who asks receives; the one who seeks finds; and to the one who knocks,
the door will be opened.
—Matthew 7:7-8, Christian Bible, NIV

*A*sking, seeking, and knocking are vital components of obtaining the best possible conventional care for our individual situations.

In Cincinnati, we are fortunate to have a support community for people diagnosed with cancer. When stymied by questions about what type of medical treatment to do next, a friend directed me to Bonnie Crawford, LISW-S, who was program director with The Wellness Community (that later became a full member of the Cancer Support Community). She was trained in a process called Open to Options, a service provided for patients. Bonnie worked with me to develop questions to ask my doctors so I would better understand my treatment choices. She provided me with my list of questions so I could take them to my appointments.

Here were some of my questions for the lung surgeon: How will having surgery affect my ability to live as long as I can? How many incisions will you make? Do you need to break a rib? How likely is it that you can get everything, given the nodule's location? Under what conditions should you remove the diseased lower lobe? Will the sarcoma spread to the upper lobe if the lower lobe is removed? What is the recovery time—how long will I be in the hospital, and how long will someone need to stay with me once I'm home? How much do these times depend upon the surgical approach? How do my complementary therapies interact with surgery?

Here were some of my questions for the radiation ankhologist: How effective is radiation when treating sarcoma? Can radiation be used as a follow-up to surgery? If so, how long is the waiting period before radiation can start? How frequently would I need radiation? What are the side effects of radiating the lung? What other areas would be damaged by radiation, such as the skin and bones? What is the recovery time from radiation? Do you radiate if there's no visible tumor? How do my complementary therapies interact with radiation?

Through this process, I ended up asking the surgeon another question: is a lung transplant an option? No, he said, because the immuno-suppression required for the procedure would allow the sarcoma cells to run rampant.

Because I made time to think about my options and discuss them with Bonnie, I felt prepared for my appointments. I sought, asked, and knocked until I was satisfied that I was making the best decisions possible for my circumstances.

Thriver Soup Ingredient:

If you are wondering about next steps and you have a Cancer Support Community in your area, make an appointment with someone trained in the Open to Options consultation process. If not, use the list of questions above as a springboard for developing your own list.

≈≈≈

Trance Fusions

Jesus said to them, "Very truly I tell you, unless you eat the flesh of the Son of Man and drink his blood, you have no life in you. Whoever eats my flesh and drinks my blood has eternal life, and I will raise them up at the last day. For my flesh is real food and my blood is real drink. Whoever eats my flesh and drinks my blood remains in me, and I in them. Just as the living Father sent me and I live because of the Father, so the one who feeds on me will live because of me."

—John 6:53-57, Christian Bible, NIV

These words of Jesus intimate that by imbibing his blood, a follower receives eternal life. Christians often enact this gift during worship services by drinking a symbolic sip of wine or juice, a ritual usually called the Eucharist. English cleric George Herbert (1593–1633) expressed his nexus with the communion cup and the crucifixion-shed blood of Christ through his poem, "The Agonie":

> Who knows not Love, let him assay
> And taste that juice, which on the crosse a pike
> Did set again abroach; then let him say
> If ever he did taste the like.
> Love in that liquour sweet and most divine,
> Which my God feels as bloud; but I, as wine.

If Herbert lived today, he might have connected swallowing the Eucharistic wine with receiving a blood transfusion from Christ; the energizing Spirit would be coursing through his veins, suffusing his body with Divine love. In the same way, when patients receive blood transfusions, we become steeped in the vitality of another human being. The one who fuses with us through his or her blood literally gives us back our lives. The energy fills our cells with life-giving nutrients and clears away what's no longer needed.

As I lay on the hospital bed, all the cells in my body thirstily sucked in a portion of a sacred crimson pint like parched dogs lapping up water. My hemoglobin count had dipped to seven gm/dl (twelve to sixteen is normal). My downhill slide had been so subtle I hadn't realized how off I felt.

My heart rate calmed and my body relaxed. My uterus absorbed the blood like a sponge. Then spurted it all out.

The red elixir of life lay useless beneath me, having filled a large pad stretched across the bed.

Starving cells, after tasting this appetizer, pleaded for more. My body tensed, its pallor telling its own tale of terror. Was there any more blood available in my type? How could I prepare for surgery when I couldn't even hold onto transfused blood? How could I staunch the flood? Would more useless units fill more pads?

How could I grasp for life when it so easily slipped away?

A nurse brought another hallowed pint. And another, and another. Fortunately, I received enough blood from four transfusions to prepare my body for the hysterectomy.

During surgery the nurses pumped in another two pints; after surgery, two more.

Oxygen flooded my body. Toxins exited my cells. Color returned to my skin. Ah, delicious nectar of life. Oh, sweet gratitude. Others had infused their life essence into me—a trance-fusion of their blood with mine. Their gifts provided more mortal time so I could continue seeking that most sacred infusion of eternal life through an inner trance fusion of the elixir of Spirit.

Thriver Soup Ingredient:

Suggest to family members, friends, and neighbors that donating blood is a great idea. It really does save lives. I lived through surgery and beyond because of the priceless gift of others' donated blood.

～～～

Levels of Albumin: Blood Will Tell

Proclaim! (or Read!) In the name Of thy Lord and Cherisher, Who created—Created man, out of A (mere) clot Of congealed blood.

—Qur'an 96:1, 2

The Islamic prophet Muhammad clearly associated blood with life—for we were formed, he said, from this precious bodily fluid. The Complete Jewish Bible forms a similar connection in Leviticus 17:11: "For the life of a creature is in the blood."

Blood is made up of red cells, white cells, platelets, and plasma. The red cells deliver oxygen and nutrients to individual cells and carry away waste products. The white cells fight infections. Platelets help blood clot so wounds can heal. All of these are carried through the body's blood vessels in plasma, a yellowish protein-containing fluid.

The most abundant protein in blood is albumin. Albumin has several functions, including transporting hormones and nutrients and detoxifying heavy metals and chemicals. It regulates fluid and helps prevent cell mutation.

When albumin levels are low (below 3.4 g/dL), the body can't properly absorb and digest protein. In studies done with a variety of cancer patients, lower levels of albumin were associated with poor survival rates. This is probably because albumin levels provide a good indication of a person's nutritional status; low levels indicate poor nutrition, which can interfere with healing.

Our blood is our lifeline. Proper eating can help our blood do its job to increase our chances of survival.

My abdomen tingled with excitement and I heaved a huge sigh when I learned, before starting chemotherapy, that my albumin level was 4.3. The sarcoma specialist at the MD Anderson Cancer Center in Houston said it indicated I was eating quite well.

Even after two years of chemotherapy, my albumin level was the same, most likely because of my diet. I am grateful for this, because maintaining high levels probably greatly improved my chances of surviving not only the chemo treatments, but also the illness itself.

Thriver Soup Ingredient:

Ask to have your blood serum albumin levels checked. If the levels are low, talk with your ankhologist and a dietitian about how to raise those levels so your body has the best possible opportunity to survive. Chlorella, a blue-green algae, can increase albumin levels, according to Donald Yance, author of *Herbal Medicine Healing and Cancer*.

~~~

Pain Management: A Time to Kill the Pain

My head aches, my body is burning, and my heart is filled with anguish. Such is the disease that has struck me; there is no medicine to cure it. ||2|| The Name of the Lord, the ambrosial, immaculate water, is the best medicine in the world....

—"Raag Sorat'h," Shri Guru Granth Sahib

Cancer gives us first-hand experience with headaches, burning sensations throughout our bodies, and anguish in our hearts. There usually is no cure available from the medical community. I was terrified of the agonizing process of dying from cancer. I later learned that not only could I call upon the Divine in my agony, I could call a doctor who specialized in pain management.

The Cancer Support Community in Cincinnati offered a talk by a professor in the University of Cincinnati's pain management department. He lay to rest most of my fears.

Three important things came out of this for me. First, it is better to see a pain management specialist when pain becomes more difficult than normal medicines can relieve. For example, a woman attending the talk said she had pretty bad neuropathy in her feet and legs (this is a side effect of chemotherapy in which the nerves set off continuous pain signals even when there is no damage to surrounding tissue). The doctor said there is a hockey-puck-sized device containing pain medicine that can be implanted in the abdomen with an attached wire that runs up the spine. With the help of a remote control, the patient can control extremely low dosages of pain medication that make the feet feel like they are being massaged. If you have experienced neuropathy, you know what a tremendous blessing this device can be.

I also realized it is better to consult a pain specialist before going into Hospice care because the specialist can provide innovative ways for controlling or eliminating pain that Hospice might not have available.

Finally, you can make your pain management choices and add them to your living will.

The professor clarified that it now is possible for someone with agonizing pain to have the pain controlled without the medications clouding the mind. Being able to call upon the Divine Doctor in our agony, and call upon our human doctors, we are blessed beyond reason. Even so, the sweet Spirit provides the best medicine in the world by filling us with the ambrosial waters from on high.

Thriver Soup Ingredient:

If fear of pain dogs your heels, know that great strides have been made toward its management. Visit www.cancer.org and search for "pain." Perhaps some of the articles will decrease some of the fear.

≈≈≈

Scanning with CATs

[A] leopard is watching their cities....

—Jeremiah 5:6, New American Standard Bible

There's a CAT keeping watch over the internal landscapes of cancer patients. CAT (Computerized Axial Tomography) scans are ordered by ankhologists every few months because they provide a window for watching structural changes within the body. The test combines x-rays with computerized technology to produce three-dimensional, cross-sectional slices of an area inside oneself. The results tell a doctor the size, shape, and exact location of any abnormal growths of at least a few millimeters in size. This lets him or her know how a particular treatment is working, or where to perform surgery.

In preparation for a full-torso scan, I would pick up a barium smoothie at Dairy (er, Bethesda) North's outpatient imaging center and store it in my refrigerator. One flavor had notes of vanilla, while another provided tones of butterscotch. Yum. The barium provided a contrast so the scan could detect structural abnormalities in my abdomen and pelvis. I needed to stop ingesting anything for six hours before the scan. Two hours before the scan I would quaff half of the bottled barium shake; the other half I drank an hour beforehand.

When I had only lung scans, I simply showed up a little early, having already pre-registered and obtained approval from insurance. No shake necessary.

I learned to wear sweats and a T-shirt so I wouldn't have to change into a hospital gown. When called back to get started, I removed all metal from my body and received an IV before entering the scan room. I lay down on a narrow cot stationed in front of a large white doughnut.

The bed was pulled through the hole for an initial check. Then I was given the other part of the contrast though the IV, which cascaded warmly from my head down through my torso. I felt warm and like I'd peed in my pants. The sensation quickly passed.

Then the real scan began, with me holding my breath for twenty to thirty seconds as the bed smoothly slid through the doughnut hole. The scanner revolved completely around my body.

The whole process didn't take long—just a few minutes.

One added bonus of the abdominal scans is that the barium shake acts as a colon cleanser. One nurse suggested I drink lots of water to flush out the garbage, so I tried to drink a good quart within the hour.

At the local hospital, scan reports normally are available within forty-eight hours. The typed-up report is sent to the doctor, who typically wants to see the patient before telling her the scan results. I can understand this, because the results are written in medicalese, which can be difficult to understand for the average laywoman, and unnecessarily frightening. After my second scan, I waited four torturous days to hear the results of my scan.

Never again.

After that fiasco, I would wait about thirty-six hours, then drive over to the medical records department of the hospital where the scan was performed. The department would not tell me over the phone when the results were available. I had to guess when the report was ready, drive over, sign a release form, and show an ID.

The big CAT was completely surrounding me, watching my internal city with unblinking eyes. My friend Marnie wrote in a touching note, "I am envisioning the CAT to have No Claws–Glinda has removed them with her magic wand and is keeping them in an airtight jar for you."

Thriver Soup Ingredient:

If you have issues with your IV veins, you can ask the attending scan operator to inject the contrast more slowly to possibly keep the vein from blowing.

Some Scans are Diamonds, Some Scans are Stones

But if we walk in the light as He Himself is in the light, we have fellowship with one another, and the blood of Jesus His Son cleanses us from all sin.
—1 John 1:7, Christian Bible, New American Standard Version

I tried to walk in the light and wanted my blood cleansed by the Divine. Instead, I got a free ride on the metastatic roller coaster. A clean scan this time. A new growth next time. Oh, and now one nodule is shrinking while another is growing.

Get me off this wild ride! All I want are clean scans. Is that too much to ask?

In December 2009, after three months on chemotherapy, I felt elated. My legs wanted to skip around the world, telling everyone that I only had one spot left to eliminate. My family and I celebrated with a bottle of sparkling apple cider.

By April, a new nodule was growing. So we started the next treatment. After four infusions, a scan showed shrinkage of the two nodules. "Impressive," said my ankhologist, because changes usually didn't show up for several months with those particular drugs. How nice to hear those words from a doctor with more than thirty years of experience administering chemosabe.

Terror preceded the next scan—which showed one nodule dying and one re-growing. Questions flooded my mind. Had I missed something important during my healing journey? Would I not survive as long as I wanted, or with as much physical comfort? If healing really was up to faith and trust, why didn't I have enough of either, and how could I increase them?

Following surgery in January 2011, I had a clean scan in March before the start of my final chemo treatment. The May scan appeared clean, so we continued with the final three drips. I thought I was home free.

By mid-July, another nodule showed up. I felt totally crushed. I slipped into self-defeating fear and self-blame. Maybe I was eating too much dark chocolate. Maybe I should have drunk more green smoothies. Maybe I hadn't drunk enough water. Maybe I hadn't done enough emotional release work.

I felt fortunate when the surgeon told me he was fairly certain he could get into the depression where the nodule sat and remove it. When he finally got into my lung, the nodule had grown to five times the size seen five weeks earlier. I wrestled with the news. Perhaps the nurse was right and it was time to get ready for Hospice. I had no more viable chemotherapy options.

On the other hand, perhaps I had made enough changes in my life that the nodule produced an extinction burst. Such a spurt occurs when previous actions that received some type of return no longer get the same response; the subject, however, continues the activity until exhausted rather than try a new behavior. In this case, the nodule might have grown rapidly in a last-ditch effort to survive, or perhaps it already was dying and had expanded because of the inflammation of its death throes.

Now I had an opportunity to become healthy. I longed to believe in the potential for my health, yet fear and doubt crept in: I must be in deep denial to think any such thoughts.

I read a newsletter published by people who follow the German healer Bruno Gröning and noted good reminders sprinkled throughout, such as giving my situation over to the Divine and letting go of results. Rejecting thoughts about illness. Trusting that if it's in Divine will, I am being helped. Acknowledging that sometimes the healing can take months, even years, and not to look at the outer evidence but instead keep the faith, keep believing. Talking about my health, rather than the opposite.

In mid-November, even without any infusions, I had a clean scan. I felt such joy and gratitude, combined with a deep sense of vulnerability, like a tender seedling that could easily be crushed underfoot. It motivated me to continue with my healing practices.

I sought to walk in the light of the Spirit, asking for my blood to be cleansed. Ultimately, all results were up to the Divine, not me. As I have already learned—this was a process of moment-to-moment living. Did it really matter what the next scan might say? I would continue with what I was doing, and if the results indicated a new course of action, I would make a decision then about what I would be willing to do.

Thriver Soup Ingredient:

Listen to John Denver's song, "Some Days are Diamonds," and sing your own refrain. Whatever your scan results are, know that all you ever have is the present moment. Make the most of it.

∾∾∾

PET Scans: Just a Silly Centimeter Longer

And it came to pass, when Joseph was come unto his brethren, that they stript Joseph out of his coat, his coat of many colours that was on him; And they took him, and cast him into a pit;
—Genesis 37:23-24a, King James Version, Christian Bible

Like Joseph, I felt naked and vulnerable, stripped and cast into a deep pit with an unknown, terrifying future.

After my hysterectomy, the doctors ordered a CAT scan to see if there were any other tumors. They found a spot on my lungs, yet were not sure if the spot was from a common local lung condition or if it was metastatic disease.

One of my first stops, a month later, was at MD Anderson Cancer Center. The ankhologists suggested getting a PET scan to determine if the lung spot that appeared on my initial CAT scan was cancerous.

A PET scan is an imaging technique that uses positively charged particles (radioactive positrons) to detect subtle changes in the body's metabolism and chemical activities.

During the procedure, I fasted from food and water for several hours, had blood drawn to check my glucose levels, and then was given an IV containing a sedative (some people inhale it as a gas). Then I was injected with a radioactive tracer and asked to wait about an hour. During this time, the tracer interacted with my body to produce gamma rays (which are similar to x-rays).

I was asked to visit a restroom and remove all metal before being led into the scanning area. It consisted of a large white doughnut with a long, thin cot running through the center and back into a tunnel. The ring detects the gamma rays being given off by the body. I was asked to lie as still as possible on the bed, with my arms resting above my head, for about twenty minutes. (For some people the scan might last up to two hours.) I felt grateful for my prayer shawl, a gift from Cathy Robbins, because it had the perfect configuration for keeping my arms warm during the procedure.

A specialist will read the scan, looking for an image indicating fast metabolism. Sure enough, the lung spot lit up red-yellow, indicated moderate activity.

It was metastatic cancer.

Sht.

Thriver Soup Ingredient:

If you chill easily, take a prayer shawl or small throw along for your PET scan and ask the scan staff to place it over your arms during the procedure. If you don't have anything with you to cover up your arms, ask for a blanket. If your scan lasts more than a few minutes, ask the staff to place a pillow under your hands and forearms to reduce neuropathy.

Getting a PET CAT

[A]mong the animals, I am the king of beasts (the lion); and among birds, I am Garuda ("lord of the skies," vehicle of Vishnu).

—*God Talks with Arjuna: The Bhagavad Gita*, 10.30b

The Divine is king of the lions and reigns over the results of any PET CATs that cancer patients might get.

After two surgeries and two years of chemotherapy, with the expectation that the cancer had been wiped out of my body, my then-husband suggested getting both a PET scan and a CAT scan at the same time. Called a PET/CT, this scan shows both functional changes, such as cellular hyperactivity (indicative of cancer), and small structural changes in one's anatomy (such as a new tumor).

I thought it was a great idea, and my ankhologist agreed to order one from the base of my skull to mid-thigh.

No eating or even gum was allowed for six hours beforehand. Not even flavored water.

I registered at the mobile unit and received an injection of radioactive glucose. "Now you're hot and sweet," the man joked. Then I rested quietly for about thirty minutes to prevent false readings of rapid metabolism in muscle tissue.

I was escorted to the restroom, then to the trailer. The machine appeared as a white tube with a cot that moved through the tube to the back, then to the front, scouting my body.

The bed moved to the back of the machine again, and I was asked to hold as still as possible while the scanning began. Eighteen minutes later, the bed had glided to its starting position at the front of the machine.

Results for this scan take about forty-eight hours. I marched over to the hospital's medical records department and received a copy of the technician's report.

"I'm baaaack," the results mocked. A half-inch nodule was growing in the depression of my lower left lung lobe. Right next to my heart.

My eyes watered. I could hardly breathe. I don't remember the journey back up the elevator and out into the parking lot, or fumbling for my cell phone to spread the news.

Despite our best efforts, despite two years of conventional and complementary treatments, despite all the prayers and meditation and visualization, I learned once again, this time more deeply: Of my own accord, I cannot control this demon. It is the Divine who helps and heals. The Spirit is the king of beasts, a great lion, whose power is not limited by the results of a PET CAT.

Thriver Soup Ingredient:

After a PET and a PET/CT scan, your urine will contain radioactive waste for about twenty-four hours, so use caution during that time. Take water along to drink after the scan to help flush out the components that were injected into your bloodstream.

<center>~~~</center>

Lung Mets or Fungus Among Us?

Exhale and inhale the essence qi, concentrate the spirit to keep a sound mind, then the muscles and the flesh unite as one.

—*The Yellow Emperor's Classic of Internal Medicine*

The importance of breath to health and longevity is taught in the ancient text *The Yellow Emperor's Classic of Internal Medicine*. This document has been the primary source for traditional Chinese medicine for more than two thousand years.

Keeping my lungs breathing freely, healthy, and clear of metastasis is an ongoing concern for me. When another woman with a uterine sarcoma and lung metastasis, who had been in remission for years, contacted me in 2014, she said a spot was found on her lung. Unfortunately, current medical science is unable to distinguish lung mets from a common condition in the Ohio River Valley called histoplasmosis. Histoplasmosis is a fungus that likes to infect the lungs. It looks just like a lung met on a scan.

Unfortunately, with a uterine sarcoma, there's no time to wait around to check if the spots shrink through weeks of standard histoplasmosis treatments. The patient scheduled surgery and had the spots removed. Fortunately, the tissue was infected by the fungus. Unfortunately, it took major surgery to find this out.

I can only imagine her terror before getting the lab results. How could I avoid this? I felt vulnerable because I, too, live in the Ohio River Valley.

She recommended staying away from caves, bat and bird droppings, compost, and construction sites, along with wearing a mask and moistening soil first if gardening. That sounded easy enough, though I had to give up on the fantasy of raising my own chickens. It is far more important to keep my lungs clean and clear so I can keep exhaling and inhaling the essence qi, or vital life-force energy.

Thriver Soup Ingredient:

Histoplasmosis is generally found in states bordering the Ohio River Valley and the lower Mississippi River, and in caves where bats live. Bat and bird droppings encourage the growth of the fungus. Construction and demolition areas can stir up the fungus in soil. A thorough resource for self-protection in potentially contaminated areas is available at www.cdc.gov/niosh/docs/2005-109/pdfs/2005-109.pdf.

≈≈≈

Radiation: The Refiner's Fire

Behold, I will send my messenger, and he shall prepare the way before me: and the Lord, whom ye seek, shall suddenly come to his temple, even the messenger of the covenant, whom ye delight in: behold, he shall come, saith the LORD of hosts. But who may abide the day of his coming? and who shall stand when he appeareth? for he is like a refiner's fire, and like fullers' soap: And he shall sit as a refiner and purifier of silver: and he shall purify the sons of Levi, and purge them as gold and silver, that they may offer unto the LORD an offering in righteousness.
—Malachi 3:1-3, King James Version, Christian Bible

The purifying nature of fire became evident to my family following the devastation of Yellowstone National Park's terrible 1988 fire. When we arrived at the park in 2005, empty stumps still stalked many hillsides, yet in the midst of the charred remnants grew green saplings.

We learned from park rangers how that holocaust benefited Yellowstone's ecosystem. Much of the park's forests are composed of lodge pole pines, whose cones are sealed with resin. It takes intense heat to melt the resin, allowing the cones to open and release the seeds inside. Only after such a conflagration are the conditions right for the seedlings to establish themselves on the forest floor, where they access plenty of sunlight without the crowding of other plants and debris.

Just as a blaze can be essential for rebirth of a forest to occur, it also can bring forth intense human spiritual activity. For the Frenchman Blaise Pascal, a "Night of Fire" in 1654 transformed his entire existence. For two hours he burned with the heat of intimate contact with the Spirit. He drew a crude flaming cross on a piece of parchment, and around it scribbled a few phrases. "From half-past ten till half-past twelve, Fire!"

His newfound passion led him to enter a monastery and abandon his former life that focused on physics and mathematics. Like the legendary phoenix bird, his Night of Fire gave birth to joy and a new mission.

Many cancer patients have not a Night of Fire, but Weeks, or even Months of Fire. One of the women I met at the ankhology office had a uterine sarcoma that ended up manifesting as a six-centimeter lung tumor. Rather than have that two- and one-half-inch blob surgically removed, she opted for a procedure called stereotactic radiosurgery. The nodule in her lung shrank to two and three-quarter centimeters in four months.

"The tumor is dead, I have my whole lung and complete function," she wrote. "If the other tumor grows, we will do the same thing. No chemo or drugs to follow up. It is a strong form of targeted radiation that only hits the tumor. I went five days in a row, and the treatment lasted eight minutes each time. The side effect was fatigue.

"You lay on a table, it is completely open, and a large disk delivers the radiation to the spot at different angles.... The machine is called Novalis."

So here was another life-prolonging option for me, if needed. It would be like the Divine Refiner's fire that burns away the dross so the gold and silver can rise like a phoenix from the flames.

Thriver Soup Ingredient:

As your body receives radiation, contemplate Malachi 3:3, put to music in movement seven ("And He shall Purify") of "Messiah," the widely known oratorio by George Frederic Handel (1695–1759).

II. Congruent Care

Introduction to Congruent Care: Making Hard Choices

They looked to him and grew radiant; their faces will never blush for shame. This poor man cried; ADONAI heard and saved him from all his troubles.
—Psalm 34:5-6, Complete Jewish Bible

An answer from the Divine—arriving as an inner knowing, the wise counsel of another human being, or an outer synchronicity—can help deliver us from our fears and bring us the radiance of inner self-confidence.

The questions, and choices to make, are especially tough with cancer, because it isn't simply a disease. The illness and its journey can encompass one's entire existence. It forced me into making numerous life-altering decisions. How was I going to approach the dis-ease? Should I stay in my marriage or leave? How was I going to view the span of my earthly existence? If my life went on the line, how did I want to be treated by the medical community? How did I want to approach death, should it become inevitable?

Throughout my experience, I sought counsel not only from others, but especially from the Divine. Listening to that still, small voice within was hard, yet I kept after it, employing a wide variety of methods. Sometimes I felt I had an answer; often I did not. Still, I felt compelled to make choices and move forward. I made one particularly bad choice—to not get into a doctor's office sooner to find out why my so-called benign fibroid was causing such pain. I nearly died as a result. My decision to delay a CAT scan by two months proved to be another big mistake. Other choices, however, proved perfect—like leaving my 23-year marriage to salvage what I could of my life.

Even though I have not been particularly prone to writing poetry, one did flow out of my pen about nine months after the diagnosis—sort of a gestational period for a smidgeon of grace. It reflected the consequences of my willingness to face my inner darkness as I scrambled to save my life.

Cancer
Uninvited indweller
Rattling the cages in my mind
Cracking the safe in my heart
Leaving a gaping wound through my *hara*
Swinging doors I'd barred shut
Widening my soul.

Perhaps with the right choices, we can turn the cancer from a foe into a source of deep healing and regeneration, especially through the hard choices we will have to make. When we come through on the other side, more Divine radiance probably will be shining forth from our faces.

Thriver Soup Ingredient:

I learned not to expect myself to always be able to make good decisions. Sometimes I waited months before selecting an option. Decisions that are huge and life-altering should be approached with caution, openness, and a willingness to try out new ideas. We are human, and we make mistakes. That can be okay, especially if we use it as an opportunity to learn so we can do better the next time. Accepting ourselves as we are, with our flaws, mistakes, and good decisions, helps us become more full and wise human beings.

～～～

DeNial: Playing the Fool

The childish, due to confusion or carelessness do not know about the emerging disorder in early stage as fools about the enemy. The disorder, though having a minute start, advances afterwards and gradually becoming deep-rooted takes away the strength and life of the foolish one.
                              —Sutrasthana 11 #56-63, *Charaka Samhita*

I thought I had been wise about the benign fibroid growing in my abdomen.

I hadn't.

July 23, 2009: I'm lying, doped up, in a hospital bed. The doctor tells me the ultrasound of my uterus shows evidence consistent with sarcoma cells. What are sarcoma cells? Why are they calling in a cancer surgeon? I don't have cancer. I'm healthy! I eat a healthy diet, exercise, maintain my weight, avoid all drugs, and meditate an hour each day. This low-grade fever arose from an internal infection, I'm sure. I can explain every symptom.

Oh, and deNial is a river in Egypt.

I take solace in knowing the pain and heavy bleeding also are symptoms of endometriosis and myomas. My sister, Roselie Bright, explained that endometriosis is a condition where endometrial cells attach to other organs. They respond to hormones and bleed during menstruation. I had mild endometriosis.

Myomas, she said, are common benign tumors of the uterine wall. They tend to grow as women approach menopause and are diagnosed with ultrasound and physical exam. These fibroids generally disappear around menopause. Unfortunately, uterine sarcomas and myomas appear alike on ultrasound and physical exam. The only way to distinguish them is through a biopsy. Since biopsies carry some risk and sarcomas are so rare (and catching one of these sarcomas at an earlier stage doesn't make much difference to survival), biopsy is not considered good practice.

I had an ultrasound a few months earlier and was diagnosed as having a myoma. I played conservative by delaying the hysterectomy.

The evening before going to the emergency room, however, my level of pain had jumped significantly. It seemed wrong to experience so much suffering from a fibroid. I knew I would hurt fairly badly for hours if I didn't go to the hospital. I kept asking myself: Is it worth going to the ER in the middle of the night for a benign fibroid? Could I grit it out for the few remaining weeks before my appointment with a surgeon?

I am grateful my positive inner masculine side proved strong enough to answer my question—yes, go to the ER, now! I'm so glad I chose to take care of myself and did not take a pain pill.

By listening to the level of pain instead of masking it with over-the-counter medications, and because I paid attention to the positive masculine principle within me, I got the help I needed—barely in time. Even after having surgery right away, world uterine sarcoma specialists expected me to die before the year was out.

If I had waited three weeks for the surgery, I most likely would have died quickly. The cancer had already spread into the bloodstream before the surgeon cut on July 24. Given its vicious nature, the cells probably would have spread all through my body. I would have moved beyond the possibility of surgical intervention.

I had played the fool, not taking my symptoms seriously enough to insist on getting medical care sooner. I had allowed the illness to grow deep roots, throwing my life on the line. Now it would take Herculean measures to save it.

Thriver Soup Ingredient:

If you are in doubt about your condition, get it checked as soon as possible. The earlier issues are addressed, the easier they are to treat and the better off you will be.

Diagnosis: I'd Rather Fight than Bitch

No kind of calamity Can occur, except By the leave of God: And if any one believes In God, (God) guides his Heart (aright): for God Knows all things.

—Qur'an 64:11

It was a complete disaster. Where was the Divine in this mess?

Only one percent of all cancers are sarcomas. Sarcomas affect soft, connective tissue. There are three main types of uterine sarcomas, but I didn't have one of those. I had one of the other two types: high-grade undifferentiated sarcoma. "Highly undifferentiated" meant the cells were highly abnormal. "Endometrial" referred to the inner wall of the uterus where the cancer had taken up residence.

Highly undifferentiated endometrial sarcomas are extremely aggressive and rare. During my two years of chemotherapy at a regional sarcoma treatment center, I only heard of one other woman diagnosed with highly undifferentiated uterine sarcoma.

After my initial surgery, four different laboratories (two in Ohio, one in Texas and one in New York City) attempted to provide a diagnosis. The first pathologist decided the tumor was highly undifferentiated; the second labeled it leiomyosarcoma. The third pathologist said it was highly undifferentiated, as did the fourth.

I learned from this process both the value of a second opinion (and in my case, four opinions) and that diagnosis is more an art than a science.

While reading my pathology report from New York's Memorial Sloan-Kettering Cancer Center, we learned that my uterus was getting around. Slides of the tumor were presented at a Gynecologic Pathology Consensus Conference. Maybe someday, somewhere, my uterus will help someone else.

The Divine had allowed this disaster to visit me. This gave rise to confusion, rage, terror, self-blame, shame, and profound feelings of powerlessness. I faced a choice: bitch by focusing on the negative and then dying, or fight by doing everything I could to live.

I chose to fight. I also chose not to reject the Power who knew and allowed this disaster. Instead, I recognized the Spirit's call to enter into unconscious realms and eventually emerge into the radiance of Divine light.

Thriver Soup Ingredient:

I think obtaining at least a second opinion—if not more—is essential in the case of a cancer diagnosis. If I'd gone with the first opinion, the chemotherapy probably would have been ineffective, and I might have died within the first year. My second diagnosis was different from the first, so I needed a third opinion. Once two specialists and two pathology reports showed agreement, I felt confident in my choice of treatment. Press for at least a second opinion, and if they differ, get a third. Check with your insurance carrier to make sure it's covered. If not, appeal your case.

∽∽∽

Curing and Healing

And as he entered into a certain town, there met him ten men that were lepers, who stood afar off; And lifted up their voice, saying: Jesus, master, have mercy on us. Whom when he saw, he said: Go, shew yourselves to the priests. And it came to pass, as they went, they were made clean. And one of them, when he saw that he was made clean, went back, with a loud voice glorifying God. And he fell on his face before his feet, giving thanks: and this was a Samaritan. And Jesus answering, said, Were not ten made clean? and where are the nine? There is no one found to return and give glory to God, but this stranger. And he said to him: Arise, go thy way; for thy faith hath made thee whole.
—Luke 17:12-19, Douay-Rheims Bible

Jesus generously cured all ten lepers by cleansing a terminal disease from their physical bodies. They were free to return to their lives. Only one of the ten returned to thank Jesus. Jesus responded to his gratitude and faith by making him whole—healing, or transforming, him on the inside. This singular man showed a willingness to fully receive all that Christ had to offer, including internal wellness within his depths. He received a full measure of grace into his core, like a thirsty traveler holding out his cup for clean, holy water. His cup would overflow with spiritual refreshment for others as well.

What about the other nine, who received cures? They exhibited no gratitude. They might be akin to water gourds with holes in them, leaking out the unrecognized, precious, liquid grace they had received. They could not provide cures to others, and without gratitude they took their cures for granted.

The urge to share the experience of healing arises from an expanded sense of communion with all life. Author Alberto Villoldo, in *Shaman, Healer, Sage,* identifies other characteristics of healing: an experience of infinity, an increased sense of well-being, a newfound peacefulness, and a feeling of empowerment.

Author Ken Wilber describes his wife in those terms in his book, *Grace and Grit: Spirituality and Healing in the Life and Death of Treya Killam Wilber.* Treya, who struggled with cancer for five years, was not only healed—she most likely reached enlightenment. While the cancer claimed her physical life, it could not touch her spirit.

Some people are neither cured nor healed. Some people are both cured and healed. I want to be among those both cured and healed. And so I did all possible conventional and complementary treatments that seemed reasonable and helpful.

While I was told the condition was chronic, I decided the word "incurable" really meant curable from the inside. I was in(a)curable state of being. And why not? Paul Brand, MD, and author Philip Yancy said our bodies are more like fountains than sculptures: maintaining their shapes, yet constantly being renewed.

Our cells are continually being replaced. The linings of our mouths can be renewed in a matter of hours; we have completely new skeletons every few years. It seems to me the key to a cure is to change the cellular patterns so new growth is healthy. And tricky it is. Sometimes this might require a healing before the body effects a cure. Whichever needed to come first, I was willing to work toward both, because I wanted both. My greatest desire was to overflow with the faith and gratitude that heals and makes one whole. I longed to be a chalice brimming over with the wine of new life so I could share it with others.

Thriver Soup Ingredient:

Use your imagination to experience your body as a vessel filled with light that renews each cell. Allow Divine luminescence to enter your body through your crown chakra on the top of your skull and to flow slowly throughout your body. As if your body is a fountain, watch fresh light continuously pour over and through you in ever-new waves of Divine glory. Feel the Spirit's love wash every cell and drain toxins into the earth where they can be recycled.

If you experience a cure, offer deep gratitude to the Divine. Then focus on shifting any patterns that might have contributed to the illness so your body receives messages for both maintaining health and experiencing healing. Share your gratitude with others.

<p style="text-align:center">~~~</p>

Eldering: Regenerpause

She is the one who reveals reality, She is the genetrix, the mother of the victorious ones.

—*The Perfection of Wisdom*

The Divine feminine reveals reality because she is the genetrix, or mother, of all matter. The word "matter" is derived from *mater*, the formal Latin word for mother. The Great Genetrix forms matter from energy, creating the reality we experience.

This creative motherly energy can be profoundly experienced by women when they encounter menopause. Chills streamed through my body when I heard futurist Barbara Marx Hubbard explain that during this stage in life, when a woman no longer produces ova, she becomes the egg—a person of pure potential. Hubbard termed this transformation "regenopause." It is a period when women can push the pause buttons on their lives, start to regenerate themselves, and begin to more thoroughly expand into the experience of feminine authenticity and creativity.

Cancer pushed my mid-life pause button and thrust me into menopause. It forced me to evaluate every aspect of my life, from how to shower to whether I should stay married. I began to see the lack of self-compassion, authenticity, and creativity that had marked my life to that point.

The egg theme rolled through my cancer journey. It started with a dream in which an unknown item was stolen from inside a beautifully carved egg. Later I dreamt that I was given an egg containing a transformative substance. After I started having clean scans, I had a waking vision of a woman rising up out of an egg.

I needed an entirely new paradigm, and the pause of cancer provided the time to sift through the ashes produced by treatments for the lovely phoenix egg that represented my rebirth into the second half of life.

Reality had been revealed to me—in all its harshness and blessedness. I had entered regenopause and become the genetrix of myself, a mother to my victory over my dead past.

Thriver Soup Ingredient:
Make a treasure map in the shape of an egg.
What you will need:
A large piece of paper or poster board
Scissors
Pencil
Glue

Pens, markers, paints, fabric scraps, stickers, old magazines for images and words, yarn, glitter, and/or other craft supplies.

Fill your paper or poster board with a drawing of a large egg shape. Cut it out. Then spend a few minutes breathing deeply while focusing on the egg shape. If you could manifest your feminine energy in a positive way for the world, what would you do? What would it look like in terms of words, colors, textures, and shapes? How would it feel? Be expansive, creative, and bold. If a sense of fear or contraction emerges, experience it in the moment. Follow it, allow it to dissipate, and then continue onward. The Divine realm knows infinite possibility.

When you feel ready, place images that arose from the process onto your egg and arrange them in a way that feels good. When satisfied, glue them to the paper or board. After your treasure map dries, get it laminated and hang your feminine creation in a prominent place to remind you of where you want to head with your life.

~~~

Why I Needed to Leave the Marriage: Be All You Can Be

For everything there is a season, a right time for every intention under heaven...a time to kill and a time to heal, a time to tear down and a time to build, a time to weep and a time to laugh, a time to mourn and a time to dance.

—Ecclesiastes 3:1, 3-4, Complete Jewish Bible

I didn't believe in divorce unless my spouse was into drugs, was an alcoholic, lied, or was cheating on me. It took months for me to recognize and accept that there also could simply be a time to weep, mourn, and kill the marriage so I could heal.

I had carried childhood behavior patterns and conditioned responses into my marriage by playing victim. I became resentfully compliant to appease my husband. This behavior on my part, however, did not stop the conflicts. I gave away my personal power and moved into resignation, passivity, and depression. These reactions covered up my sense of hopelessness and failure. Out of unacknowledged fear and anxiety, I distanced myself and went numb. My unconscious attempt at a solution probably contributed to the illness.

Dean Ornish, MD, explained part of the mechanism in his book, *Love and Survival*. One's immune system loses some of its effectiveness when a person experiences marital conflict, and women are more prone to negative changes than men.

My marriage improved after the diagnosis, yet the changes only lasted nine months. Then old patterns reasserted themselves. Gritting my teeth, I continued with the marriage. Bernie Siegel, MD, also wrote about marital discord and illness. He noted that when a woman says, "I'll make this marriage work if it kills me," the relationship might do just that.

Nine months into treatment, my then-husband said he wanted out. Terror squeezed my heart. If the marriage ended, what would become of me? I had no job, I was about fifty years old, the economy was in bad shape, chemotherapy wasn't being effective, and I was not expected to get into remission. How would I take care of myself with such an illness, how would I support myself, and how would I get medical insurance? I knew many women who walked away from their marriages with nothing.

The issue moved to the backburner. Several months later I meditated and asked: Should I stay in the marriage or leave? The answer came with conviction: "Get out of the marriage, or you will die."

My next scan a couple of weeks later seemed to show both the truth of my inner conflict and the need to get out of the marriage: the remaining lung nodule was dying while a new one had developed.

As I weighed my seeming lack of options, more clarity emerged: Did I want to stay in the marriage and have health insurance, and die, or get out, risk living in poverty with no medical insurance, and possibly live?

While I didn't expect to end up in poverty, the decision became obvious. I chose life. My marriage had drained my life energy. To be revived, I needed to leave it.

I found a lawyer.

After we told the kids we were separating, I moved into the guest room. We both thought it was best if I stayed in the house because I would be recovering from surgery and on another chemotherapy regimen. I thought I could maintain my equanimity if I stayed.

I was wrong.

Five months later another new nodule lit up the CAT scan image.

I called Maria Paglialungo, an energy intuitive, who made it unequivocally clear: Move out *now*. Even staying in the guest room was damaging my efforts to get well.

The time had arrived to weep, mourn, and kill the marriage.

Thriver Soup Ingredient:

If you are in a relationship that leaves you feeling angry, empty, afraid, hurt, and/or power-less most of the time, consider what it might be doing to your immune system and your health. Are you willing to die to stay in the relationship? If not, look to friends for assistance and find a way to get out so you can save your life.

≈≈≈

I'm Moving Out

"But ADONAI—it is he who will go ahead of you. He will be with you. He will neither fail you nor abandon you, so don't be afraid or downhearted."

—Deuteronomy 31:8, Complete Jewish Bible

To not be afraid or downhearted was impossible for me at the time.

Tense with terror, I picked up the phone with trembling hands and called my friend Mim

Grace Gieser. My voice shook. "Can I come stay with you for three days while I look for an apartment?" I knew I needed to leave my husband as quickly as possible—the new nodule in my lung was growing, the marriage was not going to improve, and my life lay on the line.

With kindness, she opened her heart and apartment to me in my hour of need.

With tightly contracted muscles and a sick stomach, I packed up a few essentials and drove away from twenty-two years marriage.

I barely slept on an air mattress in her little living room, filled with gratitude, tension, and terror. She lightened my stay with a listening ear, movies, and love.

Then my friend Laura Dailey generously took me in for a few more days. I advanced to a real bed in a guest room. By then, my friend Brecka Burton-Platt had found someone who would take me in on a weekly paid basis while I looked for the right apartment in my sons' school district.

A couple of weeks later, my husband signed the lease for a nice apartment for me that could accommodate both boys. I relaxed and prepared for surgery. Some of my siblings and their spouses had come to town and helped me move in. The apartment felt like a sanctuary for my soul, and I relished the quiet and solitude. It would become a sacred space of healing for my body.

I had moved just in time. The half-inch nodule discovered in July had grown to two and one-half inches by the time it was removed in August. If I had waited much longer, I would have lost the lower lung lobe and the cancer might have invaded my heart.

As Brecka noted, it was the hardest thing I'd ever done. I had gone back on a sacred vow and against a cherished lifetime belief. I had broken up family life and left my sons to be raised in a divided household. I faced an uncertain future with cancer growing rapidly in my weak body. I didn't know how I was going to make it financially. I didn't know how or where I would get medical insurance if I managed to live past the time the benefits through my then-husband expired.

Even though my life appeared to be lying in complete ruin, I knew I had done the right thing. I knew the Divine had gone before me to prepare the way and was with me through it all. I sensed all would eventually be well.

Thriver Soup Ingredient:

If you need to get out of an unhealthy relationship, ask your friends for assistance with finding a place to stay, even if it's only temporary. There are shelters and agencies that will help you, because many women have traveled this road before you and have given so you could have support as well. Ask until you find what you need, and then act. You are worth it.

≈≈≈

Ending of a Marriage: Braveheart
Don't be afraid, for I am with you; don't be distressed, for I am your God. I give you strength, I give you help, I support you with my victorious right hand.
—Isaiah 41:10, Complete Jewish Bible

My forehead creased with worry, my gut tightened with fear, and my heavy heart drooped with discouragement whenever I thought about trying to negotiate a fair divorce with my then-husband. Like a wet noodle, I lacked sturdiness and confidence, allowing others to manipulate me and heavily influence my choices.

My psychotherapist asked me, during one session, how I wanted to grow through the process of ending the marriage. I straightened on her couch as I realized I wanted to develop strength and personal power, becoming more like Home Tree in James Cameron's movie "Avatar"—deeply rooted, strong, reaching to the sky, bendable yet not breakable. I also wanted to enliven a greater sense of fairness, integrity, and authenticity within myself, which I found challenging due to my habit of appeasing him.

To accomplish this, my psychotherapist reminded me that I needed to practice feeling the inside of my body as I interacted with my husband. And I needed to rehearse physically experiencing the vision I was creating about my growth. I heard the assurance with which certain people spoke, and I wanted to emulate them in my negotiations. I wanted to feel in my bones what they exuded. Focusing on that sense of confidence in my whole body when it came to negotiating required that I recall how that felt when I spoke about other areas of my life, such as my writing skills. Placing this sense of sureness into my energy field during negotiations required discipline, focus, persistence, and endurance. This practice helped me grow in my ability to know what was true for me and to have the courage to stand by it.

My therapist suggested I call on my power animals—panther and snake—and to immerse myself in them to help my confidence grow. She encouraged me to breathe deeply before interacting with my then-husband and to remind myself to play on my own ball field rather than on his, as I had been doing for more than two decades.

I knew she was right. I also realized that if I let my then-husband have his way during the negotiations, I would be playing victim once again and end up deeply resentful. This would create stress and perpetuate my unhealthy situation.

I had known women who walked out of marriages, taking nothing with them—to their later detriment. I also had heard of women dealing with cancer who didn't fight for their rights and gave up, letting their husbands have whatever they wanted during their divorces. These women had perpetuated their roles as victims.

I was tired of the resignation, the appeasing, the powerlessness. It was time for me to embrace my personal power and change my role to equal partner in the process. I wanted to live free of regrets, satisfied and content. To do this I needed to acknowledge, accept, and honor my fears, my right to exist, and my legal rights to financial support and marital assets.

My therapist helped me understand that my inner experience of anger could help me find my bottom line during negotiations. It could provide a seedling for being more self-determined, more present in the moment, and strong enough to firmly stick to what I wanted and needed.

The struggle to stay grounded and strong, like Home Tree, proved difficult. How easily I sometimes slipped back into appeasing behaviors. I sometimes had to wait a few days to get grounded again in what I wanted before I could respond to his emails. I found myself groggy when I read them, indicating my desire to avoid conflict.

Because I didn't back down on everything, negotiations dragged on for years. About a year into them, I woke up with the theme song from the 1966 movie "Born Free" playing repeatedly through my mind. I sensed it was time for me to freely leave the marriage.

My therapist noted my pain around any hope that my then-husband might change. She said if I felt hopeless, then I could experience a transformation. It was better to accept where I was and to experience my feelings so I could eventually let them go. This could bring healing.

It still was too early to forgive, yet I also sensed that forgiveness would come at some point, and come authentically. When we process fully, she said, then we can naturally let things go—including in our memories.

Eventually, I realized my higher Self wanted me to go through the difficult, lengthy negotiations so I could learn to stand firm in what I needed and wanted. It also was time for me to learn to listen to my inner voice for guidance before making any decisions. By doing the Map of Emotions©, I let go of some of the fears and rage. Through prayer, practice, my therapist, and my friends, the Spirit helped me experience courage, strength, and support.

Thriver Soup Ingredient:

If you are negotiating a settlement with your spouse, and lack some confidence, think about someone you know who exudes poise, or a time when you felt buoyant. Allow yourself to feel that self-assurance in your body each day, perhaps in the morning as you dress. Let this sense of sureness overflow. Then when you enter into negotiations, recall this feeling and try to hold it in your awareness as you engage your spouse.

Another strategy suggested to me by someone is to ask your higher Self to step in and allow your ego self to step aside.

I heard about a third strategy when listening to a June 2012 TED (Technology, Entertainment, Design) Talk by Amy Cuddy, a professor and researcher at Harvard Business School. She suggested people who need to increase their internal power can stand in the Wonder Woman pose—elbows out, hands on hips, feet spread apart—for two minutes. This pose increases one's testosterone and decreases the hormone cortisol, enlivening one to feel empowered.

Legal Documentation: It's the Law

So teach us to count our days, so that we will become wise.
—Psalm 90:12, Complete Jewish Bible

If we wisely count our days, we will recognize that our time on this earth is limited, whether we have cancer or not. To protect ourselves and our bodies against the unwanted side effects of the possible and the inevitable, we need certain legal documents in place. Every hospital and treatment facility I entered wanted a copy of my living will so they would know how to treat me in case of an emergency.

This raised questions for me. Did I want to be kept on life support? Did I want both water and nutrition during the final stages of illness, or if a surgery went wrong? Who would make decisions regarding my care and my finances if I were unable to make them? And, heaven forbid, if I should pass, what did I want done with my underage children, and where did I want any possessions to go?

Important documents to have in place are an advance health care directive, a power of attorney for health care, a general financial power of attorney, and a final will and testament.

The advance health care directive, or living will, should be created and signed before you enter into treatment, but can be done at any time you are mentally competent to make decisions. Through this document you can specify exactly what sorts of treatments you do and do not want while under medical care. For example, you can stipulate that you do not want the use of extraordinary measures, such as life-support equipment, to prolong your life. You can request or deny the administration of fluids and/or nutrition. You can deny the use of cardio-pulmonary resuscitation, which can evoke long-term chest pain. I liked being able to make these decisions ahead of time to ensure they would be carried out.

A power of attorney for health care allows you to name a person (or a list of persons to serve in priority order) who will make health care decisions for you when you no longer can for yourself. Be sure to discuss all your concerns and wishes with this individual.

A general financial power of attorney enables you to name those who will handle financial matters for you. You decide if the agent will be authorized to handle your property as of the day the document is signed, or when your physician signs a letter stating that you no longer are able to handle your financial matters.

Your final will and testament will carry out your wishes after you pass away. This includes who will represent you and carry out your wishes; what this person will be enabled to do; who will inherit your belongings; when and how your property will be distributed; and who will become the legal guardians for any minor children.

While standardized forms are available, be sure you have the correct forms for your state. Read each document carefully. I think it is wisest to invest in an estate attorney to ensure that your rights and property are protected to the fullest extent possible.

If you develop legal issues around your treatments, free information and resources are available through the Cancer Legal Resource Center (www.disabilityrightslegalcenter.org/cancer-legal-resource-center). Questions and issues around insurance coverage, employment, access to benefits, and estate planning are part of the services offered by this joint program.

You might feel as though getting these documents prepared is an admission of defeat. On the other hand, you might be able to view this process as self-care and a way to relieve some of the stress of living through a cancer experience. This is one area in which counting your days exercising wisdom can lead to peace of mind and the fulfillment of some of your deepest wishes.

As my former husband liked to say, "Plan for the worst and hope for the best." Now is a good time to enact such a cliché.

Thriver Soup Ingredient:

A list of local attorneys who practice in the area for which you need assistance can be found through the American Bar Association's national Lawyer Referral Directory at apps.americanbar.org/legalservices/lris/directory/. Begin asking others for referrals as well.

≈≈≈

Aging: You're Not Getting Older, You're Getting Wiser

When the day of Pentecost came, they were all together in one place. Suddenly a sound like the blowing of a violent wind came from heaven and filled the whole house where they were sitting. They saw what seemed to be tongues of fire that separated and came to rest on each of them. All of them were filled with the Holy Spirit and began to speak in other tongues as the Spirit enabled them.
—Acts 2:1-4, Christian Bible, NIV

Tongues of Divine fire initiated the first Christians into a new phase of spiritual life. Licking flames of the Spirit filled them with the ability to speak truth to others. A similar transformational process occurs for women who enter menopause. For me, the Spirit burned in three ways: my tongue began twitching when I spoke, reflecting my growing ability to speak my truth; chemotherapy burned through my body for two years; and I sometimes felt my own heat in the form of hot flashes. How wonderful they felt on cold nights, warming me up so I could more easily fall asleep. For me, these power surges felt akin to the Spirit's flames that descended on the followers of Jesus. I later discovered that when I went off all dairy except organic butter, the hot flashes disappeared; when I ate some cheese, they returned.

My initiation into the wisdom years took other forms. I saw many new wrinkles on my face—most likely the result of chemotherapy, and perhaps enhanced by the loss of my hormone-factory ovaries. Because of the nature of the cancer I'd been diagnosed with, my ankhologist urged me to avoid ever taking replacement hormones, even natural or bio-identical formulations. Guess I'll be keeping these lines. I did earn them all. I tell my friends that sagacity doesn't come with a smooth face.

In the West's youth-worshiping culture, I can purchase creams to mask wrinkles, dyes to hide grey hair, and bras to defy gravity. They don't appeal to me as much as they might others. I love having the opportunity to grow old. It is a time to fully love and accept who I am and to follow my sacred path without regard for others' opinions. It is a time when the mysteries of surrender and death present themselves more freely. It is a time to turn inward to rediscover the gold I'd been laying away for years. And it is a time when my inner beauty, my personal truths, and Divine light can pour forth from my inner depths, outshining all the creases cracking my face.

Tough times had glazed my face to form deliberate and decorative crackle lines, like a prized piece of pottery. I am becoming a hag. Our English word hag comes from the Greek word *hagios*, which means holy, consecrated to God. As the first Christians were filled with fire and were enabled to speak truth, so am I now blazing, increasing in wisdom and holiness, and much more free in my ability to speak my truth. This, I like.

Thriver Soup Ingredient:

If you want nicer facial skin and fewer wrinkles, consider skipping expensive products containing unpronounceable chemicals and switch to an old Ayurvedic formula. The wife of Bharat B. Aggarwal, PhD, recommends the *ubtan* facial mask. It contains the brightly colored spice turmeric, so use caution around clothing, and tie back or cover your hair with something that you don't mind staining. (Turmeric's anti-inflammatory properties also make this treatment helpful for acne.)

In a sealable container, mix one-half cup chick pea flour with one and one-half tablespoons turmeric. To make the facial, mix one tablespoon of the powder with five drops of raw, organic sesame seed oil in a small bowl. Stir in just enough water to give your mixture a cake-batter-like consistency. With your fingertips, gently spread the paste all over your face and neck, avoiding the sensitive eye area. Let your mask set for fifteen minutes. It will become hard and crusty (yes, I still have enough ego to do this every so often). Rinse your skin with lukewarm water.

I also follow my showers by spreading a thin layer of jojoba oil on my face to moisten the skin.

~~~

Dying: The Terminator

When it comes time to die, be not like those whose hearts are filled with the fear of death, so when their time comes they weep and pray for a little more time to live their lives over again in a different way. Sing your death song, and die like a hero going home.

—Chief Aupumut, Mohican

I don't fear death. Really, I don't. What I mind is the process of getting to death—the physical agony. That evokes terror.

Two years after the diagnosis, I went to my post-operative appointment with a nurse who said she had seen situations like mine for thirty years. "You need to get back on chemotherapy or get ready for Hospice," she said.

I felt struck in the head.

There were no more chemotherapy agents known to benefit endometrial sarcoma patients.

If the nurse was right, I would be in Hospice within a few months. Part of me could then relax and let everything go, even the books I wanted to write. On the other hand, perhaps I had made enough recent changes in my life that I would become healthier.

Then fear and doubt crept in—I must be in deep denial to think any such thoughts.

Yet I had heard many stories of people with miraculous last-moment-type remissions. And many of the women I know with similar cancers are living for years—one even had a six-inch tumor in her lung that she got radiated down to two inches.

Perhaps I could live for years with occasional surgeries.

There were many possibilities. I kept asking for faith and trust, and to let go of fear and doubt. I was doing everything I knew to do to extend my life.

During a psychotherapy session, I did the Map of Emotions© about my fear, allowing it to intensify. It turned into anger. Tension showed up in several areas of my body. I stopped breathing except for quick gasps. Finally my therapist asked me to look at a spot on the floor to return my mind to the room. I shook and shuddered, then relaxed. I experienced tingling all over my chest and emotionally felt nothing. Then I experienced peace.

As Vince Lasorso pointed out, it's so easy to slip into feelings of hopelessness, powerlessness, emptiness, loneliness, and being forsaken. No one can face death with you—it's a solitary assignment. A dark depression, induced by the chemicals of medicine and mind, can extinguish all faith. "It is during these times when one must look to the light," he wrote.

No matter how putrid, disfigured, or close to death I might come, he reminded me that reliance on the Divine can change my course at any second. He was right. I later read about Anita Moorjani, who lay in a cancer-induced coma while her organs shut down. She had a near-death experience, during which she was cured of cancer, and walked out of the hospital within weeks.

I feel most fortunate to have had clean scans since that time. For many people, there is no hope for a life extension, and Hospice becomes a reality.

Even if we have no choice about our dying, we do have a choice about how we die. Dean Ornish, MD, wrote about one cancer patient who faced death with peace. She developed a meditation in which she saw herself entering a meadow with a butterfly sitting on one finger and a bird perched on her shoulder. Then she would become one with the sunlight.

Unfortunately, writes Bernie Siegel, MD, there often is a lengthy living death when the patient receives the message "Don't die." This can be conveyed through unresolved conflicts and unexpressed feelings. In these situations, death is viewed as a failure.

I hoped I had reached the point where I could let go emotionally and pass when it was my time. I also found it most helpful to read in the book *Anticancer* that death itself is not painful. He writes that those who are dying lose the desire to drink or eat. The body stops secreting fluids like phlegm or urine and gradually dehydrates. This reduces nausea, vomiting, and abdominal pain. As fatigue increases, the mind grows distant. The patient experiences a sense of well-being, perhaps even a little euphoria.

If you are faced with the prospect of relinquishing a decayed bodily habitation, sing your death song with a brave heart, and die like a hero going home.

Thriver Soup Ingredient:
I found Ken Wilber's account of his wife's passing deeply moving and inspirational. If you

are facing death, ask someone to read it to you, in the final chapter of *Grace and Grit*.

~~~

Death: An Exchange of Raiment

Just as an individual forsaking dilapidated raiment dons new clothes, so the body-encased soul, relinquishing decayed bodily habitations, enters others that are new.
—God Talks with Arjuna: *The Bhagavad Gita*, 2.22

An acquaintance of mine with stage IV ovarian cancer was about to forsake her dilapidated raiment. I attended her good-bye celebration two years after my diagnosis. She looked amazing for someone who would pass in nine more days. She was with Hospice, had control of the pain, was talkative and cheerful, and said she was excited about her coming transition.

What a blessing she was to me, to see her facing death with joy and gratitude, surrounded by family and friends.

Both Buddhism and Vedanta Hinduism stress the paramount importance of dying with skill, said my friend Mim Grace Gieser. "It determines the conditions of one's next lifetime. It is that important."

She has been practicing dying with skill for at least a dozen years.

My friend Kathy Nace wrote, "It's so hard facing the fact that these bodies of ours are dust—they're all we know! And yet...they are not the essence of us; they do not define, contain nor constrain us. They will crack open and our souls, the kernel of us, will fly free. At some point, it will all be made new—the heavens, the earth, and these bodies of ours. What will they be like, freed from the shadows of sin and decay? Faith is 'confidence in what we hope for and assurance about what we do not see'" (Hebrews 11:1, Christian Bible, NIV).

I agreed with her, yet experienced deep sorrow about leaving behind my children and my unfinished projects. Nothing could have resolved that anguish.

At the same time, I experience confident assurance that when I pass, my soul will move into a new, spiritual body, and my blissed-out essence will continue beyond the grave.

Thriver Soup Ingredient:

If the specter and finality of death are terrifying for you, seek a qualified mental health professional who can work with you to ease the fears and assist you with preparing for death. You might also ask someone to read to you the instruction manual for dying found in *The Tibetan Book of Living and Dying* by Lama Sogyal Rinpoche. Ask family or friends to locate someone who can walk you through the stages of death and teach you how to leave your body when there's no more point in holding on.

III. *Complementary Therapies*

Introduction to Complementary Therapies: Sow Your Seeds

Just as you don't know the way of the wind or how bones grow in a pregnant woman's womb, so you don't know the work of God, the maker of everything. In the morning, sow your seed; and don't slack off until evening; for you don't know which sowing will succeed, this, or that, or if both will do well.
—Ecclesiastes 11:5-6, Complete Jewish Bible

The Hebrew writer of Ecclesiastes encouraged his readers to put forth whatever effort was necessary to accomplish a goal because we simply don't know what will work and what won't, or how things will turn out. I found this especially true when trying to survive cancer.

Once I met a woman who clearly had undergone chemotherapy. I asked her how she was doing. She said she was waiting for her doctor to tell her the results of her most recent scan. I said, "You can get the scan results yourself by going to Hospital Medical Records and requesting them." She didn't want to.

I felt sad for her—she was letting things be done to her and for her rather than sowing her own seeds for health.

I was determined to sow my seeds, to dig in and get my hands dirty. That meant taking a multi-pronged approach to getting well. I felt encouraged in this approach by what Henry Crow-Dog, Sioux Native American, said: "You can heal one who is sick with the power of herbs or with the power of the spirit, the power of the eagle wing, the smoldering cedar, the sage. You can use certain stones for healing because they, too, have power. You can use the power of an animal—the buffalo, the coyote, the eagle, the bear, the elk. There are many ways of healing known to the *pejuta wichasha* (medicine man)."

I altered my diet, worked with my body, developed greater emotional awareness, improved my mental outlook, sought Divine guidance, practiced spiritual disciplines, and asked a community of family and friends for assistance. These efforts gave me more confidence and I felt empowered, even though the disease had spiraled out of human control. And I could also relax some, knowing ultimately everything was beyond my ability to manage anyway, for I could not see the Divine hand in all this mess.

My diet gave my body a chance to repair and eventually heal itself, as shown by my blood-protein levels and overall blood test results. One of my ankhologists, Dr. James Pavelka, once commented that he wished all his patients had blood panels like mine. As he could attest to, complementary treatments made a huge difference in my experience of the cancer journey.

My body responded to the care and attention I gave it by gaining strength and moving closer to health.

My emotions responded to my acceptance of them in the moment, which freed up previously bound energy so I could devote more resources to my well-being.

My mind grew stronger as I learned to better observe my thoughts and shift them when it would benefit my well-being.

My soul soared, with the assistance of several guides, providing me with a deep connection to the Spirit—a source of ineffable love, peace, and comfort despite the pain and discomfort I endured.

And my friends provided much-needed support with the kind of faith that could cure.

Taken together, I replaced the cancerous uterus that a surgeon had excised with a new womb for myself, filled with incredible potential for new life. This plump nesting space would eventually bring forth a vibrant new creation, a life filled with joy and health.

Thriver Soup Ingredient:

The information in this section is not intended to be complete or current, but simply what I found useful during my own journey.

Use caution and common sense when selecting complementary healing modalities. A good friend of mine who had cancer turned his back on Western doctors and chose only alternative treatments. He urged me to purchase a particular book he'd read that touted a cancer cure. I looked at the website. It used marketing ploys to manipulate people into buying the book—long lists of testimonials, profuse explanations without any useful information, and secrets available only to those who bought the book. My friend took the bait and religiously followed the book's so-called cure protocol.

Seven months later I attended his funeral.

It is wise to consult with a medical professional before trying any complementary methods. Everyone's body is different. What helps one person might be detrimental to another. Be aware that some foods are inherently harmful to those with certain pre-existing medical conditions. Dietary supplements may interact with medications or other supplements, may have negative side effects of their own, or may contain potentially harmful ingredients not listed on the label. Also keep in mind that most supplements have not been tested in pregnant women, nursing mothers, or children.

Select your complementary practitioners with care. Ask other cancer patients for suggestions, find out about a given practitioner's training and experience, and ask for references.

David Simon, MD, goes in-depth with excellent questions to ask practitioners in his book, *Return to Wholeness: Embracing Body, Mind, and Spirit in the Face of Cancer*. What are the sellers claiming about the product, service, or therapy? Do their claims make sense? Can they show you good documentation about the effectiveness of their therapy? Have they followed clients for a long period to see how helpful the treatment was for them? What are all the costs involved in the treatment? What are the potential side effects of the therapy?

David Servan-Schreiber offers important warning signs in his book, *Anticancer: A New Way of Life*: only work with providers who are willing to collaborate with your ankhologist; stay away from therapies that lack proof of their benefits yet demonstrate risks; avoid treatments with little proven effectiveness compared to their costs; and be suspicious of those whose promises are contingent on your desire to get well.

If you choose to use other healing practices, give your health care providers a complete picture of what you do to manage your health. This will help ensure coordinated and safe care.

A. Let Food be Your Medicine

Introduction to Let Food be Your Medicine: Harvesting Health

From food, creatures spring forth.
—*God Talks with Arjuna: The Bhagavad Gita*, 3.14a

Food is necessary for survival; good, wholesome food can even add a spring to one's step. Half-way through my final chemotherapy treatments—after nearly two years of infusions—my ankhologist said my blood profile looked exceptional. He wished all his patients had similar blood work, and commented on how well I must be eating. My albumin level had been maintained throughout treatment at four point three out of five, which was terrific news for my prognosis. It meant my cells were getting the nutrients they needed.

My doctor had acknowledged that diet made a difference in my experience of cancer. I did not seek nutritional advice from my ankhologists because they are not dietitians. They are trained in applying chemotherapy and killing rebel cells, not in how to bring the body back into balance. It is my understanding that physicians typically are not trained in nutrition. For that, I looked elsewhere, as you can see in the resources section.

When I mention in this section that a particular nutrient or food will affect cancerous growths, this does not mean that if I eat a large amount of that nutrient each day that it will cure me of cancer. I think nutrition works in a far more subtle way, that foods work synergistically to effect change, and that the goal of a wholesome diet is to nudge the body back into a natural balance that promotes health.

To maximize my chances of achieving health, I primarily follow an organic whole-foods diet, which means I mostly eat unprocessed foods. My starting posture is selecting organic foods as much as possible. Breakfast consists of an apple or pear slowly cooked in ginger water, then covered with cinnamon, with a side of one or two raw, soaked Brazil nuts and almonds. One snack usually involves juiced vegetables—often including a beet and carrots—poured over greens that are then pulverized by my Vitamix blender. A snack of chicken gelatin broth with mushrooms offers more nutrients. For one small meal I mix raw flax oil with cottage cheese until it's creamy.

To round out the day I might eat sprouted cooked beans, vegetables, wild-caught fish, free-range or grass-fed eggs or meat, whole grains, or berries. I take handfuls of supplements to cover my bases.

I do indulge in treats. I love popcorn, which I enjoy about once a week. When squash and pumpkin are in season, I make sweet breads, soups, and crustless pies, and sometimes add a little coconut-milk-based ice cream sweetened with erythritol.

Early in my treatment, I expressed concern about eating sugar, afraid that any would become life-threatening, since cancer loves to gobble it up. Another cancer survivor reassured me. "I do not believe that eating a little bit of dark chocolate every day makes a big difference. Just think—half a year of tough, almost life-threatening chemosabe is weaker than a little bit of chocolate.... Do you believe that? I don't."

A friend wrote, "Chocolate is healing for one's soul, along with anything else the soul desires. Now is the time to feel free, be free, follow your bliss!"

So, occasionally I will bake brownies or chocolate-chip cookies, using sprouted whole-grain flour and unprocessed sugar. Usually I have some dark chocolate each day.

My blood work continued to improve. Fourteen months after treatment ended, and after two more major surgeries, my albumin levels rose to four point seven out of five. One year later it had bumped up to four point nine. To me, this indicates my dietary choices work well for my particular body. I am grateful to have access to the food, supplements, and equipment that make it possible.

I am not, however, a dietitian, nor have I studied human nutrition. I have no particular expertise in this area, other than doing extensive reading and talking with my Ayurvedic doctor to figure out what works for me. While this section of the book contains general information about nutrition, with sources listed by entry at the end of the book, the material is far from complete, nor do I claim to have any special knowledge in this area. For more ideas, please see the Resources section for excellent books and websites on the topic that can provide a wealth of useful information.

Using this section as a starting place, I encourage you to become the expert on what works for your body. Seek the assistance of a registered dietitian or a qualified Ayurvedic physician. Be sure to advise them of any medications you are taking. Always check what they say with your doctors and with your own instincts and intuition.

And focus on eating more wholesome foods to create more of a spring in your step.

Thriver Soup Ingredient:

Ask for assistance researching various nutrients, diets, and kitchen gadgets. The Sources and Other Resources sections of this book have recommended sources to start with, though the list is far from exhaustive.

Settle on a plan that will provide the maximum nutritional benefit for the least amount of cost and time. I consider a food processor, a juicer, and a high-speed blender excellent investments, as long as you commit to using them regularly. You might find a friend or two with unused juicers you can purchase. Also consider how long you are willing to continue the discipline of the diet. If the cost of a high-speed blender is out of touch, consider finding a high-quality green powder to consume daily.

～～～

Alkalize or Die?

And We send down From the sky Rain Charged with blessing, And We produce therewith Gardens and Grain for harvests; And tall (and stately) Palm-trees, with shoots Of fruit-stalks, piled One over another.

—Qur'an 50:9-10

Blessed clean, pure water that gives life—does it also need to be alkalized for greater health? Some alternative health care practitioners urge cancer patients to alkalize their bodies due to a prevailing belief is that cancer forms in an acidic body. Alkalizing involves bringing the pH (potential hydrogen) of the body up above at least 7.0. Some claim the body's pH can be altered by drinking water alkalized by expensive machines; others urge dietary changes to bring the body's pH back to a healthy level.

Friends urged me to alkalize me body because chemotherapy drugs create an acidic environment in which cancer can thrive. What they said seemed to make sense, especially when several people in my cancer support group talked about getting more than one type of cancer. My whole body cringes when I think about those discussions.

Friends suggested drinking baking soda, raw apple cider vinegar, or lemon juice mixed in water to keep my body pH out of the acidic range during chemo treatments. While lemons and raw apple cider vinegar are acidic when we consume them, they leave an alkaline ash residue after being digested. Others urged me to purchase machines that alkalize drinking water.

While I did not purchase a water-alkalizing product (some cost thousands of dollars), I drank the baking soda, raw apple cider vinegar, and lemon juice. I bought pH-testing strips for my morning saliva and urine. I believed these theories for a while, yet was not totally sold on the idea.

The baking soda (sodium bicarbonate) did resolve the burning diarrhea caused by docetaxel, yet I later learned it could soften bones, so I switched to potassium bicarbonate powder in water. Potassium bicarbonate is used to change the pH of beer and wine, so it is available for purchase from home brewing supply companies.

While the lemons and raw apple cider vinegar supplied plenty of vitamin C and potassium, they also greatly exacerbated my chemotherapy-induced mouth sores, so I stopped using them.

Then I found a website by a chemist and learned some important information.

• Our bodies breathe out carbon dioxide to remove excess acid.

• Once water enters the stomach, highly acidic gastric juices remove the excess alkalinity. Excessive intake of alkaline substances can impede proper protein digestion.

• Pancreatic secretions in the intestines neutralize anything alkaline.

• Various parts of our bodies, and even various parts within our individual cells, have different pH values.

• Acidosis and alkalosis are serious conditions that require medical intervention and can be properly diagnosed only by measurements of carbon dioxide and blood electrolyte content.

• Blood pH remains fairly constant and we cannot change it by what we eat. Only by testing blood can the pH of the blood be known.

The reason plant-based diets help reduce the risk of cancer is not because they can change the pH of the body, but because they contain essential nutrients. The enzymes in many raw, soaked, sprouted, and cultured or fermented foods are necessary for proper digestion. If your diet does not include enzyme-rich foods, you can supplement with digestive enzymes.

The life-saving enzymes and nutrients found in healthy, wholesome, unprocessed foods naturally help protect our bodies against cancer. Keeping hydrated with plenty of fresh, clean water helps the body function properly. Our blessed rainwater, falling from the heavens, does not need to be alkalized for our health. It has always kept humans hydrated and caused seeds to sprout and plants to grow, all in Divine order. Feed on these and don't worry about whether your body is alkaline or not; it will be healthier and happier through the care you shower upon it.

Thriver Soup Ingredient:

Some people drink water with a slice of lemon in it throughout the day. The acids in the lemon can wear away at the enamel on teeth. To get bioflavonoids and vitamin C from organic lemons, I drink a lemon water first thing in the morning. I slice off a portion of the fruit, including the peel, and stick it in my Vitamix blender, along with a teaspoon of raw honey and some water. After blending, I drink it down, then eat my cooked apple to help remove the acids from my teeth.

Rather than being concerned with alkalizing your body, focus on drinking purified water and eating wholesome, fresh, organic, nutritious foods.

Amino Acids: They Will be Assimilated

Having become Vaishvanara (fiery power), I exist in the body of living creatures; and, acting through prana and apana, I digest food that is eaten in four ways.
                                        —God Talks with Arjuna: *The Bhagavad Gita*, 15.14

According to the Hindu Bhagavad Gita, the four ways to ingest food are chewing solids, drinking liquids, licking, and breathing in oxygen. Light from the Divine provides our bodies with the power to assimilate food in our digestive systems. This light works with digestion and elimination to provide the body with life-force energy.

During digestion, proteins are broken down into amino acids. I have read that people who consume specific amino acids, usually in the form of supplements, suffer from fewer specific side effects during chemotherapy.

Eric Braverman, in *The Healing Nutrients Within*, specifically recommends supplementing with an amino-acid derivative called N-acetyl-cysteine for decreasing the toxicity of the chemo drug doxorubicin. This amino acid also can help prevent abnormal hair loss. The amino acid arginine inhibits sarcoma tumors and works to detoxify the liver.

One study found evidence that the amino acid acetyl-L-carnitine might reduce symptoms of peripheral neuropathy caused by the chemo drug cisplatin. There is evidence that glutamine powder can help patients who have peripheral neuropathy and it helps repair damaged intestinal cells.

Amino acids, as the building blocks of protein, are important for keeping the body healthy. By ingesting healthy, wholesome foods, including specific amino acids for specialized purposes, we work with the Spirit to bring healing and health to our bodies.

Thriver Soup Ingredient:

As with any supplement, I urge you to discuss the use of specific amino acids with your ankhologist. If you are able, try doing some research on the internet, especially for possible contraindications. You might find some amino acids helpful for your specific issues and chemo-therapy treatments.

~~~

An Apple a Day

Iduna, the Goddess, tended the tree on which the shining apples grew. None would grow on the tree unless she was there to tend it. No one but Iduna might pluck the shining apples. Each morning she plucked them and left them in her basket and every day the Gods and Goddesses came to her garden that they might eat the shining apples and so stay for ever young.

—"Iduna and Her Apples," *The Children of Odin*

The Norse peoples considered the apple a food of the gods. They might have appreciated the more modern English cliché, "an apple a day keeps the doctor away." My Ayurvedic doctor, Hari Sharma, MD, agreed, urging me to start each day with a cooked apple.

Here's why:

One apple holds about five grams of fiber, some of which is soluble pectin. Fiber helps keep blood sugar stable, binds and removes carcinogens, and helps keep the colon clean.

Apples contain the flavonoid phloridzin, which French researchers have discovered might help prevent osteoporosis and increase bone density, especially in post-menopausal women.

The fruit also has boron, which assists the body with laying down calcium in the bones. This is good news if you have or will take steroids with chemotherapy.

Another flavonoid, quercetin, has demonstrated anti-cancer, anti-inflammatory, and antioxidant effects. Quercetin turns the twelve milligrams of vitamin C in the apple into the equivalent of 1,500 milligrams of vitamin C.

The peel includes triterpenoids, compounds that possess strong anti-cancer activity, especially in preventing breast, colon, and liver cancer.

Potassium in the apple helps regulate the balance of fluids on both sides of cell walls and regulates the transfer of nutrients into cells. It also stimulates the kidneys to eliminate toxins.

In one study, rats with known mammary carcinogens were fed extracts equivalent to one apple a day. Their number of tumors was reduced by twenty-five percent.

I learned from my Ayurvedic doctor that apples are best eaten if they are organic, sweet (not sour, like Granny Smith), freshly picked, and then cooked. They also are best eaten first thing in the morning to signal the body that it's time to start digesting food.

Apples appear in many wisdom traditions, and for good reason. They are filled with nutrients that can help us stay younger than our years. This food of the gods was set on the earth by the Divine for us to use. Prepared the right way, they can do much to enhance our health.

Thriver Soup Ingredient:

I buy organic sweet apples by the bag (no orchards around here have organic apples). Each morning I put a piece of fresh ginger root in my Vitamix blender with water, churn, and place in a pot on the stove. Then I cut a fresh apple into eighths and remove the core. I place the slices into the ginger water and cook on a low setting for about twenty minutes. This way the ginger tea doesn't boil yet the apple slices cook. I take out the slices, dash them with cinnamon, and enjoy. Later I drink the ginger tea.

For variety, my Ayurvedic doctor suggested piercing the slices with whole clove buds or cooking fresh pears instead.

∾∾∾

Ayurveda: Balancing Act

Foods that promote longevity, vitality, endurance, health, cheerfulness, and good appetite; and that are savory, mild, substantial, and agreeable to the body, are liked by pure-minded (sattvic) persons.
                    —*God Talks with Arjuna: The Bhagavad Gita*, 17.8

Ayurveda, a 5,000-year-old medical system still used today, promotes longevity and health through a variety of means. I figured if it's been around that long, there's something to it.

The system notes there are three basic body types: *vata*, that tends to run cool; *pitta*, that tends to run hot; and *kapha*, that tends toward the slow, moist, and heavy. When disease occurs, the body type is out of balance; to heal, Ayurveda seeks to assist the individual with regaining balance.

My body temperature runs cool and I've always felt more comfortable wearing more clothes than other people. Eventually I realized I was a *vata* type. As such, I was better off eating cooked foods instead of trying a raw diet. I simply needed to add digestive enzymes to my meals.

More than a year into treatment, Connie and Vince Lasorso told me about an Ohio State University physician, Hari Sharma, MD. This doctor had researched the effects of the Asian Indian supplement Amrit Kalash among cancer patients taking the chemotherapy drugs Adriamycin and cisplatin. Dr. Sharma had retired, yet was working as an Ayurvedic practitioner at OSU's integrative medicine clinic.

"Ayurvedic recommendations are personalized for use by the individual according to their specific psychophysiologic constitution and specific imbalances in their system," he told me. Any recommendations made to an individual should not be applied generally to others, nor should one self-diagnose or self-manage health issues without consulting a physician.

Dr. Sharma took my pulse, looked at my lower eyelids and tongue, and said I was pretty healthy. I laughed. Hadn't he read my chart? Yet, considering I'd been on chemosabe for fourteen months, including the hard-core, end-of-the-line goodies, I was managing extremely well. Because I was still in chemo treatment, he did not recommend Amrit Kalash for me, but rather two other types of Ayurvedic supplements.

After chemo was over, he did recommend Amrit Kalash, a blend of forty-four fruits and herbs which is at least 25,000 times more powerful than vitamins C and E. According to research, it shrinks tumors, slows tumor growth, and prevents tumors from starting. It also enhances alertness and attention, which are important when dealing with chemo brain. Dr. Sharma recommended some other Ayurvedic preparations to assist my body with letting go of stress.

He also provided me with lists of foods to eat and foods to avoid for my body type. These foods are designed to raise my vibration, something I had not realized at the time. Out of the blue, an energy healer told me the vibration of my body was high because of my diet. That felt gratifying. The foods I was consuming were promoting longevity, vitality, endurance, health, cheerfulness, and good appetite.

Thriver Soup Ingredient:

Many cancer patients rave about following a raw food or vegan diet. Yet such diets aren't for everyone—it wasn't right for my body type. That explained why I felt drawn toward soups and stews instead of salads. If you want to know your body type and recommended diet, check with an Ayurvedic physician, and if none are available in your area, try a nutritionist.

≈≈≈

Becoming Juicy

The Word is the tree; the garden of the heart is the farm; tend it, and irrigate it with the Lord's Love. All these trees bear the fruit of the Name of the One Lord.

—"Raag Aasaa," Shri Guru Granth Sahib

If we tend to and irrigate our hearts with divine love like a farmer would care for an orchard, then like the trees in that garden, we will bear good fruit in the Name of the Spirit. And just as the good fruits of spiritual endeavors in our lives yield many benefits, so the precious fruitage of orchards and gardens will provide excellent nutrition.

As cancer survivors, we need all the nutrition we can get. I believe it's best to use organic produce when possible. If not, peel the produce before juicing, as most pesticides reside in the peel.

To maximize your nutrition even more, try juicing several vegetables and using that juice as the liquid base for a smoothie made in a high-powered blender. (The Vitamix supposedly can grind peanuts into peanut butter, so I think this product is a good investment in your health.) With the fiber, your blood sugar won't go haywire and your intestines will get a little extra cleanup help. Since many chemotherapy drugs induce constipation, extra fiber can assist—yet it is best to discuss adding this fiber, and the fruits and vegetables you select, with your health care provider before starting.

It is my understanding that it's not a good idea to juice brassica vegetables, such as kale, cabbage, broccoli, and cauliflower. They are easier to digest if they are cooked, and don't provide much juice anyway.

If you are vulnerable to mouth sores, you might consider avoiding citrus and fruit with citric acid, including tomatoes.

Fruit juices might be more palatable, especially if your sense of taste has changed. I liked the combination of lemon, lime, and a full orange (with the orange-colored portion of the fruit pared off). If you want to mix fruit and vegetables, the best fruit to use probably is the apple.

Cucumbers produce a lot of juice.

My brother Walter came up with a vegetable concoction he really enjoys. "I love yellow onions, and like to stuff a small one into the juicer along with the tomatoes and carrots. My usual recipe: tomatoes, carrots, cucumber, celery, [and] small yellow onion. Mmmm! Of course, I vary it. Sometimes throw in a beet or an apple."

One disadvantage of juicing is the amount of time it takes to prep, juice, and clean up. Perhaps you could study the various juicers for one that is reliable and easy to clean. Many people I've talked to quit juicing after a short amount of time because the process is labor-intensive. Try to determine if your level of dedication to juicing matches the cost of the juicer.

When I obtained precious fruit and ran them through my juicer, the extracted nutrients provided me with tools to help my body heal. In the same way, tending my inner garden provided me with life-giving spiritual fruit.

Thriver Soup Ingredient:

As with everything, I suggest you ask your health care provider before changing any routines to ensure the maximum benefit of your course of healing. I have heard that patients with kidney disease and those on ACE inhibitors for high blood pressure should avoid juicing certain types of produce. Also, note that without the fiber of whole produce, juicing might spike blood sugar and add a lot of calories without giving you a full feeling.

I've read in a few sources that juicing raw beets, celery, and carrots creates a beneficial anti-cancer cocktail. Fresh carrot juice is both sweet and loaded with beta carotene, a key ingredient in producing those all-important white blood cells. Try using it as a base for your Vitamix smoothie with fiber-rich veggies, or by mixing it with cucumbers or tomatoes. Consume your juice right away, as letting the juice sit will cause a depletion in its nutrients, especially vitamin C. Swish the juice in your mouth to encourage your own digestive juices to join in the action.

~~~

Berries: Be the Berry Best

Medicinal plants...should be planted in unctuous, black, sweet or golden sweet soil which is also soft but unploughed. The plants should be unaffected [not over-grown by] other stronger plants.
—Kalpasthana 1#9, *Charaka Samhita*

This Ayurvedic text demonstrates the importance of taking care when growing medicinal plants. The healthier the soil, the healthier the plants, and the more nutrients they can supply for those who need their curative properties.

Years before I was diagnosed, I visited a single mother of two who was struggling financially. It was winter, and I was surprised to see her preparing fresh, expensive strawberries, raspberries, and blueberries for her daughters. I asked her why she chose the most expensive fruit, and she said she wanted her girls to get the micronutrients from the berries. I hadn't heard of micronutrients before. Too bad I didn't follow her example.

I have read about berries in a variety of sources. They most likely were eaten by our ancestors and apparently are nutritional powerhouses. They boost the immune system and provide cell-protecting antioxidants. Raspberries and strawberries contain especially high amounts of ellagic acid, a phytochemical that interferes with cancer development. Blueberries are high in flavonoids, which have powerful antioxidant and anti-inflammatory properties. The berries' anthocyanidins and proanthocyanidins force cancer cells to die. Cranberries sport proanthocyanidins and have shown antioxidant and anticancer activity. These sour berries might create issues, however, if eaten in excess or for those on aspirin or heart medications. They probably also should be avoided by those being treated for liver failure. Juniper berries are tiny pinecones, not berries. They are a diuretic, which helped me during my ifosfamide chemotherapy treatments because they stimulated my kidneys to produce fluid. They can relieve pain and are anti-inflammatory. They appear to inhibit breast cancer cell growth and provide protection for the liver. I would suggest not picking your own, as some juniper berries are poisonous. I purchased mine dried in the spice section of a grocery store and added them to my green smoothies.

Whichever berries you choose, go for the organic ones as they probably will be of greater nutritional benefit; their growing conditions most likely are better than those of berries produced by conventional practices.

Thriver Soup Ingredient:

Add colorful berries to your breakfast. When cranberries are in season, I add a handful to my morning Vitamix-blender drink with a tangerine, raw honey, and water. Juniper berries can be added to green smoothies.

During the summer months, I will dissolve a little raw honey and coconut cream in hemp milk. Then I add some chia seeds and let them absorb the moisture. I add chopped fresh berries and raw, soaked, dehydrated nuts. Even my teenager really likes this mix.

≈≈≈

Cruciferous Vegetables: Cabbage Patch Dollops

We should understand well that all things are the work of the Great Spirit. We should know that He is within all things...and even more important, we should understand that He is also above all these things and peoples. When we do understand all this deeply in our hearts, then we will fear, and love, and know the Great Spirit, and then we will be and act and live as He intends."
—Black Elk, *The Sacred Pipe: Black Elk's Account of the Seven Rites of the Oglala Sioux*

Everything created is from the Divine and has a taste of heaven within.

Even cabbage.

As a child, I savored my German mother's cooked red cabbage—smooth, creamy, mellow. She cooked it in a heavy, old pressure cooker. She cautioned me about how to open the lid after the cabbage was done cooking—no water was to touch the center of the lid. Still young and impressionable at the time, I have continued to feel trepidation around pressure cookers. That fear kept me from asking her for the recipe. No one else asked for it either, even though we all liked that dish, and to my regret, that knowledge disappeared when she passed in 1984.

It was another twenty-five years before I ate red cabbage that tasted anything like my mother had made. My stepmother had found a recipe, and voilà! Mama's red cabbage, even prepared without a pressure cooker. I had my taste of red cabbage heaven again.

After my own diagnosis in 2009, I learned that cabbage is part of the cruciferous family of vegetables—sister to cauliflower, broccoli, kale, Brussels sprouts, bok choy, radishes, turnips, and mustard greens. All of them contain indoles, which scavenge free radicals and prevent toxins from damaging DNA. Indoles communicate to individual cell nuclei that they need to slow down tumor growth. Their phytochemicals block carcinogenic growths. They are loaded with powerful antioxidants and flavonoids, along with selenium and vitamins C and E. Their D-glucaric acid assists the body with eliminating toxins.

Broccoli is a favorite sibling in the anti-cancer crowd. This dark leafy flower contains sulforaphane, which triggers the body's own means of protection against free radicals. Sulforaphane tells liver enzymes to deactivate and destroy cancerous growths.

I have read that all cruciferous vegetables should be cooked (though not boiled—steaming is best) before being eaten. The heat prevents the brassicas from interfering with thyroid function.

The Spirit has gifted us with these special cancer fighters. Women who frequently take advantage of those offered through cruciferous vegetables have a lower risk of developing breast cancer. With gratitude in our hearts for these offerings from the cabbage patch family, we can find ways to enjoy cruciferous vegetables so we can better live our lives.

Thriver Soup Ingredient:

I cannot recommend the red cabbage recipe because it contains a lot of refined sugar. However, a favorite with my children was the following: Steam a head of organic cauliflower until tender. Then blend it with real or clarified butter (ghee) and add Celtic sea salt.

It's quick and simple, and looks and tastes almost like mashed potatoes. Top with toasted, salted, hulled sunflower seeds for a special treat.

It's easy to adopt a daily dollop from the cabbage patch family. Load these beauties onto your plate each week for a heavenly treat.

<p style="text-align:center">~~~</p>

Curcumin: Go for the Gold

Yet he knows the way I take; when he has tested me, I will come out like gold.
—Job 23:10, Complete Jewish Bible

While we are being tested for our mettle during cancer therapy, we might not only emerge like gold; we can receive special assistance along the way by ingesting the gold-medal power of curcumin, the leading anti-cancer spice.

Curcumin works against cancer development in at least ten different ways, affecting each stage of the disease. It offers powerful antitumor, antioxidant, and anti-inflammatory properties. It stimulates the immune system. It blocks the formation of blood vessels to tumors while promoting the flow of blood to wounds. Turmeric intensifies the anti-cancer activity of other plant-based nutrients, especially green tea and black pepper. It enhances the effectiveness of chemotherapy.

Even though curcumin is a powerful antioxidant, it still can be taken during chemotherapy because it follows a different metabolic pathway than other antioxidants. When researchers added curcumin to paclitaxel treatments, curcumin both enhanced the drug's effectiveness and decreased the drug's side effects by protecting organs from chemo-induced damage. The golden spice guards the liver by promoting the production of enzymes that detoxify the organ. It promotes the flow of bile that cleanses the liver and rejuvenates its cells.

I don't care for the taste of turmeric, so I take curcumin in pill form. It's best to take with black pepper and green tea because of the synergistic effects of all three. Black pepper makes the turmeric 2,000 times more absorbable by the intestines.

Note that curcumin is known to inhibit blood clotting, so I would suggest not ingesting any for a two-week period before major surgery. I also suggest not consuming curcumin if you are on blood thinners or have issues with gallstones or your liver.

Thriver Soup Ingredient:

Go for the gold in your kitchen. Curcumin is the main component in turmeric, the orange powder found on grocery store spice racks. Turmeric boasts its best activity when cooked first in clarified butter (ghee) or olive oil, because this releases its fat-soluble compounds. Then add other vegetables to allow turmeric's water-soluble molecules to blend with the nutrients in the other foods. This works well if you add curry powder to enhance the flavor of your dish. Sprinkle on some freshly ground black pepper. Drink green tea with your meal.

~~~

Dark Leafy Greens: Emerald City

The righteous will flourish like a palm tree, they will grow like a cedar of Lebanon; planted in the house of the LORD, they will flourish in the courts of our God. They will still bear fruit in old age, they will stay fresh and green.

—Psalm 92:12-14, Christian Bible, NIV

Piles of organic, dark-leafy greens filled the small building with their freshly picked pungency. As part of a community-supported agriculture (CSA) program I had joined before the diagnosis, I had come to gather my share of produce—pound after earthy pound of salad greens, beet greens, Swiss chard, spinach, kale, and more.

What to do with all this verdant richness? I didn't really want it. My family wouldn't eat it. In fact, a friend's son had renamed the CSA's pickup location Kaleville after its bumper crop that none of us wanted to consume. Still, I knew it was good for me, and I had purchased part of the crop, so I dutifully filled bag after bag with the emerald produce. And later ate it all.

The CSA recipes suggested sautéing the dark, bitter, green vegetables, like kale, with fresh garlic and salt. Not real bad, if I cooked them long enough and ate them quickly. Fortunately, Swiss chard and beet greens proved slightly more tender and palatable. With the less-bitter greens I dared to make salads, adding a mixture of avocado, buttermilk, cilantro, and a bit of garlic and dill to avoid commercial salad dressings.

Much to my chagrin, I learned that the deeper and darker the greens, the greater the plant's vigor and nutritional wallop, and therefore the healthier I could become by eating them daily.

Maybe it wasn't a gourmand's dream, yet I knew my cells welcomed the valuable cancer-fighting nutrients, like beta-carotene, vitamin C, folic acid, and important trace minerals. With effort, I managed to come close to eating three to five servings of dark leafy greens daily. Later blood tests confirmed my diet was an important aspect of my recovery.

Eating plenty of fresh, dark, leafy greens each day can be boring, and it's easy to get tired of them. During the winter I sometimes find I can't stand them anymore, so I switch to cooked root vegetables or vegetable soups. Whatever your choice, the discipline of daily dietary improvements can pay off in burgeoning physical vitality. Your chances of flourishing greatly increase when you take the emerald beauties into your body.

Thriver Soup Ingredient:

I prefer to gently and slowly sauté my dark leafy greens in organic, extra-virgin olive oil. I put the heat on low. While the leaves are cooking, I finely chop a clove or two of fresh garlic. (Caution: If you are on blood thinners or anti-coagulants, talk about eating garlic with your physician.) I let the chopped raw garlic sit for at least fifteen minutes to maximize the levels of allicin that form. Allicin holds the key to the health-promoting benefits of garlic. When the kale is tender, I add the garlic and sauté lightly for another 90 seconds to preserve the nutrients.

Remove from heat, add salt and pepper to taste, and enjoy.

∽∽∽

Enlarge Your Circle of Foods

It is He Who has Spread out the earth For (His) creatures: Therein is fruit And date-palms, producing Spathes (enclosing dates); Also corn, with (its) Leaves and stalk for fodder, And sweet-smelling plants.
—Qur'an 55:10-12

According to the Islamic holy book, the Qur'an, the earth was made for the creatures upon it, with foods of various kinds to meet our bodies' needs. When we don't get our basic nutritional requirements met through a wide selection of food types, we can become ill.

Scurvy, the scourge of sailors for centuries, was caused by a vitamin C deficiency. Pellagra was caused by the lack of a B vitamin. It took hundreds of years and millions of deaths before people came to understand the connection between these illnesses and vitamins. What if cancer also is caused by a nutritional deficiency of some sort due to our consumption of a limited variety of foods?

One proposed so-called "vitamin" deficiency is "vitamin B17," also known as laetrile, amygdalin, and nitriloside. According to this theory, cancer results from a deficiency in nitrilosides, which are found in bitter edibles. Foods said to contain nitrilosides include sour berries, such as cranberries, elderberries, and wild blackberries; macadamia nuts; squash seeds; fava and mung beans; and buckwheat, flax, and millet. These foods might have been part of many of our ancestors' diets; now they typically are missing from the average American menu. Whether or not nitrilosides can help cancer patients or not, introducing these foods into one's diet will provide a wider variety of healthy nutrients.

While I don't advocate laetrile treatments, I would encourage the consumption of a wide variety of wholesome natural foods to enhance nutritional status. As always, I recommend checking with your doctor first. You might also want to check some websites listed in the Sources and Other Resources sections for information on particular foods, protocols, or products.

After reading books by Ralph Moss, PhD, I came to the conclusion that we need a great variety of nutrients from a large circle of food types to keep our bodies in optimal health. The Benevolent One has provided us with a rich diversity of plant and animal life so we can nourish our bodies. Why not enjoy more variety in your diet?

Thriver Soup Ingredient:

If you have access to sour berries, perhaps you can add them to your breakfast. Fresh, sprouted mung beans can be eaten raw, so I suggest adding them to salads or tossing them into a high-speed blender when you make a green smoothie. Try looking online for appealing recipes using buckwheat and millet. The nutritional variety will give your body more tools for returning to health.

~~~

Food Preparation: No More Nukes

Foods that are nutritionally worthless, insipid, putrid, stale, refuse, and impure are enjoyed by tamasic [self-destructive] persons.

—*God Talks with Arjuna: The Bhagavad Gita*, 17.10

While modern scientists have dissected food in search of individual nutrients and physical properties, the ancient yogis perceived the vibratory nature of food. Not only did the yogis express concern over what they ingested; they also considered how the food was prepared. They wanted everything they ate to lift up not only their physical bodies, but also their minds and spirits, because they believed all of material existence stemmed from the Spirit and contained the Divine. About 5,000 years ago, they developed a medical system called Ayurveda, combining various ingredients to bring healing energy to those with a variety of ailments.

Just as yogis created healing balms by synergistically combining and preparing various food elements, many humans can alter food to induce unhealthy vibrations. Currently, it seems to me that some foods are processed to the point they are nutritionally worthless; then synthetic vitamins are added back into the food. Stale food lacks vitality. And I don't know how microwaving food affects its vibratory nature. Britain's top medical journal reported that when microwaved food is eaten, it can cause "structural, functional, and immunological changes in the body. It [microwave cooking] converts the amino acid L-proline into a proven toxin to the nervous system, liver, and kidneys." Years before I knew about this report, energy intuitive Maria Paglialungo said she would not recommend eating food prepared in a microwave. A few years later I chose to abandon microwave cooking. Instead, I use the stovetop or a toaster oven. It takes a little more time, but the food tastes better, so it's worth it to me. Even my teenaged son now prefers reheating food in the toaster oven instead of the microwave.

According to my Ayurvedic doctor, it's best to avoid canned, frozen, and leftover foods. Everything ought to be prepared fresh each time. This is hard to follow, yet I have switched from making large quantities of a dish for future use to preparing small portions. It takes more time, yet I am assured of higher nutritional values. It helps keep the vibrations of my food higher, which is something I need to give my body the best possible chance to survive and thrive.

To minimize impurities in my food, I avoid using plastic or nonstick cooking products around heated food. When cooking in a crock pot, I use wooden spoons. Crock-pot cooking allows me to cook slowly so food is far less likely to burn. This helps preserve and mingle some of the nutrients that otherwise might be lost. I also enjoy the convenience of dropping things into the pot in the morning and having a hot meal in the evening.

I don't grill out because burned meat can contain carcinogens. Studies indicate grilling allows heterocyclic amines (HCAs) to build up on meat four minutes after it reaches temperatures above 351 degrees F. The longer the meat is cooked, and the higher the temperature, the more toxins infiltrate the food. Some studies indicate that those who eat a lot of grilled meat have an increased risk of developing cancer.

When I shop, I select organic foods when possible. Organic foods are grown or produced without pesticides, herbicides, fertilizers, genetic engineering, growth hormones, antibiotics, irradiation, or artificial ingredients. Separate research conducted by Cynthia Curl, PhD, and Claude Aubert demonstrated that conventional foods created a high toxic load in the bodies of children and in the milk of new mothers when compared to those who consumed organic food. To find organic produce, look for labels that have five numerals beginning with a "9." I decided it was worth it to me to spend the extra money so I would have fewer concerns about what I put into my body. I wanted pure, nutritionally packed food. I also joined a local organic food cooperative so nearly all of my vegetables are fresh, local, and organic.

The Bhagavad Gita makes it clear that impure and nutritionally sparse foods are not good for the spirit, much less the body. I suggest choosing an enjoyable variety of foods that are fresh and full of vitality, and prepare them in ways that preserve as much nutritional quality as possible.

Thriver Soup Ingredient:

If you are thinking about switching to more organic foods, start by purchasing organic items that, when grown conventionally, have the highest pesticide levels. For more information, check the chart on the Environmental Working Group website (www.ewg.org). Peaches have the highest pesticide levels, followed closely by apples.

Mim Grace Gieser taught me to mix a little of Dr. Bronner's Magic Soap with water and put some in a little spray bottle. When I want to eat produce, I spritz it with this solution and rinse before preparing the food.

If you eat microwaved food, consider purchasing a toaster oven. It's an energy-efficient way to prepare small quantities of food, thus avoiding leftovers so that your meal is as fresh and vitality-rich as possible. And when you eat, see if you can select a pleasant environment and chew your food thoroughly before swallowing. This will maximize digestion and feed your cells more of what they need to regain health and vigor.

≈≈≈

Fruit: It's Magically Delicious

The next full moon she [Medea] issued forth alone, while all creatures slept; not a breath stirred the foliage, and all was still. To the stars she addressed her incantations, and to the moon; to Hecate, the goddess of the underworld, and to Tellus, the goddess of the earth, by whose power plants potent for enchantment are produced. She invoked the gods of the woods and caverns, of mountains and valleys, of lakes and rivers, of winds and vapours. While she spoke the stars shone brighter, and presently a chariot descended through the air, drawn by flying serpents. She ascended it, and borne aloft made her way to distant regions, where potent plants grew which she knew how to select for her purpose.

—"Medea and Aeson," *The Golden Age of Myths and Legends*

During the cancer journey, it helps to have nutritionally potent plants to eat. Among them, select fruit that is nutritionally dense to increase your chances of survival.

Fruit is an important potent plant food to include in your diet. Fruit contain caffeic acid, which helps the body create an enzyme that aids in eliminating carcinogens.

Some fruit have additional benefits. Cherries contain glucaric acid, which can detoxify the body. Tart cherries are high in antioxidants, which help reduce inflammation. Citrus fruits have anti-inflammatory flavonoids and stimulate the detoxification of carcinogens by the liver. Modified citrus pectin from the peel and pulp of citrus fruit appears to reduce the risk of metastasis. Pomegranates are full of polyphenols, are anti-inflammatory, contain antioxidants, and have other anti-cancer components.

When you are picking up produce, select your fruit as if you are a goddess, looking for the best for your journey in the region of cancer treatment.

Thriver Soup Ingredient:

I didn't have a clue how to eat a pomegranate without spending an hour picking out each seed. I had heard one can eat the seeds, pulp, skin, root, and flower, so I tried juicing the whole fruit. Whew, that was so bitter, and the unpleasantness stayed in my mouth for hours, despite trying to saturate my taste buds with other flavors.

Then I accidently came across an online video that demonstrated how to easily get the seeds out of the pulp. Here's what I learned:

Remove the crown of the fruit by cutting a cone into the top, so you don't cut into the seeds. Slice off the end with the stem. Look at the pomegranate now from the cone-cut angle, and see the ridges rising around the center of the fruit. Score the skin from top to bottom along the top of each ridge, creating several sections. Cut into the membrane but not very deeply. Then you should be able to easily break open the fruit, peel away the membrane, and eat the seeds. If you still are unable to get the seeds easily out of the membrane, soak the fruit for about five minutes in a bowl of cold water. Strain off the membranes and collect the seeds at the bottom.

Getting Seedy

When he has leveled its surface, does he not then scatter black cumin and sow cumin? He plants wheat in rows and barley in plots, with spelt as their border.
—Isaiah 28:25-27, Holman Christian Standard Bible

Black cumin seeds have been ground and used to flavor bread and as a pepper substitute for millennia. This aromatic culinary herb has since been found to fight cancer—even pancreatic cancer—in numerous ways. It also can help reduce pain and soothe the digestive system.

Seeds symbolize enormous potential lying dormant within. On a physical level, seeds are tiny packets loaded with genetic information and nutrients. All it takes is a little warmth and water to turn a seed into a sprout, a process that dramatically increases its vitamin and enzyme content.

Many types of seeds can be particularly helpful for those on the cancer journey. Caraway seeds are full of limonene, which can stop cancer growth.

Chia seeds contain large amounts of alpha-linolenic acid, an omega-3 fatty acid. The tiny seeds are high in antioxidants and contain high levels of protein and fiber, along with the minerals iron, magnesium, zinc, and copper. When moistened, chia seeds become gelatinous, thereby releasing carbohydrates slowly, which helps the body regulate blood sugar.

Cocoa beans—my favorite—are full of flavanols that can protect cell DNA. Chocolate that's been "dutched" has lost its beneficial flavanols. Try to stick to chocolate that has at least a sixty percent cocoa content. I prefer straight dark chocolate bars that do not contain ordinary sugar. I look for brands that sweeten their chocolate with rapadura—unprocessed cane sugar—or use a sugar alcohol, such as erythritol, isomalt, lactitol, maltitol, mannitol, sorbitol, or xylitol. Because the human body does not absorb sugar alcohols quickly, sugar alcohols have minimal effect on blood sugar levels, making them less likely to feed cancer cells.

Coriander seeds appear to relieve constipation as well as help prevent colon cancer. Their anti-inflammatory properties protect against nerve damage. They also might lower blood sugar and increase the release of insulin from the pancreas.

Fenugreek seeds can help slow or stop the growth of breast and pancreatic cancer. They can be used to make tea.

Flax seeds are a rich plant source of omega-3 fatty acids which reduce inflammation, and of lignans, which can retard the growth of cancerous cells. Researchers found that women who consumed the most lignans had the lowest risk of breast cancer. Lignans also appear to enhance the benefits of the chemotherapy drug tamoxifen. Flax seeds need to be ground and immediately consumed for humans to gain access to their nutrients. Eating cereals and chips containing flax seeds probably won't provide the benefits for which you might be looking. They might, however, provide more fiber, which is useful.

Mustard seeds, from the cruciferous mustard plant, are full of glucosinolates and probably can help protect the body against the growth of cancer cells. I get black mustard seeds from an Asian Indian section of a grocery store. I gently fry them with turmeric powder in oil or butter until the seeds pop and are fragrant. Then I add veggies and start a slow sauté. I find this delicious when I add curry powder.

Pumpkin seeds are full of anti-oxidants, magnesium, iron, protein, and zinc. I collect both pumpkin and squash seeds during fall harvests. I scoop the seeds and pulp out of the gourd with a mildly serrated grapefruit spoon. Sometimes I simply add these to my veggie Vitamix blend. When I have the energy, I soak the pulp and seeds in a bowl of water, then press on the pulp to remove the seeds. I refrigerate the pulp for my next veggie Vitamix blend. The seeds get rinsed and soaked overnight. Later I mix the seeds with a little organic extra-virgin olive oil and a mineral-rich sea salt. I bake them at 350 for about 15 minutes; stir, add garlic powder, and bake for another 15 minutes. I store them in a glass jar in the refrigerator to use as a snack when I leave the house.

Sesame seeds might reduce the activity of genes linked to certain types of cancer. They are great when added to hummus or stir fries.

Getting seedy by increasing your intake of these nutritional jewels can help you on your journey toward improved health. As always, I urge you to discuss alterations to your diet with your health care provider.

Thriver Soup Ingredient:
Being a chocolate lover, I discovered I could make a thick chocolate pudding with chia seeds, bringing together two nutrient-dense food packets.

I place one-quarter cup chia seeds in one and one-quarter cup of a milk base, like hemp or coconut milk. Then I add up to a quarter cup of organic cocoa powder and a sweetener of choice. I use raw honey, letting it dissolve in the milk base. Stir occasionally while the chia seeds turn gelatinous. It will thicken into a delicious pudding.

~~~

Grab Life by the Herbs

The goddess of medicine and healing was also one of her attendants. Her name was Eira and she would scour the whole earth for powerful ingredients and rare herbs for her remedies. She taught her skills with care to the women of the Northern peoples who, following her fine example, became accomplished healers.

—"Frigga, Queen of the Gods," *The Viking Gods: Pagan Myths of Nordic Peoples*

Frigga and Eira scoured the earth for herbs to use as remedies. They might have gathered basil, marjoram, mint, oregano, rosemary, and thyme—herbs made especially fragrant because they contain fatty acids of the terpene family. Terpenes can provoke the death of cancer cells and reduce their capacity to spread.

Here is a brief overview of a few herbs that can be used as remedies. Please discuss each with your doctors before using them, as some of the plants might have an adverse effect on your situation.

Basil contains eugenol, which blocks pain-triggering enzymes. It's also anti-inflammatory and a good source of vitamin K, which helps clot blood when needed.

Bay leaf contains parthenolide, shown to slow the appearance and growth of breast tumors in mice in a Russian study. This anti-inflammatory is a potent anti-oxidant.

Carnivora, made from the Venus fly trap, might be useful against primitive tumor tissues, though not against highly differentiated cells. Carnivora is said to stimulate and modulate the immune system.

Cat's claw, which contains numerous unusual components, has demonstrated anti-cancer and anti-inflammatory effects. Most adults with cancer get a response when taking three capsules of 350 mg bark or root capsules after each of three meals.

Lemongrass has been found in several studies to have anti-cancer properties. It offers the additional benefits of possibly protecting cells from damage caused by x-rays and CAT scans, as well as calming anxiety.

Oregano is full of antioxidants. One teaspoon contains as many antioxidant compounds as three cups of chopped broccoli.

Parsley can help cleanse the kidneys, so it might be useful in combination with the chemotherapy drug ifosfamide. Parsley also is packed with apigenin, an antioxidant that helps other antioxidants perform more effectively. A side benefit is assistance with reducing constipation.

Rosemary contains the terpene carnosol, which is especially useful in preventing cancer cells from invading new tissue. It also has demonstrated effectiveness at enhancing the work of chemotherapy drugs.

Sage can improve mood and memory, possibly counteracting some chemotherapy side effects.

Thyme is another anti-inflammatory and anti-oxidant herb. It protects DNA and acts against cancer.

To help maximize these herbs in my diet, I combine equal parts dried basil, marjoram, sage, and thyme, and sprinkle them on my scrambled eggs. If you gather powerful medicinal herbs like Eira, select organic, fresh plants with potency, rich aroma, and good taste. Your body will thank you.

Thriver Soup Ingredient:

One of my favorite summer dishes is basil-garlic pesto with walnuts on whole-grain pasta. It tastes wonderful, gives comfort, and combines anti-cancer ingredients.

Start by covering one-half cup raw, organic walnuts with filtered water and a little salt, and soak them for about eight hours.

After the soaking time is up, begin cooking pasta according to package directions.

Rinse walnuts and combine in a food processor with two cups packed fresh organic basil leaves, one-third cup organic olive oil, one-half teaspoon salt, and two cloves of garlic. Blend until thoroughly combined. Add one-half cup grated parmesan cheese and blend for another five or ten seconds. Just before serving, blend in two tablespoons of hot water from the cooked pasta.

Drain pasta and serve covered with the pesto sauce.

≈≈≈

Grass is Always Greener

Within the hour the word was fulfilled. N'vukhadnetzar was driven from human society, he ate grass like an ox, and his body was drenched with dew from the sky, until his hair had grown like eagles' feathers and his nails like birds' claws. "When this period was over, I, N'vukhadnetzar, lifted my eyes toward heaven, and my understanding came back to me. I blessed the Most High, I praised and gave honor to him who lives forever. 'For his rulership is everlasting, his kingdom endures through all generations.'"

—Daniel 4:33-34, Complete Jewish Bible

A story in the Jewish book of Daniel recounts the life of Nebuchadnezzar, a neo-Babylonian monarch who reigned about 605 BC–562 BC. When this king went mad, he was driven from his palaces and lived among the wild animals, grazing on grass for seven periods of time.

My mind flew to his story in May 2010, while talking about juicing wheatgrass with a cancer survivor. I suddenly saw Nebuchadnezzar's story in a new light. This king probably had sumptuously feasted on meat and alcohol much of his life, which might well have destroyed his mental and/or physical health. Perhaps he needed a period of cleansing, a time for focusing on eating living chlorophyll-packed greens. When his time was finished, he declared that his reason had returned to him. His mind and body were restored to health.

Many cancer survivors extoll the virtues of juicing wheatgrass. Since I have trouble digesting wheat, I decided to try growing spelt grass. Spelt, an heirloom grain, is a lighter and more easily digested form of wheat. I sprouted the spelt berries, then placed them in a tray of soil and put them in front of my window. I continued spraying the berries with water each day until they grew about three inches high. I cut the grass off about an inch up from the soil and juiced them. It took a large amount of spelt grass to get a trickle of juice, so the next time I put the grass into my Vitamix blender instead. The only difference between juicing and using a high-speed blender is that juicing removes the fiber. Fiber helps keep the colon clean. I have been told by friends that both juicing and using a high-speed blender break open the plants' cell walls. This supposedly releases more nutrients, including amino acids, which are the building blocks for protein.

I left the cut spelt in the tray and continued watering, just like a lawn, until the shoots grew high enough to harvest again. Like Nebuchadnezzar, I drenched the inside of my body with spelt grass to help restore my physical health and mental clarity. Fortunately, I didn't have to go graze in fields for seven periods of time. I grazed in my own kitchen.

Thriver Soup Ingredient:

Some grocery stores now sell wheatgrass in little planters. If you purchase these, try just cutting the stems about one or two inches from the bottom so the grass can regrow over and over again.

Or, obtain organic wheat or spelt berries that can sprout. Place about 1 cup in a quart-sized glass bowl or jar and fill with water. After about twelve hours, strain off the water, rinse, drain, and let sit for another twelve hours. Rinse and drain every twelve hours until the berries sprout. Plant your sprouts in organic soil. I use a shallow planting tray and set the sprouts in the soil, barely covering them. I water twice a day until I have a tray of grass.

≈≈≈

Green Smoothies: Liquid Sunshine

By Guru's Grace, the supreme status is obtained, and the dry wood blossoms forth again in lush greenery.

—"Raag Goojaree," Shri Guru Granth Sahib

The supreme status can be obtained only by grace—and when we experience this state, we will be like dry wood that blossoms forth with lush greenery.

Going green took on new meaning for me while reading a book on sacred geometry. I stumbled upon an interesting phenomenon: The chlorophyll molecule has magnesium at its center and twelve-fold symmetry extending outward, like a rose window in a cathedral or a mandala. Human blood has a similar configuration, featuring iron instead of magnesium at its core.

Raw green smoothies became extremely important to Kris Carr, who was diagnosed in her early thirties with a rare, yet slow-growing sarcoma. In her movie "Crazy Sexy Cancer," she first tried a macrobiotic diet, yet when she got her blood analyzed by someone who advocated raw foods, she discovered that her red blood cells were clumping together too much. Then she tried a raw food diet, only consuming green smoothies for a month. She attended a healing institute and ate lots of raw fresh sprouts and other healing foods, and her blood cells looked about perfect afterward. After less than two years on this diet, her CAT scan showed that the cancer had hardly progressed. (I do think her falling in love and getting married might have contributed to her positive scan results.) It appears she has continued with her diet and is living with the cancer at an arrested state.

A raw diet isn't for everyone. I found it doesn't work for me. My body has an easier time digesting food if I take enzyme capsules with cooked meals. I did, however, adopt a diet that included a daily dose of lettuce, celery, or kelp powder (a good source of iodine and trace minerals) run through my Vitamix blender. I found this especially useful when I experienced extensive mouth sores. I could drink in liquid sunshine to keep my cells humming. I didn't have to become as a dry tree; I could become lush and green again, filling my body with minerals, vitamins, and protein. It helped me fall in with the company of the blessed who attained a measure of liberation from cancer. Perhaps not the supreme status, but close enough for me.

Caution: If you are on blood thinners, or are prone to kidney stones, talk to your ankhologist about eating dark, leafy greens.

Thriver Soup Ingredient:

If you do not have a Vitamix or similar high-powered blender, select some nutritionally potent green powder and take it daily.

If you like mint and have a high-powered blender, try this green smoothie.

1 cup unsweetened organic coconut milk

1 handful raw organic cacao nibs

1 bunch fresh organic mint leaves

1 tsp. organic vanilla flavoring

Sweetener of choice (sucanat, raw honey, raw agave nectar, stevia, and xylitol are options I've used.)

Place all in a Vitamix, whirl and enjoy. For a minty ice cream, place the smoothie in a freezable dish. Pull out of the freezer every hour and beat with a mixer to break up the ice crystals. Eat when ready.

~~~

Here's the Beef

And in cattle (too) ye Have an instructive example: From within their bodies We produce (milk) for you To drink; there art, in them, (Besides), numerous (other) Benefits for you; And of their (meat) ye eat; And on them, as well as In ships, ye ride.

—Qur'an 23:21-22

Meat is a bit controversial in cancerland. Some people urge cancer patients to go vegetarian, vegan, or raw with their diets. Certainly adding a great deal of produce to the diet is important. However, meat is important as well for many people, as the Qur'an notes. Humans have jaws designed to eat both plant and animal matter. Some people, such as the Inuit, developed digestive systems that require meat. Many Asian Indians are healthy vegetarians all their lives. Your body has its own unique needs. I believe it is more important to pay attention to your body's true instincts regarding food rather than to follow a moral or health dictate regarding diet.

I found that I did well if I followed what my body wanted. After I started making green smoothies, I noticed a total lack of interest in eating any more meat, except possibly for fish, for a few months.

On the other hand, a long-time vegetarian in treatment for breast cancer developed a craving for chicken broth. She told me she started drinking chicken broth during each chemotherapy cycle to satisfy her new desire.

Even those with digestive issues around meat have a healthy option. Edgar Cayce, a medical intuitive, provided a recipe for beef juice (not broth) that can nourish without putting meat into the stomach. A small amount of the juice is swished in the mouth for a few minutes before being swallowed.

If you purchase meat, try selecting organic, pasture-raised, grass-finished, or flax-seed-fed products. These animals will likely have more of the healthy omega-3 fatty acids in their meat and should be relatively free of hormones and pesticides.

I found nearly a year after declining all meat that I developed a craving for beef. I really wanted a juicy hamburger dripping with ketchup, tomato, mustard, and fresh onion. Alas, I had to avoid the fixings to try to limit the mouth sores I had developed during my doxorubicin and cisplatin treatments.

A week later I took my meat craving to a new level when I slowly cherished each bite of two bratwurst. YUM. The craving disappeared and my energy levels rose almost back to normal. Perhaps this was as much a craving for fat and protein as it was for meat.

A couple months later I craved beef bone broth. I found a grocery store with soup bones from free-range cattle. I had to call ahead to find out when the bones arrived. Properly prepared broths will have pulled calcium, magnesium, and potassium out of the bones, cartilage, and marrow.

During the summer months, a local 4-H participant raises free-range chickens and sells them at our community-supported agriculture pickup location. I asked him for the chicken feet, and each fall I have had bags of chicken feet with which to make gelatin. Gelatin is a great aid to the digestion of cooked foods. Just as gelatin attracts water to make desserts, like Jell-O, gelatin also attracts digestive juices to the surfaces of cooked food particles in the stomach to aid digestion. It enables the body to better use the proteins consumed in other foods.

Animals provided by the Divine can offer us nourishing food, if raised in clean, humane conditions. Similarly, how we prepare the food can have an impact on how healthy the dishes will prove for our bodies.

Thriver Soup Ingredient:

To make a nourishing chicken bone broth, I follow instructions from Sally Fallon's book, *Nourishing Traditions*. I place cold, filtered water in a pot and add a tablespoon of white wine or vinegar for every two quarts of water. I prefer to use a crock pot. Add parts from free-range birds, because they produce gelatin, especially the feet. Let stand for thirty to sixty minutes. This process enables the fibers in the animal parts to open slowly, releasing more nutrients into the water. Then turn the heat on high until the mix is boiling. Scoop off the scum that rises to the surface. Turn the control to low and let the broth simmer for six to twenty-four hours. Filter, cool, and refrigerate. After the fat collects at the top, skim it off. I then divide up the broth into pint-sized canning jars to freeze for later use.

For more information, including how to make other bone broths, see the book *Nourishing Traditions*, by Sally Fallon.

$$\sim\sim\sim$$

Little Sprouts

Take wheat, barley, beans, lentils, millet and buckwheat; put them together in one bowl; and make bread from it.

—Ezekiel 4:9a, Complete Jewish Bible

As I walked up to the tortilla shelf at a natural health food store, I noticed a package that shouted the name Ezekiel. Ezekiel? What did a Hebrew prophet have to do with Mexican tortillas?

I looked more closely and noticed that the package included this verse from Ezekiel 4:9. "Take also unto thee Wheat, and Barley, and Beans, and Lentils, and Millet, and Spelt, and put them in one vessel, and make bread of it..."

The package also explained that the grains had been sprouted before they were turned into tortillas. Why was that so important?

And then I remembered the onion. A solitary onion had been left, forgotten, in a bag in the back of our pantry. I don't know how long it sat there, overlooked—weeks, or perhaps even a month or more. When I opened the bag, I expected to see something moldy to throw into the compost heap.

Instead, I found a living onion stretching itself outward with long emerald arms, seeking the sun.

Filled with amazement at the tremendous life force expressed by this onion, I realized it had produced green shoots, which must have been at least six inches long, with no water, no sunlight and no soil. If a sprouted onion can produce so much life, perhaps the sprouted grains turned into tortillas also could impart a healthy meal—certainly far more healthy than the trans-fat, bleached-white-flour tortillas I had been used to.

Since the diagnosis in July 2009, I have chosen the path of life-giving sprouted grains, greens, and beans. I sprout my dried organic beans before cooking them. I generally sprout mung beans, clover, and sunflower seeds, all of which can be eaten raw. I toss a handful into my Vitamix blender, along with aloe vera juice, green tea leaves, rejuvelac (a tonic made from sprouted wheat berries), freshly juiced vegetables, and some salad greens. It's not a tasty treat, yet it is highly nutritious.

Sprouting provides many benefits. Digestion is easier with sprouted grains because the process neutralizes phytic acid, a substance that inhibits one's own digestive enzymes, while enhancing the body's ability to absorb calcium, magnesium iron, copper, and zinc. Sprouting can increase carotene content of food as much as eight times. Vitamin B levels grow. Enzyme activity increases six fold. Rejuvelac is rich in protein, vitamins E and K, phosphates, and digestive enzymes, as well as the probiotics lactobacillus and aspergillis.

Caution: Don't sprout alfalfa seeds, said Sally Fallon in *Nourishing Traditions*. The resulting sprouts promote inflammatory illnesses and suppress the immune system.

Thriver Soup Ingredient:

Make some rejuvelac for the liquid in your green smoothie or to drink by itself. It bubbles slightly and produces a mildly tangy, lemony flavor. I didn't think it sounded appetizing, yet felt surprised that it tasted acceptable. I found a recipe for it in Sally Fallon's book, *Nourishing Traditions*.

Rejuvelac is easy to make and doesn't require much time, though it does involve some simple steps done during a period of a few days.

To make rejuvelac, purchase dried organic wheat or spelt berries. Place one cup into a quart canning jar or glass bowl. Add four cups of filtered water and soak overnight. Keep at room temperature. Drain (I use a sieve), rinse, and drain again. Rinse and drain two or three times a day for two days. When the berries sprout, rinse them again, fill the jar with four cups of filtered water, and let them soak for two days. Remove the white foam from the top. Strain off and drink the liquid or add it to a green smoothie.

Fill the jar again with fresh filtered water and soak the sprouted berries for another twenty-four hours. Again, remove the white foam from the top. Strain off and drink the liquid or add it to a green smoothie.

Make a third batch, soaking for yet another day. Strain and drink the liquid. The sprouted berries are spent and can be added to a compost pile.

~~~

Magic of Mushrooms

Characteristics of Plants Which Should Be Collected for Medicinal Use: Those which are grown in time (in proper season), mature with taste, potency and smell. They should have smell, color, taste, touch and efficacy which is unaffected by time, sun, fire, water, air and organisms, are fresh and situated in northern direction.

—Kalpasthana 1#10, *Charaka Samhita*

The potency and efficacy of mushrooms can provide a boon for cancer patients. Bringing fungus among us can help us through a variety of mechanisms. These include enhancing our immune systems and inhibiting the growth of cancer.

Maitake mushrooms, also known as dancing mushrooms, have the strongest anti-cancer activity of all the mushrooms studied. They protect healthy cells from becoming cancerous; enhance the immune system's ability to seek out and destroy cancer cells; assist cells with regaining control of their own division and programmed death; enhance the bone marrow's ability to produce blood cells; help prevent metastasis; and decrease chemotherapy side effects. If you choose to take them in supplemental form, select maitake D- or MD-fraction (which are derived by an extraction process) on an empty stomach. The MD-fraction is more pure. I bought fresh maitake mushrooms and used them in soups as well as taking them in supplement form. I have read that maitake mushrooms may not be appropriate for those taking hypoglycemic medications or warfarin.

Polysaccharide-K (PSK, also known as PSP and Krestin) is derived from a mushroom commonly called turkey tail. Double-blind studies have demonstrated increased survival rates among those taking PSK because these mushrooms affect the malignant process in several ways. Their two primary benefits are stimulating the immune system and working against tumors.

Reishi mushrooms can increase white blood cell and tumor-fighting cell production, cut off the growth of new blood vessels to tumors, and reduce the migration of cancerous cells. They have been known to decrease the toxicity created by chemotherapy drugs. When looking for a supplement, select one with a higher level of triterpenoids, which provides the most benefit. The more bitter the tea or tincture, the more potent it is. The recommended dose is three to five grams per day, or ten to thirty drops.

Shiitake mushrooms contain lentinian, which is thought to prevent some of the damage to chromosomes caused by chemotherapy drugs. Lentinian inhibits metastasis and prevents tumor growth.

Other mushrooms to consider include agaricus, chaga, cordyceps, cremini, enokidake, kombucha, oyster, phellinus linteus, portobello, and thistle oyster. The Memorial Sloan-Kettering Cancer Center website has a rich database on complementary foods and supplements at www. mskcc.org/cancer-care/integrative-medicine/about-herbs-botanicals-other-products where you can find specific information about each type of mushroom.

By taking advantage of the efficacy and potency of mushrooms, you might experience some of the benefits they offer.

Thriver Soup Ingredient:
Cook your mushrooms before eating them. This breaks open their cell walls, releasing their

nutrients. Both shiitake and common white grocery store mushrooms contain a carcinogenic substance called agaritin, which cooking will neutralize.

~∾~

Microgreens: Behold the Power of These

Irrigate your fields with the Ambrosial Nectar, and you shall be owned by God the Gardener.... The crane is again transformed into a swan....
— "Raag Basant," Shri Guru Granth Sahib

By watering my inner garden with the nectar of the gods, the great Gardener would play a larger and larger role in my life. And this Gardener had more to offer me than dark leafy greens. Soon after the diagnosis, I learned about micro greens, which are young seedlings of many everyday green crops like lettuce, mustard, radish, and kale. They encompass the middle plant growth stage between sprouting and the formation of the leaf. They pack a nutritional wallop and add tang to main courses and salads.

A couple of months after the diagnosis, my then-husband and I flew to Colorado for a long weekend looking at golden Aspen leaves. At The Fort restaurant in Denver, I enjoyed a rattlesnake cake (similar to a crab cake) with my first taste of micro greens on top.

After we returned to Cincinnati, I decided to attempt growing micro greens, even though I wasn't known for my green thumb. Steve Edwards, a gardener at my community-supported agriculture cooperative, provided me with a few seedling flats and some rich, organic soil. Mary Lu Lageman showed me seed catalogs, and I bought organic seeds from High Mowing Seeds.

I planted my seeds, placed paper towels on top and watered with a spray bottle twice a day. One morning I noticed the paper towels over my planting were elevated. I lifted them and smiled. I had a row of one-inch sprouts. The seeds had actually grown for me. How neatly packaged each was, with just the right ingredients in its DNA, and how powerful the drive to live contained in each one.

I had watered this garden as I watered my soul's garden. Just as the gawky sprouts turned into lovely micro greens, my efforts at personal growth, while initially inelegant like the crane, slowly transformed into the gracefulness of a swan.

Thriver Soup Ingredient:

You don't need a green thumb to grow these simple plants. The right equipment and conditions, along with a little patience, can make these greens accessible.

Obtain inexpensive seed trays and a plastic tub to go underneath, or use a flower pot. Recycled plastic takeaway containers and clamshell packaging also work, especially if you don't have much space in front of a window. Use scissors to make drainage holes.

Line your pots with flattened unbleached coffee filters to help keep soil from leaking out the bottom drainage holes. Fill your container with organic soil, about two inches deep. Purchase some organic micro green seeds from a health food store or online.

Sow your seeds with about one-eighth to one-fourth inches of space between them and about one-eighth inch deep. To even out their distribution, try mixing the seeds with fine sand.

Place a single unbleached paper towel layer over the seeds and gently spray twice a day with water from a clean spray bottle. Microgreens need their soil to stay moist, not dry or soggy. They're especially vulnerable to drying out when first planted.

Leave the seed containers by a sunny window. The first leaves you will see are seed leaves because they are a part of the seed. These are the micro greens and often appear about two weeks after planting. True leaves emerge later and often look different from the seed leaves.

Use scissors to harvest your micro greens at the base of the sprout.

If you wait long enough, harvest above the seed leaves and the plants—especially lettuce—might regrow for another harvest.

～～～

Nutrient Density: Thriver Soup

Though all these plants and trees grow in the same earth and are moistened by the same rain, each has its differences and particulars.

—"The Parable of the Medicinal Herbs," The Lotus Sutra

A wide range of plants and nutrients, with their differences and particulars, have enormous healing potential. Here is a sampling.

Aloe vera has an anti-inflammatory, anti-tumor gel that stimulates the immune system and protects against the ill effects of radiation treatment. The bitter yellow portion of the leaf is a laxative, which might assist with chemotherapy-induced constipation, but I would suggest being careful and talking with your ankhologist first before trying any. My Ayurvedic doctor suggested I take two tablespoons of aloe vera juice every morning and evening.

Melatonin assists not only with inducing sleep at night, but also helps prevent cancer cell proliferation. It has shown anti-inflammatory and antioxidant qualities, can enhance the effectiveness of certain chemotherapy agents, and shows it can lead to positive survival outcomes.

Legumes contain isoflavones. Mung bean sprouts, which contain lots of protein and fiber, can be eaten raw. I like to sprout dried beans before cooking them. Check with your grocer for a brand that will sprout. I have had good success with the brand Shiloh Farms. Beans can be sprouted by soaking them in clean water for eight to twelve hours. Drain, rinse thoroughly, and drain. Keep at room temperature. Rinse and drain about every twelve hours, and sprouts should start growing after two to three days.

Vitamin B12 keeps DNA messages crisp and clear, which is vital for preventing cancer.

Some studies have shown that women who have the lowest B12 levels have the highest rates of breast cancer. The nutrient can be found in organ meats, clams, oysters, sardines, salmon, egg yolks, and tempeh. Vegetarians need to supplement with B12, as does everyone over age sixty.

When eaten raw, bell peppers provide twice as much of the anti-inflammatory vitamin C as oranges, and are a source of apigenin, which might help prevent breast cancer.

If you are on the chemotherapy drug Adriamycin, some people suggest supplementing with coenzyme Q10 to protect your heart.

Sea vegetables provide a great number of necessary minerals and vitamins. They help the body detox and are rich in iodine, which is toxic to breast cancer cells. Both wakame and kombu stimulate the immune system and encourage cells to die in a normal way. A brown sea algae called Sargassum kjellmanianum has stopped the growth of sarcoma cells. Nori, used to make sushi, contains long-chain omega-3 fatty acids that fight inflammation. If you make your own sushi, my friends Heather and Judy suggested adding raw minced garlic and ginger to the rolls for extra cancer-fighting potential. Seaweed extracts have shown strong antitumor effects on sarcoma tumors in mice.

Taking advantage of each of these particular plants or supplements can assist in different ways with fighting illness and recovering health for your body.

Thriver Soup Ingredient:

This bean and cabbage soup, which I have dubbed Thriver Soup, is inexpensive, easy, filling, tasty, and loaded with valuable nutrition. I usually start it a few days ahead of time by sprouting lentils. I try to have chicken gelatin on hand that I have already prepared (see the entry "Here's the Beef" for instructions). Use organic ingredients if at all possible.

Ingredients:
Olive oil for frying
1 white onion, chopped
1 tsp turmeric powder
¼ tsp oregano
2 cloves garlic, minced and allowed to sit for at least 15 minutes
1 cup chopped green cabbage, kale, or Swiss chard
1 cup chopped potatoes, skins on, any buds or green spots cut out
2 cups chicken broth
¼ cup chicken gelatin
1 cup sprouted lentils
Salt and pepper to taste
Chopped fresh parsley for garnish

Gently fry the onions in olive oil on a low setting. When the onions are translucent (after about twenty minutes), add the turmeric and oregano, and slowly fry until the spices release their fragrance. Add the garlic, potatoes, and cabbage, and cook until soft. Add broth, gelatin, and lentils. Bring to a boil, cover, reduce heat, and slowly simmer until lentils are done (up to one hour). Serve hot with salt, pepper (if you don't have mouth sores), and parsley.

For information on how to sprout lentils, please see the instructions above in the "beans" bullet.

~~~

Oil Protein Diet: This Budwig's for You

The Name is the celestial cow, Its milk quenches our thirst. Sacred discourse is the greatest joy, Hearing the Name, pain and suffering end.
                    —Sukhmani, *The Name of My Beloved: Verses of the Sikh Gurus*

The Sikhs compared the Divine Name to a celestial cow. The Egyptians had a heavenly cow as well, named Hathor, who symbolized motherhood, feminine love, and joy. The celestial cow provided nourishing milk to quench human thirst.

In our culture, many of us have been taught we need cow's milk to grow up with strong bones. As an adult, however, I discovered I couldn't digest cow protein, especially in dairy foods. No milk, not even from a celestial cow, for me. Occasionally I'd have a taste of ice cream or cheese, some of my favorite foods. The end product, however, told the same story—dark, constipated stools and/or brown floating stools.

I heard about the Johanna Budwig (30 September 1908–19 May 2003) diet from my friend Rusty after my diagnosis. A biochemist, she recommended thoroughly mixing cottage cheese with flax oil until it had a smooth, creamy consistency. She theorized that by eating this mixture, the body's individual cells would have an easier time absorbing oxygen. She claimed in her lectures to have pulled cancer patients back from the edge of death by placing them on this diet, and wrote a cookbook to help those who wanted to use her methods of food preparation.

At first I made a half-hearted attempt at mixing cottage cheese with flax oil using a fork. I ended up with the same end results as I did other dairy products.

A year after my diagnosis I got serious and put the one-sixth cup of raw, lignin-rich organic flax oil into a small food processor with an S-blade. Then I added one-third cup of cottage cheese. I blended it until it was smooth and creamy. As if by magic, my body digested this combination perfectly well. My resulting stool neither darkened nor floated. Eureka! Like milk from the celestial cow, this mixture might well have helped quench the hunger and thirst of my individual cells.

After following Budwig's recommendations for about a year, a physician told me Dr. Budwig's theories were controversial. Yet whether the diet does what she claims or not, for me the mixture provides a digestible form of cow dairy, supplies calcium, and offers a quick, simple, easily swallowed mix of healthy protein and fat. This might work well for someone having difficulty chewing (especially with chemotherapy-induced mouth sores) or eating healthy food. With this mixture, more people can partake of the milk of the celestial cow to obtain needed nourishment.

Thriver Soup Ingredient:

If you don't care for the taste of flax oil, yet want to try this idea, I suggest starting with Johanna Budwig's Oleolux recipe, which is a butter substitute containing flaxseed oil. It smells and tastes somewhat like fried, breaded onion rings. I enjoy it on toast with a little salt. It also works as a butter substitute to place on vegetables and other foods.

Ingredients:

8 tbsp. organic, raw, high-lignan flaxseed oil

8.8 ounces (just more than a cup) coconut oil

One medium-sized onion cut into small pieces

10 garlic cloves, sliced or chopped

Place the coconut oil on a sauté pan and gently begin melting it.

Select a container with a lid, more than one cup in volume that can stand heat and cold. Ceramic and glass work well. The container should not allow light through. I use a glass jar and put a cutoff sock lengthwise up the glass sides to protect the mixture from light.

Fill the container with the flaxseed oil and place it in the freezer for thirty minutes so it chills but doesn't freeze.

Chop the onions and garlic.

Ten minutes after placing the flaxseed oil in the freezer, gently sauté the coconut oil and onion on low heat for about fifteen minutes, until the onion is slightly browned.

Add the garlic and continue sautéing for about three minutes.

Get the flaxseed oil out of the freezer and pour the coconut oil mixture through a sieve into the jar. Stir. Keep the Oleolux in the refrigerator.

The onion and garlic give the coconut oil the protection of their sulfur compounds. This also protects the flaxseed oil when it is added.

If digesting cow dairy is a concern, try using goat yogurt instead of cottage cheese.

For my mix, I prefer cultured organic cottage cheese, when I can find it. I order Barlean's organic, cold-pressed, high-lignan flax seed oil at cost, a generous gesture made by the company for those dealing with a cancer diagnosis.

Omega-3: Precious Oils

Hizkiyahu listened to [the messengers] and showed them the building where he kept his treasures, including the silver, gold, spices and precious oils.

—II Kings 20:13, Complete Jewish Bible

Hezekiah reigned over Judah from about 715–686 BC. Apparently certain oils were precious to him, because he storied them with his treasures.

I didn't see oils or fats as precious when I entered college. My first year, I didn't gain the freshman fifteen pounds. I gained the freshman thirty. Frightened by the rapid weight gain, I became fat phobic. I didn't appreciate a university dietitian telling me that fat enhances flavor and adds to a feeling of fullness.

Years later, I learned our brains are about sixty percent fat. I began to realize fat wasn't so bad, after all.

Gradually I added more fat to my diet. I switched to cooking primarily with organic, extra-virgin olive oil, which provides omega-9 fatty acids. I learned about the importance of consuming omega-3 fatty acids, found in deep-sea fatty fish like salmon, mackerel, tuna, herring, trout, sardines or halibut, and in plant foods such as walnuts, flax seeds, chia seeds, and the herb purslane.

I learned that animal fats contain omega-6 fatty acids, and we should ideally consume only four times as much omega 6 fatty acids as we do omega-3 fatty acids.

This became especially important for me during chemotherapy. I learned that omega-3s subdue inflammation and reduce the risk of metastases. They also helped my drug-dried skin plump back up a bit. The ancients understood the importance of precious oils to help us keep healthy. Pour it on.

Thriver Soup Ingredient:

While sources of omega-3 fatty acids are controversial, my Ayurvedic doctor encouraged me to take supplemental fish oil rich in EPA (eicosapentanoic acid) and DHA (docosahexanoic acid) forms. EPA has demonstrated antitumor activity, increases drug uptake, and might inhibit metastasis. When I take it, my skin feels smoother, and during the winter, my fingers no longer chap and bleed around my nail beds.

Probiotics: Rejoice and be Glad

This is the day ADONAI has made, a day for us to rejoice and be glad.
— Psalm 118:24, Complete Jewish Bible

The Divine makes each day a day in which we can potentially rejoice and be glad. It's a little easier to be happy for those who have sufficient probiotics, or good bacteria, in their digestive tracts.

Lactobacillus acidophilus has shown promise for treating depression, anxiety, and emotional distress. It also helps the body maintain a healthy intestinal tract and can assist with digestion.

Probiotics in general can facilitate digestion, help the gut maintain regular bowel movements, stabilize the immune system, and assist with detoxification.

Cancer patients who have bouts of diarrhea, who have taken antibiotics, or who have eaten poorly could find some help through probiotics for restoring health in the digestive system. Once restored to its natural balance of good bacteria, the happy owner will be better able to rejoice and be glad in each day.

Thriver Soup Ingredient:

To gain more beneficial bacteria in your digestive system, you can find probiotics in pill form, usually in the refrigerator section of a health-food store. I suggest trying a variety of strains for more benefit. Store your pills in the refrigerator to keep the bacteria alive. Note that some brands claim their products do not need refrigeration.

If you are able to eat dairy or soy, try fermented products such as yogurt, kefir, fermented soy and coconut "yogurts," miso, and tempeh. If you choose the sweeter varieties of fermented products, I suggest avoiding those with sweeteners already added. You can buy them plain and add fruit or your own sweetener, or you can even make your own fermented foods. Sally Fallon explains how in her book, *Nourishing Traditions*.

∾∾∾

Proteolytic Enzymes: The Bigger Picker Upper

He saves, rescues, does signs and wonders both in heaven and on earth. He delivered Daniel from the power of the lions.

—Daniel 6:27, Complete Jewish Bible

In the biblical story of Daniel, this hero prayed despite knowing a decree in Babylon forbade it. Daniel was arrested and thrown into a lions' den, the penalty for breaking the law. However, he was unharmed—saved, rescued, and delivered by the Divine who performs signs and wonders.

There are many ways the Divine can work in our lives to bring about deliverance from that which devours. One is possibly through proteolytic enzymes, or proteases. Proteases break down proteins into their smallest elements. If taken with food, these enzymes help digest the protein in what you eat. When taken on an empty stomach, proteolytic enzymes enter the bloodstream to break down excess fibrin in the circulatory system and connective tissues.

When one of my ankhologists told me he would send some of his terminal pancreatic cancer cases to Nicholas Gonzales, MD, for treatment, I sat up in my chair. For this man, with decades of experience in chemotherapy, to send his patients to an alternative cancer doctor, said a lot to me.

Dr. Gonzalez has had remarkable success with cancer patients, especially those with pancreatic cancer. Treya Wilber, wife of Ken Wilber, used the protocol, noticing remarkable changes in her tumor, but was too late getting started on it.

The easiest and most useful aspect of Dr. Gonzales' treatment is his pancreatic proteolytic digestive enzyme therapy. That's a mouthful, so here's the theory behind it.

During the early 1900s, Dr. John Beard, a professor of comparative embryology at the University of Edinburgh in Scotland, noticed that the pancreas in the human fetus started se-creting enzymes on the fifty-sixth day of gestation. No fetus needed those digestive enzymes until after birth. Why was the pancreas already at work? Then he noticed that on the same day, the placenta stopped growing. He conjectured the enzymes stopped the placenta's rapid growth. Later he found that those same pancreatic enzymes killed cancer cells in mice. He theorized that many placental cells remain in our bodies and can turn cancerous without pancreatic enzymes to stop their growth.

Dr. Beard's work was followed by Dr. William Donald Kelley, then Dr. Gonzales. Dr. Gon-zales uses a three-pronged approach to helping cancer patients, and one of those involves the intake of large doses of pancreatic enzymes.

If this enzyme theory is correct, it would provide one explanation for booming cancer rates among people consuming a Western diet. Americans tend to primarily eat cooked and processed foods depleted of digestive enzymes. Raw foods contain the enzymes needed to digest food properly. The pancreas churns out digestive enzymes until it gets worn out, and then there aren't enough enzymes left in the body to digest food and chase after cancer cells.

Some researchers say cancer cells are coated with a protein lining that protects them from the body's immune system. Pancreatic enzymes can strip off those proteins so the immune system can destroy the cancer cells.

To assist our bodies in fighting cancer, we can add high-quality digestive enzymes to our meals. The most important type of enzyme for a cancer patient to consume is called protease, proteinase, or proteolytic enzyme. These tiny workers help us digest protein. If we want these enzymes to go after cancer cells, they need to be consumed on an empty stomach. If they are taken with food, they will be used up helping the body digest the food proteins.

I was cautioned, however, not to consume proteolytic enzymes for two to three days prior to or following surgery because that might increase the risk of bleeding.

Through proteolytic enzymes, we can assist the Spirit with delivering us from the power of the lions consuming our bodies. This can be one way the Divine saves, rescues, and performs signs and wonders.

Thriver Soup Ingredient:

I take six proteolytic enzymes on an empty stomach each evening before going to bed. To increase the effectiveness of proteolytic enzymes, try visualizing them surrounding cancer cells and chewing through their protein sheaths so your immune system can gain access and remove tumor cells.

~~~

Root Vegetables: Buried Treasures

Now the mixed multitude who were among them craved more desirable foods, and so the Israelites wept again and said, "If only we had meat to eat! We remember the fish we used to eat freely in Egypt, the cucumbers, the melons, the leeks, the onions, and the garlic.

—Numbers 11:4-5, Christian Bible, NET

The Bible describes an ancient tale of epic escape by the Israelites from a pharaoh of Egypt. Once free, the refugees tramped around the Sinai desert for quite some time. They complained bitterly because all they had to eat was manna, manna, and more manna—a substance similar to coriander seed, which they gathered, ground up, and cooked into cakes. They justifiably longed for variety in their diets. If I'd been traveling among them, I'd probably have been among the angriest and loudest complainers. I'd also be demanding fish, cucumbers, watermelons, leeks, and especially onions and garlic for my palate.

Garlic is by far my favorite root vegetable. I cook with it nearly every day. Its many benefits are almost legendary. I've been known to exude *ode de garlique* after ingesting bits of raw cloves to stop a cold in its tracks. The stinking white rose's most active ingredient, allicin, transforms into organosulfurs that minimize oxidation and inflammation. The cloves provide powerful antioxidants. Even better, garlic can help keep carcinogens from damaging DNA; boost the activity of enzymes that detoxify carcinogens; regulate blood sugar levels; and clean up free radicals that damage cells and cause cancer. Garlic also contains a lot of selenium. Fresh cloves are best chopped and set aside for about fifteen minutes before lightly cooked with oil. (Note: garlic can decrease platelet aggregation and should not be taken with anticoagulants or if you have platelet dysfunction.)

Garlic pairs well with onions, which are full of the antioxidant flavonoid quercetin that attacks cancer cells at different stages of growth. Red onions add anthocyanins for extra kick. Onions have the extra bonus of helping bones maintain their density. For the most potent nutrient punch, use shallots.

All root vegetables are buried treasures, virtual storehouses of potassium, vitamin C, and other minerals. Perhaps the most beneficial root vegetable for cancer patients is beets because they are considered blood cleansers and purifiers—valuable commodities for dealing with metastatic disease. Raw red beets contain the tumor inhibitor betaine and are packed with vitamins A, B, and C.

Be aware, though, that beets might turn your urine or stool orange, pink, red, or purple. Before I learned this, I got an alarming surprise a couple of times. Fortunately, my brother had experienced the same colorations, and my talking with him brought back my calm. I peel and eat raw beets in a couple of ways. Sometimes I grate one and add lemon juice and olive oil for a liver-loving salad, following the advice offered on the Baseline Nutritionals website. Other times I juice a raw beet and add the liquid to my veggie smoothie.

Many cancer patients promote carrot juice, and for good reason. These bright-orange beauties contain high levels of beta-carotene (which the body uses to create its own vitamin A), along with large amounts of potassium and vitamin C. Their lycopene provides potent anti-oxidant power. They might even help cleanse the liver. Some grocery stores have huge bags of juicing carrots, though I found the bags took up too much room in my refrigerator with all the other veggies I had in store.

If your doctor finds you low in potassium, you can make a broth with potato skins. Several web sites offer potassium-rich broth recipes. My favorite is based on a broth of potato skins, carrots, celery, and kale.

Horseradish, a cruciferous root, contains the largest supply of cancer-protective isothiocyanates, along with dozens of other cancer-fighting components.

While ginger technically isn't a root, I include it in this entry because it's commonly called a root. It grows beneath the soil, yet it's an underground stem, called a rhizome. I think ginger is the best girlfriend to have with you during chemotherapy because it calms queasiness, probably by stabilizing electrical activity in the stomach. Combining ginger with some type of protein seems to assist with decreasing chemotherapy-induced nausea. Ginger also contains zerumbone, which activates genes that lead to the demise of some cancer cells, might suppress metastasis, could prevent some bone loss, and helps stop inflammation. Usually I place a quarter-inch slice of raw peeled ginger into my Vitamix blender, whirl with water, and drink throughout the day. I gently warm the concoction on the stove during the winter. If you take anti-coagulants, I would suggest consulting your doctor before using ginger.

I love my root vegetables. They are a staple in my diet. If I had escaped from Egypt, I would be one of the loudest complainers. I'd be irreverently demanding garlic, leeks, and onions. Now. I'm grateful for such easy access to these foods for my daily dinner.

Thriver Soup Ingredient:

Baked roots make a tasty winter treat. To make the bake, chop the white portion of a leek into rings; add chopped potatoes, carrots, parsnips, rutabagas, or whatever roots you enjoy; drizzle on some organic extra-virgin olive oil and sprinkle with thyme and salt.

Chop garlic and set aside.

Stir and bake the roots at 350 degrees for 30 minutes. Stir and bake for another 20 minutes. Add garlic, stir, and bake another 10 minutes. Enjoy.

≈ ≈ ≈

Sometimes You Feel Like Nuts

The next day Moshe went into the tent of the testimony, and there he saw that Aharon's staff for the house of Levi had budded—it had sprouted not only buds but flowers and ripe almonds as well.

—Numbers 17:8, Complete Jewish Bible

The Spirit chose to cause Aaron's staff to sprout and produce almonds overnight, indicating he was the chosen one from among the twelve tribes of Israel. Almonds are known for sprouting early in the year, indicating an inner wakefulness that could be compared to the watchful eye of the Divine over our lives. This characteristic of alertness in the almond could whimsically be attributed to its eye-like shape. This sacred geometrical configuration is called a mandorla after the Italian name for almond. The mandorla is formed when two circles are drawn next to each other with an almond-shaped overlap in the center. The mandorla represents the intersection of the Divine and human, the masculine and feminine, the known and the unknown. It provides the space between seeming opposites in which transformation can occur.

Almonds hold a special ability to prevent cancer, according to Edgar Cayce, a twentieth-century psychic and medical clairvoyant. For more than forty years, Cayce would place himself in an unconscious state and then give readings that often included accurate medical diagnoses. According to the Cayce health database, he encouraged a few clients to eat sweet—not bitter—almonds because they contained a particular vitamin (not an acid) and could be used to prevent (not treat) a tendency toward cancerous growths. I am not aware of anyone knowing what that nutrient is.

About a year before the diagnosis, I visited his foundation, the Association for Research and Enlightenment in Virginia Beach, Virginia. My tour guide remarked that she ate two to three almonds daily to prevent cancer. Um, did I heed the veiled suggestion? No...

Along with a possible mystery ingredient in almonds, all nuts are nutrient-dense and contain fiber, protein, antioxidants, minerals, and healthy fats. Brazil nuts contain selenium and ellagic acid. Walnuts are a good source of omega-3 fatty acids. Pecans are rich in manganese. Hazelnuts have folate.

I find that nuts make a great snack, especially when I'm away from home, because they are compact and filling.

After the diagnosis, I located a supplier of truly raw almonds (not those steam-pasteurized and still labeled as raw). Each night I place three in a cup with two raw Brazil nuts and a little salt. I cover them with filtered water so they can soak. In the morning I drain, rinse, and eat them after my cooked apple.

Thriver Soup Ingredient:

Raw nuts provide our bodies with easier access to their nutrients than cooked nuts. However, they also contain enzyme inhibitors and phytic acid, making them hard to digest. Soaking raw nuts overnight in salted, filtered water can neutralize the acids and activate the enzymes we need to more easily digest the nuts.

~~~

Spice up Your Life

Then she gave the king four tons of gold, spices in great abundance, and precious stones; there had never been spices like those the queen of Sh'va gave to King Shlomo.

—2 Chronicles 9:9, Complete Jewish Bible

The queen of Sheba wanted to bring gifts commensurate with her meeting with Solomon, considered the wisest man in the world at the time, so she apparently included an incredible array and amount of spices. Spices were uncommon in the ancient world, and therefore were valued highly. Special boxes were made for spice storage.

Today, what we consider ordinary kitchen spices still hold great value—as potent remedies against cancer.

Cinnamon, largely due to its anti-inflammatory action, has shown promise in preventing and treating cancer. Water-soluble cinnamon extract inhibited the growth and spread of cancer in laboratory cell cultures. Be aware, however, that cassia cinnamon (the most common variety) contains large amounts of coumarin, a chemical which can be dangerous for those with liver disease. Cassia cinnamon also tends to lower blood sugar levels. I recommend seeking professional advice for determining the best dosage of cinnamon for you.

Cloves boast the highest antioxidant content among spices. They contain a large amount of eugenol that reduces inflammation and protects the body against cancer.

Allspice also has a high eugenol content.

Nutmeg contains eugenol and myristicin, a potent protector for the liver against inflammation and chemical damage. Nutmeg also can reduce pain and sedate the nervous system, making it a nice spice to add to a warm drink, such as milk or an herbal tea, before bedtime.

Black pepper contains piperine, which may assist with preventing and treating cancer. It greatly increases the effectiveness of curcumin's anti-cancer properties, especially when combined with green tea.

Thriver Soup Ingredient:

Lebkuchen is one of my favorite German Christmas cookies. My German mother made them every December, and they quickly disappeared. My sister, Roselie Bright, made some suggestions for adapting the recipe to enhance both its flavor and nutritional value, even with the sugar.

Ingredients:
1/2 cup honey
1/2 cup molasses
3/4 cup packed sucanat (unprocessed sugar)
1 egg
1 tablespoon lemon juice
1 teaspoon lemon peel

1 cup almond flour

1 cup sprouted whole-grain wheat or spelt flour

3/4 cup teff flour (an Ethiopian grain with a nutty flavor)

1/2 teaspoon baking soda

1 teaspoon ground cinnamon

1 teaspoon ground cloves

2 teaspoons ground allspice

2 teaspoons ground nutmeg

1/3 cup diced candied citron peel

1/3 cup chopped nuts (hazelnuts, pecans, and almonds work best)

Directions:

In a medium saucepan, stir together the honey and molasses. Bring the mixture to a boil, remove from the heat and allow it to cool. Stir in the brown sugar, lemon juice, lemon zest, and lastly the egg.

In a large bowl, stir together the flours, baking soda, cinnamon, cloves, allspice, and nutmeg. Add the honey/molasses mixture to the dry ingredients and mix well (I use a mixer). Stir in the citron and hazelnuts. Cover dough and chill overnight.

Preheat oven to 350 degrees. Line cookie sheets with parchment paper. Using a small amount of dough at a time, use a lightly floured rolling pin to roll out the mixture on a lightly floured surface to one-fourth-inch thickness. Cut into small rectangles and place them 1 inch apart onto the prepared cookie sheet. If you are really industrious, rub the bottoms of cookie cutters in white flour and press out shapes from the rolled dough.

Bake for 10 to 12 minutes in the preheated oven, until no imprint remains on the cookies when touched lightly.

Cool completely on wire racks. Store in plastic zipper bags with the air pressed out.

The cookies will mellow over time, enhancing the flavors. However, they also will harden. To soften the cookies, place a slice of an orange or apple in the bag overnight.

Sunshine Vitamin D

Now the Prince ascribed his escape entirely to the virtue of the sword of Murakumo, and to the protection of Amaterasu, the Sun Goddess of Ise, who controls the wind and all the elements and insures the safety of all who pray to her in the hour of danger.

—"The Story of Prince Yamato Take," *Japanese Fairy Tales*

I could hardly have been considered a worshipper of the sun goddess. My fear of the sun derived from experiences of a few family members who had pre-cancerous skin lesions removed. To protect myself, I slathered on sunblock, slipped on sunglasses, and slapped on a hat every time I went outside, even if just to drive my children to and from preschool.

Now I understand that the sun insures the safety of all who follow her in the sense that they obtain enough vitamin D. It now seems crazy to me that I'd hide from the sun, giver of life, all this time, and I hadn't been supplementing with vitamin D.

Some studies suggest the sunshine vitamin might provide some protection against colon, prostate, and breast cancer, probably because it helps control cell growth and maintain a strong immune system. Vitamin D is crucial for bone health, enabling the body to absorb calcium, and assists the body with maintaining normal blood levels of phosphorus.

High levels of vitamin D, however, have been associated with higher rates of pancreatic cancer.

Half a year after my diagnosis, and after taking 1,000 to 2,000 international units of vitamin D each day for months, I had my blood level checked. It was thirty-four, fairly low (seventy-five is much more optimal). A cancer survivor told me her doctor wanted her to take 50,000 international units per week following her diagnosis. That seemed fairly high to me, yet she had remained cancer-free for a decade.

Biochemist Johanna Budwig urged getting sunlight directly into the eyes. That meant removing my glasses while outside in the sunshine. So I began taking walks in the middle of the day with my glasses ensconced in a pocket.

I haven't used sunscreen since the diagnosis. I welcome the sun on my skin because it helps insure my safety now, in my hour of danger. I also supplement with vitamin D and occasionally enjoy salmon, a good food source for this cell-safety nutrient.

Thriver Soup Ingredient:

Some experts recommend getting a test that measures the concentration of 25-hydroxyvitamin D3, or 25(OH)D in the blood. If your levels are not at least in the normal range, talk to your doctor about supplementing and about exposure to the sun. The Canadian Cancer Association recommends taking 1,000 international units per day of vitamin D during the fall and winter and for those over age sixty-five. *LifeExtension* retail magazine recommends taking vitamin D supplements with the heaviest meal of the day to increase the amount your body will absorb. Some chemotherapy drugs make the skin more sensitive to sunlight. If the doctor permits sun exposure, this can be done by sitting or walking outside for about twenty minutes a day with skin available to catch some rays.

Tea: Fill it to the Brim

Remaining in a sequestered place, eating lightly, controlling body, speech, and mind; ever absorbed in divine meditation and in soul-uniting yoga....

—*God Talks with Arjuna: The Bhagavad Gita*, 18.52

During the winter, I love to sequester myself in a comfy chair, read a good book, and sip tea. I've never been a coffee drinker because the caffeine leaves me jittery. The taste of coffee, even the good stuff, is bitter without cream and sugar. If I'm going to add those, I figure I might as well have a much more delicious hot chocolate instead.

If I need a little lift, I go for green tea. It provides me with just enough energy to help me out when I prefer a gentle, even boost. The main advantage of green tea lies in its polyphenol, EGCG (epigallocatechin gallate). EGCG influences what DNA codes are expressed inside cells. Green tea has been shown to stimulate the immune system, inhibit metastasis, reduce inflammation, provide anti-oxidants, promote the effectiveness of radiotherapy, and detoxify the body. It can even help increase bone density. I purchase organic sencha green tea leaves (the gyokuro and matcha varieties also are rich in EGCG). Each morning during the cold portion of the year, I place a fat pinch of leaves into the top portion of a double boiler, add water to both parts, and place the pots on the stove burner at a low setting. I might add licorice tea, tulsi tea, a slice of ginger, or some dried fruit tea to enhance the flavor. After at least half an hour, the tea is ready and lacks the bitterness of green tea shocked by boiling water. Green tea needs to be steeped for at least five minutes, though preferably about ten minutes, to release its EGCG. Drink it within the hour for maximum benefit. Avoid drinking green tea two weeks before surgery.

My friend Lois Clement learned how to make stinging nettle infusion and invited me to join her in becoming a nettlite. Nettles are anti-inflammatory and good for the kidneys. They reduce anemia and improve lymph system function. I imbibed daily during my ifosfamide infusions. I later learned it might protect the body from cisplatin-induced toxicity.

When I was not involved with my chemotherapy cycles, I turned to a few detox teas—licorice, dandelion root, and rosemary. Licorice root makes a sweet tea and has anti-inflammatory properties. According to Donald Yance, herbalist and certified nutritionist, licorice also blocks tumors and enhances the immune system. If you have any high blood pressure issues, I suggest using licorice in which the DGL (glycyrrhetinic acid) has been removed. Dandelion root tea contains significant amounts of antioxidants and reportedly detoxifies the liver and kidneys. The best benefit, though, appears to reside in its apparent ability to thwart cancer. Rosemary can reduce the amount of heterocyclic amines, which are cancer-causing chemicals created in flesh foods (including fish) that are cooked at high temperatures. Rosemary contains rosmarinic acid, carnosic acid, and carnosol—when blended together, they are powerful antioxidants. Rosemary also fights inflammation. I make a rosemary tea by slowly heating 1 tablespoon of dried leaves in two cups of water, then straining before drinking.

You probably will hear about Essiac Tea from others. I never drank it. For safety and efficacy information on Essiac Tea, I defer to the following: medical writer Ralph Moss, PhD, who gives an informative presentation on the tea and its history in his book *Herbs Against Cancer*; the Memorial Sloan-Kettering Cancer Center website; The University of Texas MD Anderson Cancer Center website; and the Livestrong Foundation website.

Drinking tea, whether when you are sequestered or not, can be part of eating lightly and of raising your body's energy levels to enhance your meditation experiences.

Thriver Soup Ingredient:

Want to be a nettlite? Purchase the dried herb in bulk from a health food store to make an infusion. Place one cup of the leaves into a quart-sized mason jar. Fill the glass to the top with boiling water and cover tightly. The heat from the boiling water opens up the cells, releasing the nutrients into the water. Let steep for at least four hours; overnight is fine. Strain out the herb and drink the remaining liquid. Its taste is similar to spinach broth, so seasoning it with salt might improve the flavor. Or use it as the liquid in your veggie smoothie, which is what I did. Store leftovers in the refrigerator no more than two days.

～～～

Treat Yourself Right

Then he said to them, "Go, eat rich food, drink sweet drinks, and send portions to those who can't provide for themselves; for today is consecrated to our Lord. Don't be sad, because the joy of ADONAI is your strength."

—Nehemiah 8:10, Complete Jewish Bible

I watched as someone handed Connie Lasorso, a cancer survivor, a McDonald's Happy Meal. She saw my jaw drop and eyes widen at her rich food, then said, "I figure I do more damage by not eating it than by eating it."

She had a point. Resentment depresses the immune system; joy revs it up.

To borrow a Christian metaphor, I don't think Saint Peter is going to meet me at the pearly gates of heaven and say, "Tsk tsk, shouldn't have eaten that extra chocolate bar. Had to call you up early because of it."

So maybe having a treat every so often is a way to increase the joy in life and give a little boost to the immune system. Denying myself an occasional treat isn't terribly nurturing for the soul.

Cancer cells feed off sugar; sugar also depresses white blood cells. It's best to avoid it as much as possible. Those with Western diets high in refined foods and sugar have five to ten times more hormonally driven cancers than those on Asian low-sugar diets. Becoming draconian about removing sugars, however, probably isn't the best idea. About every two or three months I will make a batch of cookies or bake some sweet bread (like zucchini) or pie with about half the sugar called for in the recipe, and only using unprocessed sugar, like sucanat. I share with others so I'm not tempted to eat all of it. I usually include real vanilla flavoring. Vanilla beans contain vanillin (not the synthetic flavoring found in the grocery stores), which has shown anti-cancer properties.

For a few years, two of my cousins mailed German *Lebkuchen* (Christmas cookies) to my family for Christmas. I would eat one cookie each week, savoring every bite.

I enjoy a little raw honey now and then.

My favorite treat (besides dark chocolate) is coconut milk ice cream sweetened with erythritol. I think a quarter cup of it now and then is acceptable—I eat it slowly and savor the flavor.

Mica Renes, a naturopath, summed it up: "Perhaps we came into a body to eat ice cream and chocolate and get the giggles."

I agree—especially because dark chocolate contains polyphenols that slow cancer growth. There are times when it is right to eat rich food and drink sweet drinks, relishing their deliciousness with joy and gratitude.

Thriver Soup Ingredient:

I make "fudge" based on a recipe in Sally Fallon's book, *Nourishing Traditions*.

Mix together:

1 cup organic coconut oil, gently warmed to a liquid (or try ghee, which is clarified butter), or use a nut butter instead

1 cup raw honey

1 cup carob and/or cocoa powder

1 teaspoon vanilla flavoring

1/2 tsp. sea salt

If you like, stir in some raw, pre-soaked and ground nuts for healthy fiber and protein. Combine and refrigerate. YUM! Even my teenage boys think it's great. The challenge: to only nibble a little....

~~~

Weighing In

Truth is the food of the Gurmukh; his body is sanctified and pure.
> —"Raag Basant," Shri Guru Granth Sahib

A *Gurmukh* is one who practices a guru's ways instead of following one's basic animal instincts and desires of the mind. This helps the individual become "sanctified and pure" because his or her food is truth. Such a person emphasizes the sacred in life rather than what's for dinner. With such a focus, the importance of one's body weight fades in comparison.

I concluded that excessive attention on how much one weighs during cancer treatment is usually a waste of energy. Instead, paying attention to spiritual nourishment can feed our souls while we wait things out.

My ideal weight was 135 pounds. I had nourished myself well for years, listened to my internal intake needs, and weighed about 140. When I emerged from the hospital after my hysterectomy, I looked like a skeleton with bags of skin sagging off my body. I was jealous of anyone who was overweight. Never dreamed I'd feel that way, but I figured being overweight was far better than being a skeleton. I have heard that forty percent of cancer patients die of malnutrition. I understood why—like carnivores at a carcass, cancer cells in the body dominate the feeding frenzy by snatching up the energy and nutrients before healthy cells have the opportunity.

The doctor wanted me to eat forty grams of protein per day to regain my strength so I could withstand chemotherapy. How was I going to do that without eating meat or dairy, foods I couldn't easily digest? The popular protein drink many suggested to me was loaded with dairy protein and sugar; cancer gobbles up sugar, its main source of energy. It's hard to gain weight when one loads up on veggies and lean proteins for every meal.

A few weeks out from surgery, I got tired of hiking my shorts and pants up to my ribcage so they wouldn't rub on the scar. My then-husband took me shopping to find some jumpers.

During the month after chemo, I stuffed my face as often as I could stand it. Six weeks later, I had managed to gain ten pounds and I could start chemo.

Two years later, I was fifteen pounds overweight. "That's great news," said the ankhologist that day. "Your healthy cells are getting nutrients." She suggested I not look at the numbers, and indicated my body weight would eventually plateau.

Uh, not that time. Back on the weight roller-coaster. I lost another twenty-five pounds because of chemo-induced mouth sores. I was glad when my weight finally stabilized with the final chemosabe, than stayed at a healthy level afterward.

I came to the conclusion that it is a pointless waste of energy to feel concern about my weight while in treatment. I chose to focus on eating healthy meals and to allow my weight to land where it needed to stabilize.

During times of medical intervention, I could let divine knowledge be my nourishment and compassion be my treasure. I could listen to my internal melody so I could move toward the experience of true rapture. In the spiritual experience of Divine bliss, my body's weight would be insignificant.

Thriver Soup Ingredient:

Don't worry about your weight unless your doctor makes it an issue. Instead, focus on eating healthy foods to keep up your energy and maintain or improve your health.

~~~

Whole Foods: Taste the Whole Rainbow

They ask you what is permitted to them. Say, Wholesome foods are permitted to you.
—Qur'an 5:4, Cleary translation

Before my initial surgery, I already followed a whole-foods diet—brightly colored produce, along with occasional eggs and meat. I'd become such a compulsive label-reader that I pretty much stopped buying any processed food. I learned to shop the perimeters of grocery stores, except for herbal teas and, of course, chocolate. When it makes sense to me, I prefer organic foods.

For about five months of the year, a local community-supported agriculture program at a women's conference center, called Grailville, provides our table with fresh, organic produce that's in-season—vegetables of many colors, including purple eggplants, red beets, leafy greens, white garlic, and plenty of golden butternut squash.

This change has paid off handsomely, as the food has shared its vitality with me. Before starting chemotherapy, my blood albumin level was 4.4. Albumin levels indicate how well nutrients are being transported through the blood and into the cells. People with a poor prognosis generally have a level of 2.5 or less, and those with 3.5 or higher usually have a good prognosis. The ankhologist commented that I must be following a good diet to get such a great level. So even though I had gotten some flak about my rigid diet for four years before the diagnosis, it just might have saved my life.

As I moved through treatment, I did not put a lot of attention on the foods I left behind to stay healthy. Instead, I focused on the positive by receiving the energy, the nourishment, and the power of fresh, organic, whole foods, so I could feel, in my cells, wholesome new life.

Thriver Soup Ingredient:

See if you can find a local community-supported agriculture program you can join. Some require members to work. I put in my hours by doing the weekly newsletter, and perform sit-down jobs like cleaning garlic bulbs and preparing onions for distribution.

B. Minding the Body

Introduction to Minding the Body: Feel the Flow

And a woman was there who had been subject to bleeding for twelve years, but no one could heal her. She came up behind him and touched the edge of his cloak, and immediately her bleeding stopped. "Who touched me?" Jesus asked. When they all denied it, Peter said, "Master, the people are crowding and pressing against you." But Jesus said, "Someone touched me; I know that power has gone out from me." Then the woman, seeing that she could not go unnoticed, came trembling and fell at his feet. In the presence of all the people, she told why she had touched him and how she had been instantly healed. Then he said to her, "Daughter, your faith has healed you. Go in peace."

—Luke 8:43-48, Christian Bible, NIV

*J*esus could feel healing energy leave his body and enter another human. That kind of body awareness had eluded me.

Not long after the diagnosis, I learned I was considered co-dependent because I was so focused on others that I rarely experienced emotions in my own body. That definitely needed to change if I was to have any hope of surviving. It was time I learned to pay attention to and trust my body's signals because they provided valuable messages.

Both my psychotherapist and Maria Paglialungo, an energy intuitive, taught me to focus on how my body felt on the inside. I needed to develop the capacity to listen to physical sensations while learning to trust my inner voice. When my body had a message, my first order of business was to notice that prod. Next, I needed to make time to trace the feeling. I could watch for muscles tightening, posture shifting, and other physical sensations, such as a sinking feeling in my gut.

My psychotherapist suggested when I realize I'm not paying attention to sensations because I'm busy with my thoughts, I can pause and feel the four corners of each foot. I found that quite easy—remembering to do it, however, was a challenge.

A couple of months later, I woke up with a sense of more kindness, gentleness, and friendliness toward my body—I had dropped some of the forcefulness and self-discipline I'd inflicted upon myself all my life. My body felt warm and good, and I sensed a deepening into inner creative pools.

My psychotherapist also suggested I try a gentle movement class, such as yoga or tai chi, to set aside time to really focus on my body. I ended up taking a Lebed class for people with lymphedema (swelling that results from lymph vessels that are unable to move lymphatic fluids back into circulation), because it was offered free to cancer patients at the local Cancer Support Community. Later I added tai chi with Vince Lasorso, a tai chi master.

One year after the diagnosis, I talked with Vince and Charley Sky, a supporter, on separate occasions within a matter of days. Both reminded me of the desperate woman who received healing energy from Jesus' body. Okay, I realized, there was a definite message for me in this story, and it was time to learn it.

As I reviewed their conversations about her, I realized that if Jesus could experientially, even if unwittingly, transfer healing energy into a woman's body, then I have that same potential healing energy in my own body. Did not Jesus say his followers would do more than he? By Divine grace, I am my own greatest healer. Perhaps simply experiencing that energy within myself was the best thing to do. Or, demand that energy from the Divine the way that impertinent woman did. By living in the present moment, breathing deeply all day long, and letting go of ego-driven thinking, I might begin to experience Divine energy flowing in my body.

Well, my pilgrimage began. I added numerous modalities to my attempts at healing—dance, hand yoga, detox regimens, chiropractic, acupressure, Reiki, breathing experiences, and art. Still, it took nearly two years for me to locate the vibrations within my body when I chanted. Vince and I laugh about it because when he does healing vibrational work on my body, I don't feel anything, yet I see the results.

That powerful woman whom Jesus healed is still way ahead of me. Yet, I've started, and I'll keep moving and exploring.

Thriver Soup Ingredient:

When I have difficulty getting into my body, my psychotherapist suggested I try focusing on my breath. I can't force myself not to think, but I can refocus the thinking. Set the intention of staying in your body at all times. Take up a physical discipline, such as yoga, and focus entirely on how your body feels on the inside while practicing.

Perhaps placing signs or symbols around your living space as reminders can help you get started, though I found they didn't work after a few days. Shift your reminders around once a week to keep them fresh.

~ ~ ~

Acupressure: Get to the Point

All things have their backs to the female and stand facing the male. When male and female combine, all things achieve harmony.

—Tao Te Ching, 42

According to the Tao Te Ching, all things carry feminine, passive facets, yet hold to masculine, active features of nature. When the two are brought together they bring stability and wholeness. According to Oriental medicine, when the two complementary aspects are out of balance in a human, he or she can become ill. The ancient Chinese developed acupuncture as a means of maintaining or restoring equilibrium in the body.

Acupuncture involves inserting fine needles into the skin along meridians, or energy pathways that course throughout the body. The goal is to help one's energy move more freely and to bring oneself into greater balance.

If seeing an acupuncturist is not your cup of tea, you can apply pressure to specific points on your body to achieve similar results. I didn't find acupuncture a panacea, yet I believe it does help.

After the diagnosis, I did some online research and learned how to use acupressure on myself to help boost my immune system and keep my white blood cell counts up for chemotherapy. I used the pressure points I could easily reach, though there are more on one's back.

You will know you have found the proper acupressure point when you feel a bit of discomfort in the area you press. Here are some spots that can help reduce nausea, strengthen the immune system, and provide other benefits. As you press or massage each point for about a minute, breathe slowly and deeply.

To reduce nausea, you can purchase Sea-Bands at a pharmacy. They are elastic wrist bands with a plastic nob used for seasickness. I have heard they work to reduce queasiness for much of the population. The pressure point is on the center of the underside of the forearm, three finger widths back from the wrist crease. Place the bands around your wrists with the knobs facing the acupressure point.

To improve immunity, place your right heel in the juncture between the bones that attach to the large and second toes. Rub, then switch sides.

To help regulate the thymus gland, which produces white blood cells, and to decrease anxiety and depression, place your palms together. Situate the back of your thumbs firmly against your sternum, three thumb widths up from the base of the bone.

To reduce inflammation, constipation, and congestion, and to relieve arthritic pain, press on the webbing between the thumb and index finger at the highest spot of the muscle when the thumb and index finger are brought close together. Caution: Do not press this point if you are pregnant.

To relieve constipation, gas, and abdominal muscle pain, place your fingertips between your belly button and pubic bone. Gradually press one to two inches deep into your lower abdomen.

For swollen feet, rub your right heel between your left inner anklebone and your Achilles tendon. Then switch to the other leg and do the same. Caution: Do not attempt this if you are pregnant.

To fortify your internal organs and relieve lower back issues, sit forward on the lip of your chair and place the backs of your hands against your lower back. Briskly rub up and down, creating heat from the friction. Caution: If you have disintegrating discs, fractured bones, or a weak back, discuss this method with your doctor first.

For constipation or fever, bend your arms in front of you with your palms down. Place the palm side of your right fist on top of the elbow crease of your left arm. Press. Repeat on the opposite arm.

For additional energy, press four finger-widths below your kneecaps and one finger width to the outside of each shinbone. When you find the location, you can feel a muscle flex as you move your foot up and down.

To strengthen the respiratory system, firmly press your middle fingers on the depressions directly below the protrusions of your collarbones outside your upper breastbone. Hold.

After pressing these points, take a few more slow, deep breaths and feel your body.

As you work with acupressure points, you will assist your body with coming into greater balance, which will help create internal harmony.

Thriver Soup Ingredient:

Make a daily routine out of pressing on the acupressure points mentioned above. Look online for more points to press for specific concerns, and discuss pressing on them with your doctor. You can tap points for rage, fear, and grief, and many other issues.

~~~

Art: Draw it Out

The Light is in the mind, and the mind is in the Light.
—"Raag Raamkalee," Shri Guru Granth Sahib

Light streaming through beautiful stained-glass windows always held a fascination for my mind. Soon after the diagnosis, I bought markers and started coloring stained glass window transparencies in the *Dover Stained Glass Windows Coloring Books*. My favorite image was the Bible Window (1270–1275) in the *Ritterstiftskirche* at Bad Wimpfen, Germany. It depicts a lion roaring at his three-day-old stillborn cubs. The roar brings the cubs to life. This image is a symbol for the resurrection of Christ.

I found drawing to be therapeutic while going through cancer treatment. It occupied my hands while my body endured various assaults and my mind ground through grief, terror, rage, and feelings of powerlessness. It also assisted me with staying inside my body.

At the start of chemotherapy, I began drawing images from my visualizations. First I depicted my power animals (animals with whom I feel a strong connection and that symbolize strength for me) and Glinda (the good witch of the north from the movie, "The Wizard of Oz"). They shot the chemo drugs docetaxel and gemcitabine at a black spot in the middle of a pink area. The next day I added images of family and friends shooting the drugs at the black cancer.

As my treatments progressed, I developed mental ideas about what to illustrate next, yet didn't feel it was the right occasion. Then I received a dream at night and knew it was time to create a new image. On the left side of the paper I portrayed healthy cell lungs with an empty space in the center that was filled with golden light radiating outward. Glinda was standing next to it with her magic wand. She reminded me of what she said at the end of the movie when

Dorothy wanted to go home: "You have always had the power within you." The empty space at the center represented the absence of the sarcoma cells that were being replaced by divine healing light. (Something has to fill in the gap.) On the right side I depicted healthy lung cells filling in the same spot, all saturated with divine light.

Eventually I felt the impulse to create paper cut-outs of people and place them inside the sarcoma nodule, attacking the cancer cells. I covered the black cancer blob with bright yellow smiley faces. Vince Lasorso said because that image arose organically for me, it most likely indicated that the nodule was ready to break up and die. He said in the beginning, cancer patients typically view the chemo attacks only on the outside of tumors because it feels safer to the patient. To be brave enough to enter the nodule, risking the spread of the cells, indicates in itself that the nodule isn't spreading—it's breaking up and dying.

Interestingly, this discussion was followed by a dream in which I was traveling along an interstate highway near my home. Traffic came to a halt and I had to wait a long time. During that wait, I learned that a dead man's body had to be removed from the highway. Once the body was removed, we began moving freely again. I see this dream as symbolic of a dead part of myself that was being removed so my energy could move more freely within my body.

Do art in a way that draws you, not in a way imposed upon you by others. Engage the senses that you want to use, allowing the light of the Divine to be expressed through your body. If you feel excited, the end product probably will feel satisfying for your mind and your heart.

Thriver Soup Ingredient:

Purchase some art supplies. Be playful with them; have fun. Draw, paint or sculpt whatever your heart desires. Feel the freedom to fully express yourself, no matter what forms from your hands. It can be bright and beautiful, or it can be angry and dreadful with dark, foreboding colors. It can feel like a masterpiece or a piece of crap. No matter. It's the process that counts, not the product. Simply give your soul some space for self-expression.

There's no need to show it to anyone. Allow it to be exactly what it is. As your creativity flows, you might find yourself refining your work and heading in a fulfilling direction.

~~~

Ayurveda: Have it Your Body's Way

O Arjuna! The gourmand, the scanty eater, the person who habitually oversleeps, the one who sleeps too little—none of these finds success in yoga. He who with proper regularity eats, relaxes, works, sleeps, and remains awake will find yoga the destroyer of suffering.
                    —*God Talks with Arjuna: The Bhagavad Gita,* 6.16-17

Our bodies enjoy the innate ability to heal themselves, always seeking health rather than suffering when we give them the opportunity. Anything we can do to assist our bodies on this quest should bring positive results. The 5,000-year-old Asian Indian health care system called Ayurveda provides guidance on how to bring our bodies back into balance.

About a year into my treatments I found out about Hari Sharma, MD, a retired pathologist at Ohio State University in Columbus. He had conducted studies with cancer patients for the university before joining the university's integrative medicine clinic to work as an Ayurvedic doctor.

Along with highly personalized dietary and supplement recommendations, matched directly to my psychophysiologic constitution and specific imbalances, he urged me to meditate twice daily.

I returned to him after finalizing treatment. He suggested I do a sesame oil massage every morning to strengthen and balance my whole physiology, improve circulation and vitality, and rejuvenate my skin. (This should not be done if your white blood cells counts are low or in danger of dropping.)

On most mornings now, I dry-brush my skin. Meanwhile, I pour one or two tablespoons of raw organic sesame seed oil into a wide-mouthed glass jar and place it into a little water in small pan on the stove. I use a low heat setting and give the oil a little time to warm up.

I place a hand towel on the bathroom floor to catch drips. Starting at my feet and moving up to my head, I gently massage the warm oil into my skin with my hands (not just my fingertips). Dr. Sharma recommended using rounded motions at joints and on the head, but stroking motions on the long bones. I also like to massage the pressure points on my ears.

Because he suggested leaving the oil on the skin for five to fifteen minutes after the massage, I use that time to practice some qi gong and draw a warm bath. The warm water opens skin pores so the sesame oil can penetrate into the skin.

Getting in and out of the tub can be a bit tricky because I am slick all over. I use a mat in the tub and hold onto a sturdy towel rack for balance.

During the recommended fifteen-minute soak, I do the balancing breath exercise, explained below. I keep an old clock nearby to watch the time.

I finish by washing and rinsing, then cleaning the tub with a grease-cutting detergent.

I hated baths as a child, yet now enjoy them. They provide one relaxing aspect of the regularity with eating, working, and sleeping recommended by yogis for thousands of years.

Thriver Soup Ingredient:

My Ayurvedic physician recommended a breathing exercise to do each morning before eating. The purpose is to help balance and calm the body.

With a straight spine, use your right thumb to gently close off your right nostril.

Exhale through your left nostril, slowly and gently.

Inhale through your left nostril, slowly and deeply.

Close off your left nostril with your right index finger.

Release your thumb to clear your right nostril.

Exhale slowly through your right nostril.

Breathe back in through your right nostril.

Repeat this process for five to ten minutes.

≈≈≈

Body Fullness Meditation

Further, bhikkhus, a practitioner who is aware of body as body, feels the joy which arises during concentration saturate every part of his body. There is no part of his body this feeling of joy, born during concentration, does not reach. Like a spring within a mountain whose clear water flows out and down all sides of that mountain and bubbles up in places where water has not previously entered, saturating the entire mountain, in the same way, joy, born during concentration, permeates the whole of the practitioner's body; it is present everywhere. This is how the practitioner is aware of body as body, both inside the body and outside the body, and establishes mindfulness in the body with recognition, insight, clarity, and realization. This is called being aware of body as body.

—Sutra on the Four Grounds of Mindfulness

Maria Paglialungo, an energy intuitive, introduced me to the idea of feeling the inside of my body. It had never occurred to me before to try it, and I certainly didn't take it up as part of my meditation practice. I meditated in my head, without any awareness of my body.

After the diagnosis, I took seriously the practice of experiencing how my body felt while I meditated, since learning to live in my body was a major goal of my psychotherapy sessions.

Mim Grace Gieser, an Emotional Freedom Technique practitioner, suggested I feel the spreading of Divine healing light as if the sun were warming my face. Then I could spread the glow into my heart, enlivening every cell with love.

Perhaps I was helped along the way by Vince Lasorso's "Bone Marrow Healing" CD. By following his guidance, I attempted to feel, not visualize, my bones lighting up from my toes to the crown of my head as a way to increase my white blood cell counts. It really seemed to help.

After about a year of daily practice, focusing on my body as I meditated, I began to experience all aspects of myself tingle during meditation. I was beginning to understand what the Buddha talked about in his teachings on the body as a ground for mindfulness. After three years of practice, I found I could be fully aware of my whole body while focusing my attention on my third eye. I had met the "recognition" stage and was beginning to move into the insight stage of body mindfulness meditation.

Thriver Soup Ingredient:

This meditation combines some visualization with some mindfulness concentration. If it feels like a useful practice for you, try it out.

Starting with the toes of your left foot, imagine you can feel every bone lighting up, progressing slowly up your leg. After focusing on your left thigh, shift your attention to your right toes and do the same. Then imagine you can feel all the bones in your torso, starting with your left hip, lighting up. Follow this to your left shoulder blade and move your attention down your left arm to your fingertips. Then move to your right shoulder, and feel your right arm bones lighting up. Continue up your neck to the top of your skull. Now your bones are completely lit up with white light. Continue to experience your bones as light while you gently focus your eyes on the area between your eyebrows. Maintain a soft focus on this location for as long as you are able, while still experiencing all your bones as light. When you are done, slowly wriggle your fingers and toes, then your hands and feet, and gently return to full waking consciousness. See if you can start to carry this energy throughout your day.

<center>~~~</center>

Breasts: Cleaving the Cleavage

This mother of yours is the great hwrt-*serpent, white of head-cloth, who dwells in Nekheb, whose wings are open, whose breasts are pendulous.*

—Utterance 703, Egyptian text

The hieroglyph of the vulture was used in ancient Egypt to represent "mother"—in this case, mother goddess of the southern half of Upper Egypt. Other cultures worshiped the vulture image as a reflection of the supreme, all-powerful mother goddess who both granted and took away life. She had pendulous breasts, a symbol of her nurturing, life-giving qualities. Even Jesus implied that breast milk symbolized rivers of living water coming from the Divine.

People living in Western cultures tend to worship breasts. While I visited Germany in 2001, I saw numerous poster-sized ads featuring topless women with products for sale. There is a pervasive attitude that a woman's femininity is defined, in part, by breasts. Losing them can feel completely devastating for a woman.

My mother lost both of hers to breast cancer. It was something she never discussed with me.

While my body is covered with scars and has been marred by cancer, I still have both breasts. I don't know what it's like to lose them. I have seen a photo exhibit of women after mastectomies, and I cannot imagine their emotional agony.

Breasts typically symbolize the nurturing side of a woman's experience. For some women, losing them to cancer might represent the emotional fallout of losing a young child or living in an unhappy, unsupportive partnership. Bernie Siegel, MD, points this out in his book, *Love, Medicine, and Miracles.*

Tami, a metastatic breast cancer survivor, disagrees with Dr. Siegel on this point. She experiences a high degree of spousal support and says many of her friends with metastatic breast cancer are in good marriages. Plenty of single women, including nuns, and even some men develop breast cancer.

Yet I think for some women this theory might hold validity, and could be worth exploring with a psychotherapist. One woman I know developed breast cancer shortly after learning her husband was having an affair. I met another woman in 2011 who was on chemotherapy for breast cancer. I told her Dr. Siegel's theory, and she freaked. One year later she passed away. After her funeral, I learned from a mutual friend that when I had talked with her, she had just discovered her husband was having an affair. That was hardly a supportive or emotionally safe environment. She had chosen to stay with her husband, which probably depleted her so much she could not survive cancer's onslaught. Perhaps if she had moved out, she might have had an opportunity to survive and heal. Now her young daughter has experienced severe abandonment and has neither a mother nor a good example for setting healthy boundaries.

Fortunately, accessing the living stream of Divine light and moving toward wholeness within ourselves is always possible, even if we are in bad relationships, are missing important body parts, or are covered with scars. Sometimes we have to radically change our outer environments before we can experience cures. Often healing involves altering our internal environments. Accepting our bodies as they are, even with the mutilations, can help us move into an experience of inner peace and wholeness.

Perhaps one way we can alter our internal landscapes is by snuggling with the Divine feminine, suckling at her pendulous symbolic breasts, and feeling her soft, loving wings enfolding us. We can draw on her strength and courage and lean toward greater self-acceptance and self-nurturing. This can enhance our abilities to heal.

Thriver Soup Ingredient:

If you are thinking about having reconstructive surgery after a mastectomy, here is a list of questions you might want to ask your doctor.

1. What types of procedures are available?

2. Do I have enough tissue available to make the necessary flap grafts?

3. How much will insurance cover?

4. What size implants do you recommend?

5. What are the chances of having the skin, flap, or transplanted fat tissue survive the procedure?

6. How much physical sensation will I have in the reconstructed breast?

Breath: In-spiring

Next he said to me, "Prophesy to the breath! Prophesy, human being! Say to the breath that Adonai ELOHIM says, 'Come from the four winds, breath; and breathe on these slain, so that they can live.'"
—Ezekiel 37:9, Complete Jewish Bible

In Hebrew, the word *ruach* means breath, wind, or spirit. The three intimately connected words are often interchangeable in the Jewish Bible. *Ruach* is used for the life-force energy breathed into humans, possibly indicating an infusion of consciousness or a soul into a physical body. Here, the Hebrew prophet Ezekiel was told to prophesy to the breath to breathe on those who were dead so they could live again. In Greek, the word *pneuma* could mean both breath and spirit. Even in English the connection between breath and spirit remains. To inspire means not only to breathe, but also to arouse by Divine influence.

It is awareness of our breathing that grounds us in our bodies, and at the same time, helps raise us up into more spiritual space.

Jungian psychoanalyst Marian Woodman tells in her book *Bone: Dying into Life* how she learned there is more oxygen in the air twenty minutes before the sun rises. This is why birds sing at dawn. The person who told her this had cancer and practiced deep breathing outdoors every predawn morning. He went into remission.

Perhaps part of the reason he went into remission is because deep breathing aids the lymphatic system. On a symbolic level, lungs represent the ability to take in life. Ezekiel was directed to prophesy so the Spirit would breathe new life into dead bodies. Breathing deeply is indicative of living more fully. Inspire yourself with deeper breathing throughout your days and see if it increases your vitality.

Thriver Soup Ingredient:

My friend Judy Merritt inspired me to place little colorful signs around my house that simply say "Breathe." They are helpful reminders, placing me back in my body—a part of my healing process. An added practice can be to imagine breathing in love and breathing out gratitude, an idea contributed by my friend Maria Paglialungo.

〜〜〜

Chakras: Raising Life-force Energy

Fire, light, daytime, the bright half of the lunar month, the six months of the northern course of the sun—pursuing this path at the time of departure, the knowers of God go to God.
                    —*God Talks with Arjuna: The Bhagavad Gita*, 8.24

This veiled stanza in the Bhagavad Gita was written for devotees who were learning the science of yoga, according to Paramahansa Yogananda, founder of Self-Realization Fellowship. The first stage of the path involves following the fire, which means learning to control one's life-force energy. The light refers to the opening of the divine eye, which is the sixth chakra, located in the center of one's forehead. Daytime is when the yogi awakens from the common lot of humanity—our sleep of delusion. The bright half of the lunar month is when one's consciousness is attuned halfway to the material world and halfway to the spiritual realms at the same time. The six months refer to the six lower chakras, or energy centers in the body, and the northern course is about moving the energy up the spine to the seventh, or highest, chakra.

While the verse might be difficult to understand, most of us have experienced the life-force energy of another person. If you have ever met someone who gave you the creeps, your body responded to the energy of that person. Likewise, if you ever met someone who opened your heart, you experienced an opening of your fourth, or heart, energy center, often referred to in Eastern spiritual teachings as a chakra.

The seven chakras, according to Eastern teachings, start at the base of the spine and continue to the crown of the head. They are part of what's referred to as the subtle body (another vehicle of consciousness associated with the physical body). There is one at the base of the spine; one in the pelvis; one near the belly button; one at the heart; one at the throat; one at the center of the forehead; and one on the crown of the head. Energy can run either up or down, or both, through these centers.

Meanings, colors, and symbols are attached to each chakra, and vary depending on the teachings. Tuning into and following your inner guidance is critical in vitalizing and raising the life-force energies in your chakras. Options for boosting one's overall vital energies are abundant, including creative self-discipline, beholding goodness and beauty all around you, giving to others in healthy ways, befriending the wisdom of your shadow-self, genuine self-acceptance, wise nutrition and exercise choices, and taking joy in life's surprises and wholesome pleasures.

My second, pelvic chakra needed to heal, my psychotherapist explained, because that was where the cancer originated. This chakra represents personal power, sexuality, and creativity. In my original family I experienced some neglect, disconnection, and disempowerment. With my personality type, this led to dissociation and fear of attachment. I continued that pattern in my marriage, in which I allowed myself to be dominated. I blocked my life-force energy, particularly in my second chakra.

My psychotherapist worked with me to heal the tear in my energetic fabric. Before I could heal my second chakra, I needed to heal my first chakra issues—to reclaim my right to exist, to feel safe and secure, and to resolve family-of-origin issues.

My progress showed up in dreams, particularly dreams about bathrooms. That made sense, since the first chakra is located where the body releases waste. At first I dreamed about sitting on toilets; then about toilets overflowing; then I cleaned bathrooms for low pay. Next I dreamed the bathrooms were cleaned for me. I realized there still was overflowing emotion, yet I could manage it. Finally I dreamt about a pit in a cave from my childhood that had been transformed into a modern bathroom with flushing toilets, purified water, a sink and a light switch.

I had made my first step toward opening up my spine so the energy could begin flowing upward. Learning to manage my fire—my life-force energy—now had a better possibility of occurring.

Thriver Soup Ingredient:
My psychotherapist recommended the following yoga posture to invite my second chakra

to open up. Sit on a floor in a butterfly position, so your knees are away from your body and the bottoms of your feet are together in front of you. Keep your back upright and straight. Visualize a diamond at the base of your spine, spreading up to your sternum and lung tips; then another diamond reaching up to the area behind your nose. On the in-breath, see a light rising to fill the diamonds. During the out breath, observe the light going back down. Do this for a few minutes each day as a meditation practice.

$$\sim\!\sim\!\sim$$

Chiropractic: Make Straight the Way of the Lord

He said, "I am a voice of one crying in the wilderness, 'Make straight the way of the Lord,' as Isaiah the prophet said."

—John 1:23, New American Standard Bible

John the Baptizer, cousin of Jesus, tells his first-century questioners to "Make straight the way of the Lord." Making the way of the Lord straight can be interpreted to mean keeping one's spine tall, erect, and relaxed during meditation. This posture is essential for uplifting one's energies and communing deeply with the Divine. When viewed from the front or back, one's spine should ideally be straight. When viewed from the side, a healthy spinal column has three curves that make it strong, flexible, and resilient. Perhaps the most critical of these spinal curves is the cervical curve at the top of the spine because these vertebrae house the brain stem. A healthy spinal column, therefore, is not literally straight; rather, we typically use the term straight to describe posture which is erect and well-aligned.

The spinal way of the Lord is a two-directional energetic highway that connects Universal Intelligence with the innate intelligence within each person. When the spinal pathway is free from obstruction, its downward flow feeds nourishing life force into every aspect of our bodies and minds. Through prayer, meditation, and other approaches to spirituality, a healthy spine also facilitates withdrawal from outward activity and preoccupations. This focus helps us collect and uplift our vital energies toward the higher spinal centers of the heart and brain, often depicted in pictures of saints with radiant sacred hearts and halos of divine energy around their heads.

The brain stem, which sends signals from the brain throughout the body, sits within two upper cervical vertebrae at the top of the spinal cord. When I attended a talk at my local Cancer Support Community about chiropractic, I learned that the health of the brainstem at the cervical curve affects the health of the rest of the body. If either bone moves out of alignment, the signaling capacity and life-force energy that travels from the brain into the body is reduced. If the life-force energy flowing into and from this battery is weak or blocked by misaligned vertebrae, the body cannot function properly, which results in less than optimal health, illness, or even death.

I decided to see if my spine needed realignment. It did, including the two topmost vertebrae. I had chiropractic adjustments the length of my spine, which helped to realign my vertebrae, thus allowing a fuller measure of life force to flow throughout my body.

Within a couple of months of starting my spinal adjustments, my back started tingling while I meditated, and eventually the sensation spread throughout my body. It felt pleasant, which encouraged me to meditate more. It's nice, after meditating for twenty-five years, to finally have positive feedback like that from my body. The way of the Lord had been straightened, enhancing my vitality and my connection both with my body and the Divine.

Thriver Soup Ingredient:

With the help of a mirror and/or a caring friend, check out your posture, which is a critical indicator of overall well-being. When viewed from the front or back, is your posture vertically straight? When in a still and comfortable upright position, does your head jut forward and/or slightly tilt or rotate to one side? Does your torso rotate slightly to one side? Is one hip or shoulder slightly lower than the other? When you stand against a wall in a normal upright yet relaxed posture, do the back of your head, your upper back, your buttocks, and your heels all simultaneously touch the wall? If not, a chiropractic assessment might be a good idea. Of course, talk with your physician first.

To find a good chiropractor in your area, check with the American Chiropractic Association (www.acatoday.org) or the International Chiropractors Association (www.chiropractic.org). Ideally you want a chiropractor who does more than just offer relief from pain and other symptoms. You want a leading-edge chiropractor who also promotes prevention, peak performance, and optimal health. Make sure any chiropractors you select are board-certified. Check among your friends as well for references. Cross-check names with your insurance plan to see if any are covered.

~~~

Daily Routine

No discipline seems pleasant at the time, but painful. Later on, however, it produces a harvest of righteousness and peace for those who have been trained by it.
—Hebrews 12:11, Christian Bible, NIV

Discipline during and after treatment can produce a harvest of peace and health. As part of my discipline, I developed a routine. Here is one I used when not in conventional treatment, which you can borrow as a starting base for your own. Many of these are explained in other entries.

Do the oil pull.

Add a lemon quarter in the Vitamix blender with water and a little raw honey.

Cook an apple and top with cinnamon, followed by three raw, organic, soaked almonds and two raw, organic, soaked Brazil nuts.

Make ginger tea and add apple cider vinegar and aloe vera juice.

Down some supplements.

Do Bruno-recommended sitting time.

Dry brush, followed by sesame oil massage. Do some tai chi, take a warm bath, do the balancing breath. Shower, clean the tub.

Do a few things, like Reiki, exercising, and stretching.

Juice carrots, celery, and beets (this is a drink for detoxing); add to Vitamix with dark leafy greens, ground black pepper, and sometimes kelp powder.

Try to get more protein—chicken, fish, or sprouted beans with brown rice. Add a handful of supplements.

Attempt a visualization (I usually ended up napping).

Make soup with mushrooms, chicken gelatin, chicken broth, and a little parsley and thyme.

Eat the cottage cheese/flax-oil mix.

Take a handful of supplements.

Do a few things.

Eat a veggie meal.

Make a treat of some kind—corn on the cob, popcorn, goat cheese on sprouted-grain bread...add more supplements.

I'm trying really hard to avoid sweeteners except a little raw honey, as cancer loves sugar. That means only a little chocolate (sniff).

I prepare food for the next day, like getting raw nuts ready to soak in salt water, rinsing sprouts, or baking squash.

Take proteolytic enzymes (when my stomach is empty) and spend another fifteen minutes meditating.

Is your head spinning yet? It keeps me too busy... The discipline isn't pleasant, especially with the diet I have chosen, yet I know it is producing a harvest of peace and health.

Thriver Soup Ingredient:

Come up with a daily routine that makes the most use of what you know to be helpful for you and that you believe you can maintain for months, or even years. It will take determination and discipline. If you find your zeal flagging from mental fatigue, alter your routines and express gratitude for whatever you can.

∾∾∾

Detox Baths: You're Soaking in it

Then I will sprinkle clean water on you, and you will be clean; I will cleanse you from all your uncleanness and from all your idols.

—Ezekiel 36:25, Complete Jewish Bible

Cleansing in the Bible took the form of sprinkling clean water on someone as well as ritual immersion in a collection of water.

I took to the tub for my cleansing ritual during chemotherapy treatments to both detox and absorb nutrients.

I started with Epsom salt baths during the week after the die-off phase. I'd learned it's a great way to absorb magnesium and sulfates (with all their health benefits) and strengthen my nails, while possibly drawing out heavy metals and other toxins.

One day I was out of Epsom salts, so I took a rosemary bath. I'd heard rosemary is a gentle detoxer, energy booster, and skin softener. I poured six cups of boiling water over three tablespoons of dried rosemary leaves and let them steep for about fifteen minutes. I strained the tea before adding five of the cups to warm bath water and drinking the remaining cup.

Next I moved to a seaweed bath to absorb iodine, potassium, and numerous other minerals and vitamins. I boiled kelp fronds for about twenty minutes before adding them to my warm bath (keep the lid on until you pour them into your tub—the smell is unpleasant). The large fronds stayed strong and felt silky as I rubbed them over my scars and bruises. The hot water opens skin pores so your body can absorb the nutrients.

When you want to sweat out toxins, a ginger bath might provide a solution. Instructions I found online suggested grating half a cup of ginger, placing it in a cheesecloth bag, and adding it to a hot bath. Soak for at least twenty minutes. I had a really hard time staying in the hot water because the ginger made my skin prickle. I sweat after getting out of the tub, and my clothes stank when I took a shower an hour later. I took that as a sign that I had been sweating out toxins. I felt weak and jittery for a few hours afterward.

I chugged water and used rejuvelac (sprouted wheat water), beef juice, chicken bone broth, and lots of micro-greens to help replenish what I spent sweating.

Months later, after another ginger detox bath followed by an hour of sweating, my wet bathrobe smelled perfectly clean. I suppose that meant there was no need to do any more detoxing of my skin before starting the new type of chemotherapy.

Thriver Soup Ingredient:

Be sure to consult your physician before taking hot baths. During my second type of chemotherapy, my abdomen looked red all the time. My ankhologist suggested I stop the hot baths during chemo because my skin was extra sensitive. It could have gotten irritated enough to form blisters. This was a big disappointment for me, but I lived with it.

~~~

Detoxing: Kill Bugs Dead

But those will prosper Who purify themselves, And glorify the name Of their Guardian-Lord, And (lift their hearts) In Prayer.

—Qur'an 87:14-15

I am in the guest room and see a roach. I kill it. Then I see another, and another. Soon I realize the house is full of roaches. I need to clean out the house—get rid of stuff—so the roaches have no place to hide.

After I had this dream, I knew it was time to purify my house—which was the dream symbol for my body. It had filled with little nasties and by cleaning out the clutter, I would get rid of whatever helped the roaches spread around.

Early in my process, I received a qi gong DVD. The one practice from the DVD that I have continued is to imagine my hands are rakes with light streaming out of my fingertips. Starting with my feet, I imagine golden luminous streams from my hands pulling imaginary black gunk, collected from my body, up through my head, and then tossing the muck out a window.

My friend Mica Renes, a naturopath, provided some important tips for me. Detoxing the body out of fear is not a healthy motive. I needed to recall what a clean internal body looked and felt like; and to make it the focus as my intended result.

We have five organs our bodies use to get rid of toxins: the skin, liver, kidneys, intestines, and lungs. Mica suggested I meditate and breathe, and then start helping my body by telling my feet, "Hello feet, how are you feeling today?" Then I could bring my attention to my ankles, then on up my body, not judging, not thinking, and just giving each part some attention. Then I could focus on my healthy cells. Ask for a vibrant stem cell in my body, one that can become anything and everything, to assist me. Focus on where it is located (which can be anywhere inside me). Then put my attention on the volunteer and ask it to teach all of my cells to be healthy. Breathe into the stem cell and let it travel throughout my systems, feeling it move rather than visualizing it. Allow it to teach all my cells to do exactly what they are supposed to do and reminding other cells how to be healthy.

Two years after starting chemotherapy, I decided it was time to do a slow, gentle colon detox. I had been through enough physical stress, so I wanted to be as kind to my body as I could. By day three I could see the cleanse was working. Twice my stool burned on its way out, just as it had done until I finished with the docetaxel eighteen months earlier. I felt a little lethargic, slept a bit more, and experienced some muscle soreness. I have read that when one begins to detoxify, headaches, nausea, malaise, and even vomiting might occur because toxins are being released from their storage spaces. Since I was already fairly clean from my organic diet, filtered water, and intense emotional work, and because I was taking my cleanse rather slowly, my symptoms were easily manageable. For some people, symptoms are distressing enough that they would be better served by backing off the program for a while before slowly easing back into it.

I did the gentle internal cleanse for a month, took a couple of months off, and considered doing it again. Then I dreamt I was attempting to clean a large bathroom drain pipe, but it already was pretty clean. I woke up and knew there was no need to do a colon cleanse. Instead, I decided it was time for a slow, month-long liver flush. With my drain pipe pretty clean, my liver could dump its toxins into my colon, which could help them exit more easily.

I began doing dry skin brushing right before heading into the shower or tub. The skin is our largest organ, so it is a main detoxification pathway for the body. I didn't buy the recommended vegetable brush because my skin is thin and sensitive. Instead, I gently brushed with a hand towel, starting at my feet and working everything toward my heart. Then the towel went into the laundry and I stepped into a soothing tub of warm water.

Philip, a friend, said he detoxed in 1984 and hasn't needed deodorant since—and he really doesn't. He follows every meal with a salad to move things through his colon. I suppose the measure of my need to detox is whether I need deodorant or not. So, if you are strong enough, talk with your doctor about whether he thinks a detox is a good idea for you. If yes, purifying your body probably will eventually help you feel better, opening a doorway to experiencing more happiness.

Thriver Soup Ingredient:

Beware of detox scams. Research them thoroughly before purchasing products. Retired chemistry professor Stephen Lower (www.chem1.com/CQ/) explains why the detox foot bath is a scam and how it works to fool consumers. I had wondered about it, having seen it at a local psychic fair. It looks really convincing...and the vendors of these products most likely are not aware that their products are scams.

≈≈≈

Energy Work

During the days I lay in the prison of Tihrán, though the galling weight of the chains and the stench-filled air allowed Me but little sleep, still in those infrequent moments of slumber I felt as if something flowed from the crown of My head over My breast, even as a mighty torrent that precipitateth itself upon the earth from the summit of a lofty mountain. Every limb of My body would, as a result, be set afire. At such moments My tongue recited what no man could bear to hear.

—Bahá'u'lláh, *Epistle to the Son of the Wolf*

A torrent of Divine energy flooded Bahá'u'lláh (1817–1892), founder of the Bahá'í Faith, while he lay chained on a prison floor. The powerful flow became so intense he compared it to being set aflame. People of the Bahá'í Faith consider Bahá'u'lláh's experience to be purely Divine and incomparable to other human experiences of energy.

Other people have reported powerful spiritual energies flooding their bodies. Some described physical sensations like fire, such as the Frenchman Blaise Pascal during his "Night of Fire" in 1654.

As human beings made in the image of the Divine, all people have access to Divine energy within themselves. Some equate this energy to the natural flow of the life force in our bodies. This vitality, however, can be blocked by emotional and physical trauma. Such disturbances can eventually manifest in physical illness, according to Dean Ornish, MD.

Some theorize that if these blockages last long enough and are severe enough, blood flow to those areas of our bodies is reduced, depriving cells of oxygen and nutrients. The end result can be dis-ease.

In the book *Cancer is Not a Disease: It's a Survival Mechanism*, writer Andreas Moritz poses a theory developed by Otto Warburg, MD, 1931 Nobel Prize winner in medicine. Warburg discovered that cancer cells have a lower-than-normal respiration rate compared to normal cells. Moritz quotes him as saying, "Cancer has only one prime cause. It is the replacement of the normal oxygen respiration of the body's cells by an anaerobic cell respiration."

I find this interesting because when both Maria Paglialungo and Vince Lasorso worked on my body to loosen blocked energy, I felt the tingling of increased blood flow into the areas where they held their hands. If blocked energy prevented proper blood flow to my uterus, I think this could have influenced the development of the cancerous growth.

Maria says she can intuitively feel those energetic blocks in someone's body, and can pull out the obstruction. She worked on my body for years. Often her hands grew intensely hot as she opened up pathways and reduced the inflammation that had run riot in my body.

Sometimes her pulling on the energy caused a lot more pain for a while. At times I experienced an aching tingle, like the stimulation of one's funny bone.

I knew I needed to continue moving blocked energy, which also can be done by working on emotional issues. When emotional healing occurs, one opens up to a greater capacity to love one's self and others. Like the chicken and the egg scenario, the opposite also can be true. Ornish wrote, "[O]ne of the most profound factors that enhances the free flow of energy is love."

By creating healthy, loving conditions throughout my body, the sarcoma cells would have no place to live.

While I didn't experience fire in my bones, I know a lot of inflammation and blockages have been removed, allowing my body to return to balance and to bring healing into my cells.

Thriver Soup Ingredient:

If you find an energy worker you trust, try to remember to set an intention about your treatment before you arrive. As you settle onto the treatment table, practice taking slow, deep breaths, and continue them throughout your treatment. This will help you stay in your body and keep your focus on your intention.

~~~

Exercise: Have a Ball

How beautiful are the feet of those who bring good news!
                    —Romans 10:15b, Christian Bible, NIV

Exercising your feet, and the rest of your body, can bring you good news on the health front. If your weight is above the healthy range, exercise can help reduce fat. Fat cells are our bodies' main storage units for carcinogens. Moving our bodies can help balance our hormones, reduce blood sugar levels, reduce inflammation, decrease fatigue, protect our immune systems, and reduce the risks of recurrence.

There are many options available that are gentle and helpful.

Someone invited me to a Lebed class, and I enjoyed it so much I kept returning. The Lebed Method is a medically based, therapeutic program of movements and dance done to music. Participants experience gradual and gentle improvements in range of movement, along with an increase in energy and strength. The exercises are designed to gently open one's lymphatic system and help the nodules drain. We do this by blowing bubbles, tossing balls, playing air guitar, and much more. The group environment energizes me and participants provide each other with emotional support.

Kris Carr, in her movie "Crazy Sexy Cancer," recommends using a trampoline to help the lymph system circulate and drain. I got a trampoline a few years ago through the online sales site Craigslist, so lucky me, I was already with the program. I did stop when I was on doxorubicin and cisplatin because I quickly developed hand-foot syndrome. When I tried using the trampoline, even gently for a few minutes, I developed blisters between my toes.

Large, inflatable balls can be used in all sorts of ways for exercise. You can sit on one to do sit ups and leg raises; roll your belly over it to do push-ups and to lift your legs up behind you; or lie on the floor and lift it with your legs.

Exercise bands are long, rubbery tubes or bands that create resistance when used for a variety of exercises. They come in several colors created for different levels of fitness.

If you are able to walk, it's probably the best exercise. If you are slow, and can afford to, purchase walking sticks. They will help you walk faster and will give your arms a little more exercise.

Whatever method of exercise you choose, have fun, and let it become a beacon of good news to others, showing them that even someone undergoing rigorous medical intervention cares enough to take care of her body and can have the discipline to exercise.

Thriver Soup Ingredient:

Consult with your doctor before starting any form of exercise, as some methods of moving might be dangerous for certain conditions.

Find a fun way to exercise on the days you feel up to it. Look for exercise classes or walking groups that can provide fun, companionship, and emotional support. Check your library for exercise videos or DVDs that might be of interest. Vary your methods and add music if you like. Karen Drucker has a CD of healing affirmation songs called "The Heart of Healing." I find listening to it while exercising provides a great way to focus my mind on affirming statements.

～～～

Hand Yoga: Your Health is in Your Hands

One day you will see the believing men and the believing women with their light streaming before them and by their right hands: "Good news for you today: a garden with streams flowing below, to abide in forever." *That is the greater success.*

—Qur'an 57:12, Cleary translation

There is power in our hands, which can be like light streaming outward, more than I had dreamed of before the diagnosis. Sure, like so many other kids, I believed if I crossed my fingers I'd have good luck. What I didn't know was that various places on my hands and feet mirrored other parts of my body. A system of hand and finger gestures was developed long ago in India to stimulate those areas for enhanced health and specific results. They are called mudras, or hand yoga.

Here are some mudras that can help bring relief during the cancer journey. While doing the gestures, try to keep your hands as relaxed as possible, and maintain gentle pressure. Sometimes you might need one hand to help the other hand hold its position. These gestures can be done while walking, sitting in a waiting area, or waiting at your computer.

To improve immunity and aid with neuropathy: Bend your ring finger and little finger and touch them with the tip of your thumb. Keep the remaining two fingers stretched out and touching each other.

To reduce nausea: Join the tips of the middle fingers and thumbs of each hand while keeping the other three fingers straight. Face your palms upward. Put a little pressure on the joined tips and keep the rest of each hand relaxed.

For stress or constipation, or to gain weight: Touch the tips of the thumb and ring finger together, then extend the index, middle, and little fingers. Rest the backs of your hands on your thighs.

To reduce insomnia and to sharpen your memory: Join the tips of the index finger and thumb and keep the other three fingers stretched and joined.

To lose weight: Place the tips of your ring fingers at the bases of your thumbs. Gently rest the thumbs on your ring fingers. Extend your other fingers.

To decrease your body's toxic load: Join the tips of your ring fingers, middle fingers, and thumbs on each hand while keeping the other two fingers straight.

These mudras can increase your flow of healing energy, like light moving through your hands. This can stream good things toward you, like water running through gardens to bless the world.

Thriver Soup Ingredient:

Select a mudra and practice it daily for twenty to thirty minutes, using gentle pressure. Do it while in a peaceful, relaxed state, such as when meditating. Add an image, say an affirmation, and/or breathe deeply to increase the effectiveness of your practice. See if you can notice a shift in energy or an energetic flow from your hands.

~~~

Inflammation: Smother the Fire

He was invincible, except to a woman. So the gods created Durga for the express purpose of defeating Mahishasura. This goddess was a beautiful golden woman adorned with a crescent moon. She had ten arms and rode on a lion. She was created out of the flames that came out of the mouths of the gods Brahma, Vishnu, and Shiva. She held weapons and emblems in each of her ten hands, each one a symbol of the power given to her by a specific god.

—*Kali: The Black Goddess of Dakshineswar*

The fierce Hindu goddess Durga was created by other gods to vanquish the evil buffalo demon Mahishasura. Forged by flames and riding on a lion, she represents transformative wrath that can bring healing.

Flaring heat can bring transformative healing within the human body as well. When threatened by wounds, irritation, or infections, cells inflame to assist with the transition back to health. A molecule called nuclear factor-kappaB (NF-kB), which normally resides in cell cytoplasm, moves into the cell's nucleus (hence the name "nuclear factor") and generates redness, heat, swelling, and pain. When the body heals, the NF-kB molecules return to the cell cytoplasm.

NF-kB, however, also provokes the genes involved in creating chronic inflammation, which generally does not help the body heal. Instead, long-term heat and swelling becomes an open invitation to cancer. One-sixth of all cancers are directly linked to chronic inflammation. Most, if not all, cancers have unusually high levels of active NF-kB. This protein is considered their missing link. Researchers, for example, found that NF-kB regulates the inflammatory cascade necessary for breast cancer cells to proliferate and metastasize.

Fortunately, inflammation can be smothered through diet and supplements. NF-kB can be suppressed by phytochemical-rich spices, vegetables, and fruit. Antioxidants can block the proteins so they don't move into cell nuclei. Vitamins C, D, and E, curcumin (found in the spice turmeric), the herb ashwagandha, pomegranate extract, garlic extract, ginger root, green tea, omega-3 fatty acids from fish oil, and isoflavones found primarily in beans can be effective cellular firefighters. I found such a diet helped reduce my discomfort during treatment, decreasing my need for pain medications.

When brought back under control, NF-kB provides the body with important healing mechanisms, as did the fires used to forge a goddess of righteous rage. Keep the chronic flames doused with an anti-inflammatory diet to help preserve your internal landscape.

Thriver Soup Ingredient:

Ask your doctor to measure inflammation markers in your blood (C-reactive protein and albumin). "Patients with the lowest level of inflammation were twice as likely as the others to live through the next several years," according to long-term studies by ankhologists at the Glasgow Hospital in Scotland.

Talk to your ankhologist about what anti-inflammatory foods and supplements work well with your treatment choices.

~~~

Qi Gong: Ancient Chinese Secret, eh?

A journey of three thousand miles begins with one step.

—Tao Te Ching, 64

One footfall made with graceful movement and a focus on the body and the spirit moves a person one step further along the journey of a thousand miles toward health. The ancient Chinese developed qi gong (or qigong, chi kung, or chi gung), a method of slow, fluid movement combined with rhythmic breathing and mindfulness to assist the body with maintaining or returning to health.

These practices were created out of an early understanding that our bodies are made up of energy. This basic life-force became known as qi (also chi or ch'i). Qi is like a field or pattern of energy, just as magnetism has a field of influence around it. When this subtle energy flows, the body is healthy. When the energies are blocked or thrown off-balance by illness, stress, or injury, disease results.

The practice of qi gong assists the energy flow, helps the body stay calm, can improve cellular regeneration, and slows the aging process. The practice is linked to improved bone density and better immune responses. Qi gong sometimes is recommended to cancer patients for regaining balance in their bodies.

Part of the practice might involve identifying a variety of symbols and sounds with specific organs in the body. Practitioners might use varied symbols as well. A teacher, for example, might identify the tiger, the color white, and the sound "see-ah" with the lungs, while the deer, the color green, and the sound "sheoo" is connected to the liver.

Vince Lasorso, tai chi master, invited me to an introductory qigong class. Each class involved learning one basic movement, with great attention given to exactly when and how specifics parts of the body moved. Each exercise brought me one step forward on the thousand-mile journey back to balance and health—especially because I experienced the movements as a terrific method for getting into my body and experiencing it from the inside.

Thriver Soup Ingredient:

If you have the energy, see if you can locate a local qi gong class. Ask the teacher if students generally learn one movement per class or if they learn an entire series of movements at once. Then decide what works best for your body.

∾∾∾

Re-treat

Whoever dwells in the shelter of the Most High will rest in the shadow of the Almighty. I will say of the LORD, "He is my refuge and my fortress, my God, in whom I trust."
—Psalm 91:1-2, Christian Bible, NIV

I needed a new shelter, a way to spend my nights in the shadow of the Almighty, a time of refuge from family life. When my psychotherapist saw how excited I was about taking a nine-day silent retreat, she said I had full-nest syndrome.

A few days later, the House of Joy, an old Victorian home at the nearby Grailville retreat center, enfolded me in her sheltering arms. My goals were to recover from chemotherapy and prepare for surgery through meditation and prayer, exercise and rest, and eating nutritious foods.

I allowed my body to lead everything. I stayed in bed until my arms pushed aside the blankets. I waited until my legs carried me into the kitchen when I felt hungry. My feet set the pace as I walked the labyrinth through the snow.

Spending time simply resting and being brought rejuvenation to my exhausted body. I didn't even do much praying or meditating. Sometimes I simply sat for hours and stared mindlessly out the window or at a wall hanging. During the evening, I spent hours circling from room to room around the open first floor, a walking meditation that allowed much to froth up from the unconscious into my mind.

Memories of those nine snow days of silence elicit a smile, and I feel again the warmth of the sheltering arms of Joy. My meditations and prayers deepened my trust in the Spirit. The restful, quiet refuge provided a womb where I could prepare for surgery and gave me the strength to endure another eighteen chemo infusions.

Thriver Soup Ingredient:

If you take a retreat, make sure you ask plenty of questions. Find out if they offer filtered water. If not, bring your own or purchase a water filter pitcher. Make sure they have a sufficient supply of sharp knives. The building where I stayed was quite old and had no humidifier, so I placed pots of hot water on the radiator in my room to ease the dry air. If you are sprouting seeds while on retreat, ask if you can have a room with a sink, and bring a sieve.

∾∾∾

Sound Healing: Good Vibrations

Durga's lion and a mere sound—a Hum from the lips of the goddess—destroyed armies of the demons.
—*Kali: The Black Goddess of Dakshineswar*

How can a lion and the sound "hum" destroy armies of demons? Mythical tales often veil truths behind metaphors, yet I learned there was a kernel of literal truth in this one piece of the story. Shortly after the diagnosis, I was listening to Deepak Chopra, MD, talk about primordial healing tones developed by the ancient yogis in India. One of them is the low-frequency sound "hum" that vibrates the lungs when drawn out through a long breath. Oooh, I thought, I need to give that a try. I could barely, barely feel my chest vibrate as I began to practice.

I didn't know how humming could heal. Perhaps it involved helping the cells become more unified and coherent. I had read in one of author Lynn McTaggart's books that a woman with cancer had incoherent bio-photonic emissions. No clue what that meant, but hey, if she needed coherence, so did I, and if humming could create more coherence, sing it on.

At about the same time, I purchased a WholiSound Serenity Box developed by Vince Lasorso. It's a wooden box, containing a speaker, which is placed under a body part that needs healing or is experiencing pain. The box is connected to a CD player and amplifier. Vince created a set of CDs with sounds that, when played through the box, communicate healing tones into living tissue. Cells begin to pulsate at a healthier frequency, which can assist with reversing and preventing disease and decreasing the sensation of pain.

It was like having a little lung hummer I could activate whenever I sat or lay down.

I used my Serenity Box whenever I reclined in a chemotherapy infusion chair. According to Vince, the vibrations would open up the spaces between the cells in my body so the drugs could gain better access to the nodules, making chemosabe more effective.

When I experienced pain, I would sit with the box for about an hour, and it took the edge off the sensations, making the experience more tolerable.

A hum coming out from my lips and a vibrating box made it more possible for me to destroy the armies of demons camped out in my lungs. I needed all the help I could get, for these armies were highly aggressive.

Thriver Soup Ingredient:

The word "hum" is synonymous with "amen," "om," "amin," or "aum." They are based in a Sanskrit (the classical language of India) root word for the Divine vibration that creates and sustains our universe. If you listen closely while meditating, you might begin to hear it as a background buzz—the sound of your inner silence. The hum is a primordial healing tone that causes the cells in your body to vibrate.

So if you pray, try adding a sound like hum, amen, amin, om, or aum. Raise and lower your voice to experiment with what body parts vibrate with the sounds you produce. Then tone regularly for the body part(s) affected by cancer.

~~~

Stress Trek

Who knows to stop Incurs no blame. From danger free Long live will he.

—Tao Te Ching, 44

I hadn't known when enough was enough, or when to stop, and it put me—literally—in grave danger.

A year after the diagnosis, I came across a nighttime dream I'd written down nine years earlier conveying the message to slow down or get punched in the gut.

Sht.

How was I supposed to slow down when I was caring full-time for two highly active preschool boys who hardly slept at night and rarely napped, while also working to maintain a freelance writing career? Yet I could have heeded the warning and insisted on loving myself enough to occasionally do something kind for me.

It was more than two years after the diagnosis, and about six weeks after my second lung surgery, that I heard a talk on stress. I learned that when we are under stress, our bodies respond with a fight-or-flight response by dumping a lot of sugar into our bloodstreams. Since cancer loves sugar, I began to more fully understand why stress can be such a culprit. In addition, sugar in the body leads to the production of molecules that increase inflammation and stimulate cells to grow.

I also found out that stress depresses the immune system by repressing the white blood cells. Under conditions of chronic despair or anger, the body secretes inflammatory hormones in preparation for wounds that usually don't occur in our modern world unless a cancer patient has surgery.

Vince Lasorso had urged me not to stress over emotional issues that flared during treatment. "Relax," he said. "Everything doesn't need to be resolved for you to be cured. The Shah of Iran had lymphoma, recovered, and was well for years until he was deposed, got depressed, and the illness returned to kill him."

Okay, if my life depended on it—and it did—I could learn to relax more, to pay attention to what was enough for me, and then to stop. It was one of the paradigm shifts I needed to make to get out of the danger zone.

Thriver Soup Ingredient:

If you are experiencing a spike in stress, exercise, if possible, to work out the physical tension so it doesn't get trapped in your body and cause a sugar dump into your bloodstream.

Also you can try the Map of Emotions© as explained in the entry in the section Mapping Your Emotions.

Other options include sharing your feelings with a trusted individual; if possible, avoid stressful situations by planning around them; invest in a hobby; do something that elicits laughter, such as watching a comedy; and possibly find a constructive way to accept things you cannot change.

∽∼∽

Synesthesia: Raiders of the Lost Art

And all the people are seeing the voices, and the flames, and the sound of the trumpet, and the mount smoking; and the people see, and move, and stand afar off.
                    —Exodus 20:18, Christian Bible, Young's Literal Translation

The Hebrew Bible records a scene in which the Israelites *see* the voice of the Divine and the sound of a trumpet at Mount Sinai. How could they have seen a voice and the blast from a trumpet?

According to Hasidic Jewish teachings, when an individual enters a heightened spiritual state, such as when hearing the voice of the Divine, the soul's capabilities flow through all bodily senses. The Israelites probably experienced what is now known as synesthesia. This condition involves a blending of one's perceptions so that when one sense is stimulated, another sensation is simultaneously triggered.

Some individuals have this cross-over already wired into their brains. For instance, they might hear something orange, or feel something pungent.

Alberto Villoldo, author of *Shaman, Healer, Sage*, wrote that South American shamans refer to synesthesia as "common sense." He suggested developing this ability to cross over between senses.

I thought he provided an interesting idea for experimenting more with staying in my body. Stepping into this exercise, I found it easiest to draw what something tasted like. For several minutes I savored a German Christmas cookie before inspiration for drawing the taste dawned. The process moved more easily with a fruit smoothie.

I still haven't seen any voices or trumpet sounds, yet I found the process a helpful practice for staying present and experiencing my body more fully.

Thriver Soup Ingredient:
The following is an exercise in staying present in the body, rather than creating art.

Gather a blank piece of paper, something to color it with (such as crayons), and a favorite prepared food with an eating utensil.

Sit quietly and inhale deeply and slowly, then gradually exhale. Take a few more similar breaths. Try a bite of the food. Close your eyes and chew slowly, savoring the flavor. Does it have a texture, shape, or color you can draw? Does the flavor change as you chew, bringing out more visual cues? Open your eyes and draw the taste.

∽∼∽

Uterus: Seat of Compassion

Therefore, my womb trembles for him; I will truly show motherly-compassion [rahem 'arahamennu] upon him. Oracle of Yahweh.

—Jeremiah 31:20, Jewish Bible

In both Hebrew and Arabic, the root consonants for the words "womb" and "compassion" are the same—*rhm*. For the Abrahamic religions, then, the uterus provides the physical basis for one who shows mercy or is compassionate. In both the Hebrew Bible and the Qur'an, the Divine is referred to repeatedly as merciful and compassionate, traits that are generally considered feminine.

Because the sarcoma started in my uterus, I thought about the womb as a metaphor. Perhaps part of the reason the dis-ease manifested in my uterus was because my compassion function had gone awry. Events in my life and my natural personality structure led me too far into niceness—I had become overly merciful in my interactions with others, while not extending enough care for myself.

My friend Mica Renes, a naturopath, also pointed out that the uterus represents safety and nurturing for new life. I had not been nurturing myself sufficiently.

Did my excessive niceness and compassion for others cause the cancer? No. Even dinosaurs had cancer. Did it place me in a position where I would be more vulnerable to cancer? Possibly, especially considering my mother had an aggressive, fast-growing breast cancer. Take one genetic predisposition, stuff it with a measure of unrecognized needs, stir in some niceness disease, and Voila! The body bubbles over with cancer.

The cancer probably was caused more by "what was eating me" than by what I was eating. It was time I developed motherly compassion for me.

Thriver Soup Ingredient:

If your uterus is creating difficulties for you, try lovingly drawing it as if it is a gorgeous flower, such as a lily, within you. Perhaps place something else that's beautiful in the center and draw light radiating outward. Create your own ritual around offering gratitude for what it represents—the power to give life and the love to offer compassion for yourself as well as others.

≈≈≈

Yoga: May the Force be with You

The state of complete tranquility of the feeling (chitta), *attained by yoga meditation, in which the self (ego) perceives itself as the Self (soul) and is content (fixed) in the Self; The state in which the sense-transcendent immeasurable bliss becomes known to the awakened intuitive intelligence, and in which the yogi remains enthroned, never again to be removed; The state that, once found, the yogi considers as the treasure beyond all other treasures—anchored therein, he is immune to even the mightiest grief; That state is known as yoga—the pain-free state. The practice of yoga is therefore to be observed resolutely and with a stout heart.*

                  —*God Talks with Arjuna: The Bhagavad Gita*, 6.20-23

The word *yoga* comes from the Sanskrit word for yoking, and infers the bringing together of body and soul. While the text above refers to yoga meditation, yoga postures also can be practiced to bring about a deeper state of inner tranquility. Studies have demonstrated that the postures lower the stress hormone cortisol, reduce fatigue, and improve emotional well-being among cancer patients. A study at Washington State University found these changes within eight weeks for patients practicing Iyengar yoga. This type of class employs supportive apparatus, including straps and blocks, to assist patients with getting into yoga postures. Randomized clinical trials have shown that yoga may help relieve anxiety and depression. Dean Ornish, MD, founder and director of the Preventive Medicine Research Institute, said yoga helps raise the threshold for what causes people to feel stressed.

Yoga has other benefits. For those who have had lymph nodes removed, the postures help the body move lymphatic fluids through tissue. Those who carry scars from surgery or radiation can regain more range of motion through yogic stretches.

For me, yoga helped with accessing emotions stored deep within my body. Energy intuitive Maria Paglialungo showed me how to do the fish pose to help open up my rib cage so I could breathe more deeply. She suggested I think about the word "acceptance" while breathing in and about the word "gratitude" on the out breath. Soon afterward, while breathing in the fish pose, I suddenly felt angry. Angry that I had to do that pose. Angry that I ate such a Spartan diet while others could eat a much wider variety of food, especially getting to eat lots of junk food without serious consequences. Angry that I spent all my time trying to regain my health.

After holding the feeling for a while and experiencing it within my body, my muscles relaxed. The emotions had dissipated and I felt a measure of peace.

I wasn't anywhere near forcing myself into a firm, resolute yoga practice and didn't have a stout heart for it, yet I had a renewed sense of the value yoga offers and an appreciation for the discipline it might involve to practice regularly. I practice some poses at home, and if my friend Mim Grace Gieser's light-hearted, restorative yoga classes were closer to where I live, I'd be there every week. I visited a couple of times and always felt better when the class was over, experienced a reduction in pain and stiffness, and enjoyed the camaraderie of being with other patients.

Thriver Soup Ingredient:

If you decide to practice yoga, try to find a class that features gentle, restorative postures that feel helpful and positive. I have taken free yoga classes offered by the local Cancer Support Community, an international network of centers that offers free programs to cancer patients and their caregivers. Yoga therapy also might be available through individual sessions for specific needs.

~~~

Your Physical Environment: Freeing Yourself from Chemicals

Do not conform to the pattern of this world, but be transformed by the renewing of your mind. Then you will be able to test and approve what God's will is—his good, pleasing and perfect will.
—Romans 12:2, Christian Bible, NIV

The pattern of Western culture is to bombard people with advertisements for chemical-based products that simple household ingredients can do nearly as well and without any endangerment to our health.

I never liked cleaning my house with industrial-strength chemicals, being forced to breathe in "air fresheners" in public restrooms, or allowing someone to spray chemicals on my grass.

After the diagnosis, I cleaned my home with lemon juice, white vinegar, and baking soda; when I encountered air fresheners in restrooms I used on a regular basis, I went to building management and objected to them; and I stopped getting my lawn sprayed. I also learned that dry-cleaned clothes should be aired out for twenty-four hours before being placed in a closet or worn; and to avoid skin-care products that contained estrogens or placental by-products.

I chose not to purchase products containing the phthalates BBP and DEHP and the parabens methylparaben, polyparaben, isoparaben, and butylparaben. I started purchasing my soap from private farmers' market vendors and my shampoo from health food stores.

I also learned I could make pesticides from essential oils, boric acid, or diatomaceous earth. While in Alaska one summer, my former husband and I tried dabbing clove essential oil onto our skin when we encountered mosquitoes. It worked extremely well—even when going through rather dense patches of the insects, we received only one or two bites each. I much preferred those few bites to spreading chemicals on my skin.

I have chosen not to conform to the pattern of this world when it comes to my environment. I might be on the fringe of our Western culture, but I like feeling safe when I walk into a public restroom, put shampoo on my hair, and wash my countertops.

Thriver Soup Ingredient:

If you have a specific cleaning or insecticide need, do an online search for alternatives to see what will work for you without spreading poisons or killing beneficial creatures. I like to soak orange peels in white vinegar for ten days, then remove the peels and store the liquid in the refrigerator. I also clean with lemon peels and baking soda.

C. Mapping the Emotions

Introduction to Mapping the Emotions: Linking Heart and Body

The thief comes only to steal and kill and destroy; I came that they may have life,
and have it abundantly.
—John 10:10, New American Standard Bible

To have a full, or abundant, life, one needs full access to internal emotional energy. Keeping emotions out of awareness can deplete us of huge amounts of vitality. If we repress the sensations of anger, we can sink into moods of hostility or resentment. Fear left unaddressed deteriorates into anxiety. Unacknowledged hurt draws us into victim and martyr roles. If we ignore feelings of powerlessness we might end up desperate or resigned to "fate." These are only a few of the silent mood thieves that can steal, kill, or destroy life-force energy. While I used such defense mechanisms during my childhood, they did not serve me as an adult. Instead, they sucked me dry, threw me out of balance, and made me vulnerable to illness.

After the diagnosis, I wanted to experience the free, healthy flow of my emotions and energy—not to act out or cause harm, but to allow the feelings to be what they were, to move through my body, and to dissipate. I wanted to link my heart with my body.

That meant I needed the guidance of a psychotherapist.

I asked around among a variety of people until the same person's name came up a couple of times. Sure enough, Sheryl Cohen, PhD, assisted me greatly by teaching me the Map of Emotions©. I found it an excellent method for me, a person hiding in my head, to begin the long journey into my heart and body. It provided a firm foundation from which my healing could begin, a rock to which I could cling for support, and an effective companion for guiding my inner journey. For me, all the other systems for dealing with emotions mentioned in *Thriver Soup* were deeply influenced by this core practice. The map provided a crucial tool for facing one crisis after another, enabling me to better cope with all the trauma I encountered.

When I started therapy, I wanted to be healed immediately. My body was a time bomb and the clock relentlessly ticked. My friend Marilyn Moore Hudson, however, reminded me that the process of dealing with childhood issues is like peeling an onion. I would have to take my time removing layer after layer—I could not simply rip to the center. Our unconscious minds know about what we can handle and what we can't, and in its infinite wisdom waits until we are ready before revealing new bits of our forgotten puzzles. Otherwise we might become overwhelmed. The slow progression builds a stairwell step by step, preparing the ground for each successive level of understanding. This gradual descent, like the deliberate yet tedious process of approaching an archaeological dig, allows us the time to explore and process what we find, and enables us to discover and gather the gems glistening in our depths.

The descent had to start in the present moment, with my checking my body to see what was happening in each moment. If I sidestepped the process, thieving moods of resentment, anxiety, victim mentality, and confusion would continue to steal away and destroy my life and my health. Now it was time for me to embrace my emotions in the now so I could begin to transform all of the domains of my life and finally begin to live abundantly.

Thriver Soup Ingredient:

If you have not had psychotherapy, I highly recommend it—if you can find a professional who can be of service to the needs of your mind, emotions, and soul.

If you have insurance, obtain a list of providers who are covered by your company. Create a list of your own, based on recommendations you receive from your health care providers, those in your spiritual network, friends, colleagues, and anyone else you think might have an idea. See if there is any overlap among the lists.

Narrow down your choices. Conduct an initial phone interview with your top options. Ask about their methodology and fees.

Narrow your list to three options. Make appointments and go see them. Ask about their strengths and weaknesses. Note how your body responds to the conversations. It is important that you feel comfortable with and can trust the therapist you select, as you probably will be sharing intimate details about your life with this person. Make your final selection, but if you later feel uncomfortable with your choice, gather the courage to switch to someone else.

≈≈≈

Anger: Eggs of Wrath

With the ferocity of a rampaging lioness, she slaughtered humans, tore their bodies apart, and drank their blood. The carnage went on. Her rage fed on itself and she became intoxicated on human blood. Then the gods realized she had to be stopped before she destroyed all human life, but none had the power to restrain her.

—The Goddess Sekhmet

The goddess Sekhmet displays fierce, lionhearted feminine fury, the type that gives rise to sayings like William Congreve's oft-quoted "Heaven has no rage like love to hatred turned, Nor hell a fury like a woman scorned." I, however, was out of touch with my rage. I had a long history of smiling while telling someone I was angry. This was incongruent and inauthentic, sending mixed messages not only to others but also to my own body. This propensity may have contributed to my uterus developing cancer, as research shows that repressing threatening emotions depresses the immune system.

One of the important tasks I faced in psychotherapy was actually feeling the rage in my body. Where was it manifesting? How did it feel? Did it move around?

I learned to allow the emotion to be where it was inside me, then watched it move, intensify, and finally dissipate. Even with my high degree of motivation, I found this process difficult to remember, and even more difficult to implement.

After two months of therapy, I became enraged about a situation and took a mile walk to relieve the tension. Halfway through my walk I realized I was not in my body—I was in my head, reverting to my lifelong survival mechanism. I chose to stay in my head because I felt it was too difficult, dangerous, and overwhelming to attempt to experience the anger inside.

When I discussed this experience with my psychotherapist, she said if I can think and walk at the same time, I can also feel my body and walk at the same time. During those two months I learned how to experience physical sensations when I took walks, yet when overwhelmed with anger I fled into the safety of my mind. This way I could avoid taking care of myself, and instead could create a story to justify my reactions.

To supplement my work on letting go of anger, I wrote dozens of nasty letters and burned them. I hit pillows and kicked cushions. I screamed and shook.

Gradually I improved at remembering to stay in my body while interacting with others. One weekend I went into my usual pattern of ignoring a negative situation because it was not about me. However, in less than a minute I decided to check in with my body. Sure enough, my muscles had tensed. I sat down for a couple of minutes and simply allowed myself to feel the physical sensations. Then the emotion dissipated, and I got up and felt free of anger. I was reminded of author Eckhart Tolle's example of two ducks fighting. When they are done, they flap their wings to release the tension and peacefully float away. They move on as if the conflict never happened. It was a beautiful image of what I needed to do.

Being mad is not the problem. Even the Bible says it's okay to be angry. The problem is what we do with the emotion. Do we experience our feelings or tell ourselves stories about an incident? By loving myself enough to experience the energy moving in my body, without dropping into thinking, I can allow it to harmlessly shift around until it evaporates. Then I am not hurting anyone with it—especially myself. There will be no sin, and the sun won't get a chance to go down on my rage.

Thriver Soup Ingredient:
What you'll need:
Soft felt-tip marker
Raw eggs
Write what you are angry about on a raw egg. When the ink dries, hold it in your palms. Use your imagination to move your anger through your body toward your hands and into the egg so it can become the container for your rage. Go throw the egg at a wall or tree trunk to watch it burst. Imagine your anger dissipating as the egg splatters.

∽∽∽

Authenticity: Be the Real Thing

There is a Light in all, and that Light is You, By that Light we are all illumined. The Light is revealed through the Guru's teaching, Whatever pleases You is worship of You.
—Rag Dhanasri Mahalla 1, "Hymn of Praise"

My illness brought illumination into my life on many levels. As I coped with cancer treatments, I kept a blog on CaringBridge.org. I confessed online that I was afraid to be authentic about my spiritual practices and beliefs because I didn't want to sound bizarre. I did not want to alienate my more traditional friends of many years, nor did I want to let go of income sources upon which I had depended. I thought about the crisis that Christian writer Sue Monk Kidd went through when she moved away from conservative Christian beliefs into a feminine paradigm (she tells her story in *Dance of the Dissident Daughter*). Part of my healing, however, involved my moving more strongly into my new paradigm and letting go of my compulsion to make things sound okay for all of my friends.

The outpouring of support for my becoming more authentic lifted my spirits. Gary wrote, "Let's all choose to live and express our truths so that when the end eventually comes, we know that we have faced the world with our truth, eh?" Kathryn wrote, "Good for you! We are not placed on this planet to live our lives to please others and/or conform to their beliefs. We are here to live our lives with fierce authenticity. That includes being willing to risk the disapproval of others to remain truthful to ourselves and our beliefs."

Their wisdom took my mind back several years. In my efforts to please others, I had shut down my own voice. My first publisher selected the title *Hidden Voices* for my 1998 book. Energy intuitive Maria Paglialungo immediately saw the connection with my own life. A few years later I had a benign lump removed from my neck. At a superficial level I acknowledged my niceness disease, my own hidden voice, yet did nothing serious about it.

Nearly two years after the diagnosis, I read *The Power Principle* by Blaine Lee. He explained that we have integrity when our thoughts, feelings, words, and actions are aligned and cohesive. I had faltered at having integrity because I often had not been aware of my emotional experience in my body. All my life I tried to do the right thing because I believed it was the right thing, yet had failed because my actions—or my silence—weren't in line with my feelings. I hadn't been entirely honest. I had not been authentic.

As I wrote this entry, I felt the familiar urge to start stuffing food into my mouth. I wanted to deny my experiences so I didn't have to feel vulnerable around others. I wanted to push the fear down with food.

Fortunately, more than two years of practice with the Map of Emotions© (a system for dealing with my feelings) paid off. I stopped writing and checked in with my body. Yup, there was a lot of tightness in my abdomen. I sat with the tension for a minute or so, until it wanted to let go. I shook the remainder out and continued writing. I sighed. A moment of clarity.

I wanted to be illuminated by Divine light, and share that light with others through an authentic presence.

I thought about Jesus—how completely genuine he was, always speaking the truth, loving all with whom he came in contact. He did not count the cost, even though he probably knew the price would be his life.

I wanted to emulate this ability to be authentic, and every day I ask it of Jesus, my supreme example.

Thriver Soup Ingredient:

My friend Kathryn told me that author Anna Quindlen was asked by a young mother, "What am I to do with my 7-year-old daughter who is obstreperous, outspoken, and inconveniently willful?" Quindlen's reply? "Keep her!"

Have the courage to be obstreperous, outspoken, and inconveniently willful. It might help you, in the words of poet Jalāl ad-Dīn Muḥammad Rūmī, a 13th-century Sufi mystic, to brush your mirror clean so the truth can shine forth.

~~~

Body Releasing Emotions: Shake Your Boody

In the same way the Spirit also helps our weakness; for we do not know how to pray as we should, but the Spirit Himself intercedes for us with groanings too deep for words; and He who searches the hearts knows what the mind of the Spirit is, because He intercedes for the saints according to the will of God.

—Romans 8:26-27, New American Standard Bible

When we are in pain, it is natural to groan. These sounds can reflect deep emotions and prayers, the Spirit within our bodies interceding for us. How comforting to know my moans are prayers for help.

Before starting psychotherapy, a therapist from another state came by to do a healing journey with me. Such experiences can bring up groans and images that words cannot express. Judy Merritt, PhD, worked on all of my chakras (energy centers in the body), starting at the base. She asked me to watch for any spontaneous images that arose during the process. When she worked at the bottom of my rib cage, I saw myself standing in front of a fortress. I experienced nothing after that.

When she finished, she suggested I draw the fortress with me in front. I did, and she noticed that the door to the fortress had no handle. Also, the crescent moon I drew was the opposite of the balsamic moon (the final phase of the moon cycle), the moon under which I was born. I recognized the building as a fortress of feelings. I needed to go inside the door and consciously experience all my emotions. I asked if it would interrupt my process to draw a handle on the door while we were talking. She said, "Not at all." She encouraged me to enter and join the party waiting for me inside.

I had to enter the fortress of my emotions to help my body let go of what it had locked away for decades.

It took time. As I lay on Maria Paglialungo's massage table month after month, I gradually began to experience the impulse to shake and moan as she worked on loosening up trapped energy in various parts of my body. I later learned from my psychotherapist that stuck emotions are released from our bodies through four spasmodic activities: anger, grief, laughter, and orgasm. We all know that laughter is good medicine. I realized I was letting go of emotional trauma through a physical experience. My body groaned too deeply for words.

My friend and naturopath Mica Renes wrote, "What you call spasms are called kriyas (it always helps to have a name for something). It is an electrical release, very well known in tantra and other Buddhist practices. It resets the body-mind."

Through my spasms and groans, the Spirit helped me in my weakness. I didn't know what was being released, and didn't need to know—the Spirit knew and interceded on my behalf.

Thriver Soup Ingredient:

I recall hearing author Deepak Chopra, MD, suggest lying on one's bed before going to sleep and simply allowing the body to sigh in whatever way it wants for about ten minutes. This process allows the body to let go of stored or blocked energy. I find this method simple, easy, and worthwhile.

～～～

Breaking Childhood Contracts: Silence of Lambs

For the Spirit God gave us does not make us timid, but gives us power, love and self-discipline.
—2 Timothy 1:7, Christian Bible, NIV

My psychotherapist clearly saw I had a spirit of timidity. She noticed gaps in my life around having the courage to experience my emotions and trust my intuition. She gave me a couple of cassette tapes featuring the teacher Lazaris. Through healing visualizations on the tape, I could learn about childhood contracts that might have influenced my timidity, let my contracts go, and access my internal spirit of power, love, and self-discipline.

According to Lazaris, there are different types of shame-based contracts that children make with the adults in their lives to stop pain and survive.

1. The child becomes a clone of a parent or defies the parent and becomes his or her opposite.

2. The child chooses to never grow up, to always seek the parent's approval, to live out the parent's dreams, or to be perfect.

3. The child becomes an abuser to justify the abuse already received; punishes herself or another; chooses never to have a negative impact on others; chooses never to admit to being wrong; or chooses not to feel.

4. A child develops an intense connection with the parental figure through cords connecting their energy centers (a symbolic representation of any contract) and surrenders her life.

My therapist suggested my contract might have been, "I won't know what I know."

Another psychologist said an ongoing bad situation can have worse effects than one clearly defined trauma. The child will not remember much but will just form expectations for life accordingly, such as "Living = being neglected; that's just how it is." This puts constant stress on the body.

I listened to the tape and wrote down a few contracts I probably made. The main contract stemmed from abandonment—I agreed never to hurt anyone as a way to prevent abandonment and to stop psychic pain. Of course, such an agreement doesn't work—it creates niceness disease and only induces more pain for everyone.

Lazaris included a discussion about associated energy leaks in the body. One signal for an energy leak is constant tension. I had experienced continuous tension in my abdomen ever since I could remember. It had decreased recently with other emotional work I'd done.

I found the visualization powerful—I had to stop and start the cassette tape three times to get through it. During the exercise, I went to a beach and saw the source of shame as a dark cloud. I had cords coming out of all but my crown chakra and also from my hips, attaching me to this cloud of shame. The experience brought up much emotional release for me, even though I had no mental memories of the causes for this shame. Different points on my body produced different emotional and physical responses. After cutting the cords, I yanked out the roots and threw them into the ocean. The holes were repaired and sealed with the pink light of love. I found the symbolic childhood contract in the sand and burned it, then walked away.

After finishing the meditation, I burned a piece of paper outlining the contract I had made.

My naturopathic friend Mica Renes suggested that rather than yanking out the cords, I could ground them somewhere in the middle between myself and the source of the cord. I could allow the energy to flow toward the center of the earth. The cords would come loose gently and I wouldn't have to yank them.

With a spirit of self-empowerment, of self-love, and of self-discipline from the Spirit to finish the process, I was able to overcome timidity and heal old wounds through the visualization.

Thriver Soup Ingredient:

If you suspect a childhood contract is influencing your adult life, spend some time considering what it might be. Write it down. Then, with the assistance of a mental health professional, do an active imagination exercise with the contract's elements and cut the cords that have been binding you.

～～～

Childhood Issues: Get a Little Closure

For hatred does not cease by hatred at any time: hatred ceases by love, this is an old rule.
—The Dhammapada 1.5

Hatred ceases by love. That includes hatred of one's self.

Nine months into cancer treatment, my face fell when a family member grabbed a giant bag of corn chips and walked off. I was conscious enough (a marked improvement for me made possible by the psychotherapy I'd had up to that point) to notice my immediate reaction—"Oh, no! They'll all be eaten, and I won't get any!" I recognized this reaction as a leftover from childhood, a dark, unexplored psychic room where fear, lack, and limitation lurked. The corn chips weren't even bought for me, and were harmful to eat. But oh! I suddenly wanted them.

I took the new awareness into meditation, and connected it to some incidents when I was five or six years of age. My self-hatred became evident when I realized I had minimized those incidents when my five-year-old self expressed anger toward me.

I meditated again on my five-year-old self. This time she was angry with me for a few minutes, and then moved into sadness and hurt. I did a small amount of crying and physically felt sorrow at the top of my throat under my left jaw. I touched it with my hand and the discomfort grew. I wanted to leap out of my chair and write about this experience rather than stay with the sadness. When I recognized that I was trying to escape from the emotional pain by writing about it, I stayed in the chair with the pain for a few more minutes. Gradually, my five-year-old self began feeling a bit better. At that point, she wanted to go wander into the woods by herself, so I let her go.

It would take some time for my inner child to trust me. While this process cannot be forced, I made myself available to her and worked to establish a better relationship.

A few months later, my therapist and I looked at a photograph of myself from childhood. She asked how I perceived that girl. The first word that came up was "sad." Then "lonely." My therapist reminded me of the Map of Emotions© and said I probably no longer needed to spend so much time on anger; I had moved into the underlying emotions of hurt and fear.

By choosing to love my inner child, I was able to let go of hatred and anger, pacify her, and find some closure.

Thriver Soup Ingredient:

Think back through your childhood and see if you can recall an incident that evoked some unhealed emotional pain. Try to imagine yourself as that child, and see if you can re-experience her feelings. Then write a letter to her, asking her how you can help her manage her emotions. Be sure to follow through if she makes a reasonable suggestion.

~~~

Childhood Issues: Invisibility Cloak

ADONAI is rebuilding Yerushalayim, gathering the dispersed of Isra'el. He heals the brokenhearted and binds up their wounds.

—Psalm 147:2-3, Complete Jewish Bible

Wounds from my childhood raised their ugly heads and cried out for healing during the summer of the diagnosis.

Right before my hysterectomy, I realized how abnormal it had been for me to pull out my hair when I was a toddler, instead of crying or screaming out my feelings. My psychotherapist and another psychologist said there might not have been a traumatic incident in this lifetime that led to my issues. It might have been a combination of my temperament, my position in the family, and my response to my situation. None of my four other siblings, after all, had cancer. It's me. What was it about me and my situation that caused me to pull my hair out when I was two, rather than throw fits or act out?

As a toddler, I would not have been able to understand the full extent of my pain or confusion. So rather than feel the pain on the inside, I became anxious and fearful. To externalize the pain, I began pulling out my hair. This activity also reminded me that I was alive. I learned to go numb and leave my body when the emotional pain became too much to deal with. My survival strategy was to become tentative and plaintive, not expressing my life force.

After the diagnosis, I understood more fully my need to move back into my body. I realized I responded to messages from my body like hunger, pain, and fatigue, but tended to discount my feelings of anger, fear, hurt, and powerlessness. Much of the time I was not even aware of those emotions. I had become invisible to myself, and found it easy to slip into being invisible to others.

I attended a "No Hidden Voices" meeting with Fran Hendrickson, a professional development coach. She outlined the fears that keep people like me silent. They are fears of abandonment, worthlessness, rejection, failure, and loss of control (internal and external).

I came to realize my fears were rooted in a deep-seated sense of unworthiness. I needed to learn to value all of my emotions and feel at home in my body. Then the lost parts of myself would have a home to whom they could return.

With help from my psychotherapist, my friends Maria Paglialungo and Brecka Burton-Platt, and my Emotional Freedom Technique teacher Mim Grace Gieser, and ultimately the Spirit, I gathered up the outcast parts of myself to rebuild my inner city. My wounds and broken heart healed.

Thriver Soup Ingredient:

If you have lost parts of yourself along life's journey, work with a mental health professional to bring them back. One technique you can use in conjunction with psychotherapy is to dialogue with those parts through journaling with your non-dominant hand. First, place yourself in a meditative state. If you feel you are ready, and the professional agrees, take yourself out of non-ordinary reality through a meditation CD or other technique. Breathe deeply and slowly. Invite along one of your spiritual guides for assistance. Ask for help locating one of the lost parts of yourself. Without attempting to control anything, write out questions with your dominant hand. Pay attention to any responses and write them down with your non-dominant hand. Take your time and see what treasures arise to help you rebuild your inner city.

≈≈≈

Codependency: Unequal Exchange

It is cowardice to fail to do what is right.... If you have faults do not fear self-improvement.
— *The Sayings of Confucius*, 2:24, 9:25

I'm at a conference center. I help others get to the dining hall by assisting them into a vehicle that needs to be pushed through deep mud. I am wearing flip-flops and get muck on my feet. Later, I walk into the eating area and there is no food left. Even though I have helped others get their meals, no one bothered to think about my need for food. I feel deeply hurt and go outside and sob.

This dream, which appeared a couple of months before the diagnosis, pretty clearly showed my co-dependent behavior patterns. I had a tendency to help others at my own expense, yet they didn't respond by helping me. I played the martyr in close relationships and ended up becoming the despondent victim.

Codependence is characterized by three modes of operating that form a triangle: persecutor, martyr/victim, and rescuer. Martyrs might sacrifice themselves for their mates, their children, or their jobs, then become ill. Then they use the illness to persecute their mates into having to take care of them. Victims play helpless and believe they have no choices, or choose not to make them. They fall into resignation and like to blame persecutors and look for rescuers, yet ironically resent it when others do assist them. Persecutors exact penance from victims and martyrs through veiled anger and guilt or resentment.

Co-dependents usually behave in one mode, yet tend to switch positions around the triangle with other significant people in their lives.

I primarily played the role of victim/martyr, and I know I'm not alone. Women in our culture have been taught to be kind, flexible, considerate, codependent, and selfless givers. This role stems from a time in Europe when five generations of women healers and mediums, along with some children and men, were tortured and burned by clergy in the Catholic Church for being witches or in league with the devil. Whole villages were exterminated. It was so terrible people deliberately forgot their gifts as a survival mechanism. Women trained themselves to under-express themselves, which developed into codependent behavior and evolved into an addictive tendency to need the approval of others. For me, codependence took the form of resentful compliance as a little girl that showed itself again in my marriage as excessive accommodation. The victim/martyr pattern had repeated itself in adulthood. It was time for healing.

I went to Mim Grace Gieser for help using the Emotional Freedom Technique around this stubborn issue. We worked on two incidents from my childhood that reflected my tendency to play victim, times when I thought I had no choices and was punished. I had gotten the message to be "an obedient little girl" as a perceived survival mechanism. Not following this prescription for my life created loads of anxiety.

Mim and I spent a lot of time tapping as I experienced the fear in my body. We got rid of a lot, yet the tendency still lurked in dark corners of my mind.

A year later, while still working on this victim tendency, I felt enraged and flipped from the comfortable victim role into the persecutor role, in a vain effort to avoid being a victim. At least I had the awareness of my victimhood, yet playing persecutor was no better, since it's simply another position on the triangle.

My psychotherapist explained that true power is not power over someone through domination, but power to, which empowers. Again I was reminded to take care of my needs first and to stay centered in my body instead of fuming and analyzing. Practice, practice...

With practice, I fell into self-doubt about myself and my power. My therapist explained that self-doubt is a mood created by thinking about fear. I realized I was afraid of my ability to make and stand by my choices. My payoff had been avoidance of taking responsibility for myself.

I stretched myself by learning to make more choices in my marriage. It felt frightening, as I learned that strength can be as scary as powerlessness.

I gradually accepted that I can feel empowered, I have choices, and I can act assertively. Yes, I still slip into victim/martyr-persecutor-rescuer roles, and often experience resignation, yet it happens far less frequently. When I do, I realize my mistake more quickly. I feel grateful.

There is a principle of reciprocity, which involves the equal exchange of energy between people, except when someone is volunteering. Like a barter system, people can choose to give and receive things or services of equal value. This prevents the victim/martyr-rescuer-persecutor triangle from forming. We can avoid playing victim by understanding that we always have choices. Even Viktor Frankl, MD, PhD, a Nazi concentration camp survivor, wrote that he had choices while imprisoned. He could choose to behave either with kindness or cruelty.

As we set healthy boundaries, positive masculine energy rises. The feminine needs this structure to flow true, like a river needs its riverbank. We can move into true strength, which is not power over others, but the ability to proceed. We learn to take care of our own needs first and to stay in our bodies rather than resenting and creating stories to defend or justify our unhealthy roles in situations.

We can do what is right and face our fears so we can improve ourselves. We can take courage, envision fresh ways of being in the world, experience emotional healing, and set new paths for our lives.

Thriver Soup Ingredient:
If you sense you have an inner martyr, inner victim, inner rescuer, or inner persecutor, and

you feel ready, set aside some time to meet this inner personality characteristic. Bringing it into your awareness gives you more ability to change the pattern.

Breathe deeply and slowly, gradually entering into a contemplative mental state. When you are ready, ask this inner tendency to show itself. When you are in touch with this aspect of your personality, begin interacting with it just as you would a real person. Ask questions, if possible, and treat with respect. When I did this exercise, I saw a woman bleeding while hanging from a cross. I interacted with her and others around her. We took her down and to a healer, who placed green poultices on her wounds. Through more active imagination sessions, she got well and began wielding a knife, setting clear boundaries. No more victim here!

≈≈≈

Courage: Saddling up Your Horse Anyway

Be strong, and fill your hearts with courage, all of you who hope in ADONAI.
—Psalm 31:24, Complete Jewish Bible

Having hope in the Divine can help us be strong and courageous. I like how actor John Wayne (1907–1979) described courage: to be scared to death, yet saddling up your horse anyway.

Someone once said being cured of cancer can require total engagement in the physical, mental, emotional, social, and spiritual aspects of life. People kept telling me I showed courage on the cancer journey by coming at it from all angles. I wanted to believe them, but in truth, it was not courage. It was abject terror of what cancer does to people's bodies. If I had done only what the doctors suggested, I might have died a horrible death in less than a year. It was my dread of the cancer demons that drove me to add every complementary treatment I felt might help.

Bernie Siegel, MD, provided me with some helpful insight about courage on the cancer journey. "Not many people are willing to become empowered and participate in their health and life, since if they take responsibility and don't do well, they experience guilt, shame, and blame."

Perhaps there is a fine line between courage and fear. I was running away from the terror-izing specter of death. For me, it seemed far easier to face my history, my inner terror and pain, my emotional work, my self-loathing, and my shame than it would be to deal with the agony of a body eaten up and breaking down by its own deranged cells. And I had to give it the old college try and be fully responsible for the outcome. Yes, I risked failure, with its attendant self-blame, shame, and guilt. But I had to at least try.

Perhaps this was the paradigm shift Vince Lasorso was telling me I needed to make when we talked right after the diagnosis. To saddle up my horse every moment, and to courageously follow my heart, my love, my passions. To let go of the need to please others. To not worry about the source of my financial support. To let go of needing to control the end results. If I was following my soul's purpose, everything else would fall into place.

Well, maybe I was courageous, though in a back-door-sort-of-way; doleful dread fueled my courage and gave me the strength and self-discipline to do everything I needed to do to stay above the ground. I also maintained hope in the Divine's ability to rescue me from this trap. I can go to my eventual grave knowing I did my best to survive. There's no shame in that.

Thriver Soup Ingredient:

I heard about a woman who knew that whenever she felt a tremor of fear in her body, she knew she had to move toward whatever was the source. Perhaps it's courage; perhaps it's simply the wisdom of life experience. Feel the fear in your body without thinking, and allow it to dissipate. You might find yourself saddling up your horse and moving toward the cause, like John Wayne in one of his Western films.

***

Crying for a Mother

The Great Spirit is in all things, he is in the air we breathe. The Great Spirit is our Father, but the Earth is our Mother. She nourishes us, that which we put into the ground she returns to us.
—Big Thunder (Bedagi) Wabanaki Algonquin

My mother had many good qualities. She survived breast cancer for many years beyond what her doctors expected. She possessed a strong will and persistence. Yet, like all mothers, she had her shortcomings.

While I was entering the cancer crisis, I felt the need for a mother figure—someone to wrap me in her arms and tell me everything was going to be all right. Mine could not—she had passed nearly a quarter century earlier.

I had to look to other people for the mothering I desired. It needed to start, however, with me. My psychotherapist encouraged me to become a better parent to myself so I could develop into a healthier person.

My sister, Roselie Bright, pointed out that informal adoptive part-mothers can be excellent choices because they have all chosen and wholly embraced their respective roles. My sister played an important role after the diagnosis by carrying me through the first months of research and decision-making, lending unconditional love and support. Many other women assisted with food, hugs, help with the kids, and other loving gifts.

Some of those who gave in maternal ways were men—a long-time friend who exudes the compassion of Divine Mother, and a store manager who always gave me warm hugs like one I'd want from a grandmother.

Mother earth herself nurtured my soul.

Even within myself I could find the "good mother"—she was my inner observer. She could feed me positive messages, such as "What would be fun to do right now?" During meditation I demanded, "Fill me with Your love."

Allow women and men to mother you. Soak up the comfort and compassion. Seek—no, demand this nourishment from within as well—where the Great Spirit dwells inside you was your inner witness.

Thriver Soup Ingredient:

Read the children's classic *The Runaway Bunny* by Margaret Wise Brown (illustrated by Clement Hurd). It begins with a young bunny who decides to run away: "'If you run away,' said his mother, 'I will run after you. For you are my little bunny.'" In this imaginary chase, the baby bunny becomes a fish, a flower in a garden, and a rock on a mountain. Yet no matter how he hides, his steadfast, adoring, protective mother finds a way of retrieving him. Like this mother rabbit, Divine Mother is always looking for us and loving us. Allow yourself to feel some sense of peace and security with this knowledge.

~~~

Daily Excitement: You Deserve a Break Each Day

Beings will enjoy the various enjoyments and pleasures on earth and will experience blessings. And may they enjoy all the various foods, drinks, nourishment, clothes, beds, seats, dwellings, residences, palaces, parks, rivers, ponds, springs, lakes, pools and tanks, these and similar varieties of aids and blessings existing on the earth, manifest on the earth and dependent upon the earth.

—*The Sutra of Golden Light*

The Buddhist goddess Drdha, source of all enjoyment, well-being, and prosperity, tells all beings they will find enjoyment and blessings. It took me a year following the diagnosis to really get this message. It was time for me to let go of any resistance to pleasure, to enjoyment, to life. Gary Matthews, a shamanic counselor, urged me to find the little girl inside of me who wanted to be happy; I needed to make every decision with her in mind. I needed to continue the practice of putting myself first.

And I needed to wake up each morning excited about something I was going to do that day, even if only for a few minutes.

I picked up old hobbies and started a few new ones. I lost my ego in the present-moment joy of creation.

I did some scrapbooking.

I bought markers and finally colored stained-glass window coloring books I'd purchased years earlier. I hung the transparencies in a window and admired the sun filtering through the colors.

I dug out my old horse figurines and started painting them, and felt inspired to add wings, unicorn horns, and sacred geometrical designs, eventually obtaining a copyright on them.

I purchased some modeling clay and made impressions with angel cookie molds, then painted them.

I wrote more chapters in a novel I'd set aside several years before due to overwhelming family responsibilities.

I called friends to do some activities with me, like touring stained-glass windows in local churches.

I read books that had been collecting dust for years.

I guffawed at laughter yoga.

And I went belly dancing.

During the process, I recovered a deep well of forgotten creative energy that longed for expression. I connected more closely with my friends and made new friends. And I had fun. I learned these elements of life were not frivolous. They opened a valve so life energy could more easily flow through me. My mourning over the loss of health turned into joyful dancing, bringing numerous blessings into my life.

Thriver Soup Ingredient:

Love yourself enough to do something nice for yourself each day, especially something you find exciting. Ask yourself daily, "What would be fun to do right now?" Ask it, even if all you can manage is a hug or a smile. You deserve it, and your body will thank you.

Depression: The Pause that Depresses

The first peace, which is the most important, is that which comes within the souls of men when they realize their relationship, their oneness, with the universe and all its powers, and when they realize that at the center of the universe dwells Wakan Tanka, and that the center is really everywhere, it is within each of us. This is the real peace, and the others are but reflections of this. Above all, you should understand that there can never be peace between nations until there is first known that true peace which, as I have often said, is within the souls of men.
— Black Elk, *The Sacred Pipe: Black Elk's Account of the Seven Rites of the Oglala Sioux*

My soul was not at peace. I understood mentally the concept that I was one with the universe and its powers, but that's all it was: an intellectual assent. It didn't bring me what Black Elk called the "first peace," and it wasn't anything I experienced within my body, which the Oglala medicine man said is the center of the universe for me.

Even worse, my friend Maria Paglialungo had suggested to me several times that I probably was depressed. Depressed? I wasn't depressed!

It took about nine months from the time of the diagnosis for me to finally acknowledge that I had been depressed for years. Perhaps not a clinical depression, but a definite lack of joy.

As I began to explore this a little further, I realized I had not really been living my life. I had been getting through life. Then it dawned on me—I had been afraid to live my life.

What! Afraid to live my life? I wasn't afraid! I had the courage to stand up to my parents, scowling small-town residents, and jealous, spit-wad-hurling teenage boys during high school to run my way to state championships; I had the courage to pursue my dream of writing for Arabian horse magazines when my mother told me it was too narrow a goal; and I had the courage several times to leave everyone I knew and journey alone to unknown cities to begin new ventures, including starting graduate school with no job and almost no money.

That vibrant, courageous woman, however, had faded away with the passing years. I buried part of my soul under the weight of overgrown responsibilities, along with unacknowledged anger, fear, hurt, and powerlessness. I had stopped doing all the things I loved. To cope, I had gone numb, dissociating and separating from my experiences—so numb I was not even aware of the depression, much less the emotions at the root. I had become an automaton, clumping down the hallway of years.

By becoming aware of the depression and numbness, I could begin to do something about it. I needed to find that lively woman with a zest for life. And I needed to find a measure of peace within. If I am truly the center of my universe, then the Spirit dwells inside, and that Spirit can help me see my relationship with the universe and provide a measure of peace.

Thriver Soup Ingredient:

If you are feeling depressed, set aside a period of time, such as an hour each day, to really get into the blah's. Don't do anything else. Simply feel as sad as you possibly can, without causing damage to yourself or anything else. When your time is up, leave the negativity behind and do something you enjoy, even if it's simply gazing out the window or listening to a piece of music that provides some peace, or even pleasure.

∾∾∾

Embracing the Feminine

O Mother! Thou art present in every form; Thou art in the entire universe and in its tiniest and most trifling things. Wherever I go and wherever I look, I see Thee, Mother, present in thy cosmic form. The whole world—earth, water, fire and air—All are thy forms, O Mother, the whole world of birth and death.

—Rama Prasada, *Devotional Songs: The Cult of Shakti*

The feminine nature of the Divine is ever-present, from the most trifling of things to the entire universe; the earth, water, fire, and air give witness to her bounteous goodness.

When it came to the matter of a feminine attitude toward clothing, I've never been a fashion plate. Goodwill is my kind of shopping place, and I don't own a sewing machine. After my first surgery I bought some old jumpers at the thrift store because my shorts were putting too much pressure on my abundance of abdominal stitches.

I must have been a site showing up at Tracy Lilly's home in Houston—frumpy old jumpers hanging off my bony shoulders, bags of skin still hanging from my arms, and bras too big since I'd lost about thirty pounds. I probably looked like a concentration camp survivor.

She took me in anyway, then took me fashion shopping. What fun we had! She and my sister, Roselie Bright, grinned with delight as they selected swishy low-cut dresses and push-up bras for me to try out. Okay, I decided. Time to enjoy the new me. My alter-ego came alive as I posed for photos with the two new outfits Tracy had just purchased. She called me Heidiva. Fashionista Heidi. Whoa...

They encouraged me to wear one of the new outfits on my return flight home. I felt surprised by my lack of embarrassment by what I wore.

Next I got to play girly-girl during an American Cancer Society program called "Look Good, Feel Better." Without thinking, I volunteered to be the woman modeling the makeup. We received some nice skincare and makeup gifts. I actually started wearing makeup more often.

Soon I dreamt that my shoes were worn out, and it was time to get a new pair of ladylike shoes (a new feminine standpoint). Obviously there was much work for me to do in the womanly realm.

My psychotherapist explained that the female stance includes an openness to my own experiences and emotions. Feminine alchemy involves creatively forming something beautiful from the imagination. It is receptive, emotional, willing, playful, sensual, and vulnerable—qualities I needed to develop. It was time I relaxed more, did what I wanted to do, and let go of concerns about getting through my daily list of healing activities. I found this challenging.

Later I dreamt I was wearing a pink bridesmaid's dress, yet was barefoot—I'd forgotten to bring my shoes. Since in dreams clothes generally represent the persona, or what one presents to the world, it appeared I had developed a more feminine persona. My feminine standpoint or foundation, however, had been forgotten. At least I wasn't wearing my worn-out shoes, so there was progress.

While my emotional work needed to go deeper, I had invited the Divine feminine to encompass me and to seep more deeply into my bones. One day it will drip down into my toes.

Thriver Soup Ingredient:

Buy some fun pink feathers from a craft store. Use one for a bookmark in this book and/or in your journal. Spread the others around your home as reminders to honor your creative, receptive, playful, sensual, feminine nature.

~~~

EMDR: Eye Movement Desensitization and Reprocessing

He who knows others is intelligent; he who understands himself is enlightened.

—Tao Te Ching, 33

Gaining insight and understanding into ourselves to bring about inner healing can be accomplished in numerous ways. One I liked using is called Eye Movement Desensitization and Reprocessing. This gentle yet powerful technique helps clients gain insight and deal with trauma. EMDR reduces, and sometimes eliminates, the emotional distresses triggered by particular memories.

During a session, the client might be asked to pay attention to moving lights or alternating audio tones, or to tap on opposite sides of the body. Simultaneously, the person is asked to focus on an appropriate thought or emotion suggested by a trained mental health professional. Often during the process, a client will discover new insights and might experience changes in memories.

I asked my psychotherapist to use EMDR to help me work on a particular childhood fear I'd carried all my life. I wanted to let the fear go so I would have more energy available for healing.

She placed a slender, horizontal bar in front of my eyes. When she turned on the device, tiny lights flashed from left to right and back again. She instructed me to follow the movement of the lights with my eyes, then asked me a question related to my fear. I tracked the lights for a short while. She turned off the device and asked me a question. Through my answer, I realized I was harshly judging myself. She asked me to focus my attention on that judgmental attitude while watching the lights again.

As we repeated this cycle several times, with each set raising a new area of focus, my initial awareness of my tendency to judge myself transmuted into feelings of anger at having been pushed too hard as a toddler. I recalled photos taken of me on a child's potty when I was only sixteen months old. My body responded to these images with mild sensations of abdominal cramping and acid reflux, which subsided as we continued with more light cycles and new foci.

As we completed the process, she asked me to find a place in my body that felt comfortable so I could establish a new emotional set-point. When we finished, she noted that I had observed myself judging myself—becoming my own silent witness or inner observer. This indicated I had released some of my fear and experienced increased self-awareness. She also pointed out that I had laughed at myself when I noted my self-judgment—a sign I had let go of some of the hurtful thoughts I had harbored. She encouraged me to continue witnessing and having compassion for myself.

By encountering myself through the EMDR experience, I learned more about my emotional experiences as a child and got to know myself a little better. It strengthened my access to my inner observer, allowing me to see better who I am. It also healed part of an old wound, giving me access to more energy that could be channeled into healing my body.

Thriver Soup Ingredient:

If you have traumatic memories, consider seeking help from a mental health professional trained in EMDR. Emotional baggage can weigh you down, draining your physical and mental vitality—which are needed by the body to deal with illness. Bless your body with the relief of letting go of these energy leaks so you can more directly invest your limited energy into healing your body.

～～～

Emotional Freedom Technique: Free at Last, Free at Last...

Just as a mighty mango tree is hidden within the stone of the mango, even so, old man, divinity itself is hidden within you. Rest not until you uncover it.
—Bhagwan Mahavira, 24th prophet of Jainism

The Spirit resides within each of us. And, like the stone of a mango fruit, that divinity can sprout and grow mighty. Unfortunately, the inner Spirit often is covered over with layers of anxiety, resentment, self-pity, confusion, disgust, or resignation. Beliefs that support these moods probably were unconsciously adopted during our childhoods, when we were most impressionable. Becoming aware of these moods and trying to fix them with positive attitudes, affirmations, and intentions doesn't usually change the underlying programming.

My friend Mim Grace Gieser introduced me to a simple, quick, easy method that can re-record our internal messages so we can grow past the early recordings in our minds. Emotional Freedom Technique involves identifying and acknowledging an issue, pinpointing a specific experience that triggers emotions in the body, tapping the ends of energy meridians on the body while speaking about the specific event, and gradually moving the dialogue from the problem to a solution.

During my emotional processing of childhood issues, I recognized that quite early in my life, possibly as early as my time in the womb, I did not want to be a female. How interesting that I would end up with a gynecological cancer. I wanted this issue healed as a part of my overall journey toward improved health.

Mim, a certified EFT practitioner, helped me clarify the presenting issue with a statement about it—"I don't want to be a female"—followed by a positive affirmation—"I enjoy being a woman." She asked me to think about a specific event in my life that highlighted this issue for me. On a scale of one to ten, with one representing virtually no problem and ten indicating the worst possible issue, I chose a high number for the emotional charge associated with the particular experience.

We selected a statement about the issue and began tapping on the sides of our hands at what's called the karate-chop point. I repeated after her: "Even though I didn't want to be born a female, I still deeply and completely love and accept myself." We said that three times, all while continuing to tap. This provided a set-point for the process.

Then, starting at the tops of our heads, we said a short version of the set-point statement and tapped seven times. We proceeded to tap at the ends of the energy meridians as used by EFT practitioners. An internet search for "EFT tapping points" will bring up numerous images that can be referenced for guidance.

When we got to the meridian points on my body where rage can get stuck, my body wanted to start shaking and my breathing got hard. I allowed myself to experience the emotion in the moment, without thinking about it. We continued tapping that point for a while, as apparently I was holding a lot of old, stuck energy that needed to be set free. When I sensed enough blocked energy had been loosened from that spot, we continued tapping through the EFT sequence. At the end of each cycle, Mim suggested I take three slow, deep breaths.

We managed to get the set point dropped a few numbers, yet I knew much more work needed to be done on the long-standing issue.

A couple of weeks later, Mim and I returned to the issue. This time, I focused on being willing to consider forgiving myself for being born female. I also wanted to let go of any associated rage, terror, or grief that still clung to a specific experience that represented the problem for me. After I was done tapping, I ended up doing some heavy breathing while my body shook out a lot of emotional tension that had been residing in my body for most of my life. I simply allowed my body to do what it wanted to do, yet held my inner observer accountable for making sure I kept myself safe. I also burped three times, which Mim indicated was a good signal that stuck energy had been moved out of my body.

It took a few hours in all, and we managed to get the set-point number for emotional intensity down below a three. I began to experience more acceptance of my femaleness, and eventually to cherish it. The process helped me recognize more deeply the feminine aspect of the Divine that resided within me. My buried and hidden female nature, like the stone of the mango, had finally been allowed to sprout and grow. Two years later, I dreamt that I had a mango tree in my back yard. It was dripping with big, ripe mangoes.

Thriver Soup Ingredient:

After working with Mim several times, I attempted to do EFT on my own. Often I didn't experience much success. I discussed this with Mim, and she explained that I wasn't asking the right type of question or being specific about the presenting problem. She was right. Doing EFT for "feeling empowered" didn't produce much benefit. Yet when I switched my statement to "I feel powerful and make good decisions when I am interacting with my husband," I found that I set better boundaries.

Cancer patients can tap for the emotional aspects of treatment, such as shock from the diagnosis, dread of treatment, fear of outcomes, rage at the Divine for allowing cancer to exist, hurt at not receiving sufficient long-term support, feelings of powerlessness in the face of the disease, or any other associated emotion. The more feeling you can allow yourself while tapping, the more effective the outcome for you. EFT is not for tapping away uncomfortable feelings, but for giving yourself space to process stuck emotions in a safe way.

EFT also can provide support for physical issues, such as raising blood counts, improving immunity, protecting certain organs from chemotherapy, increasing the effectiveness of chemo, and cleansing the blood. I used EFT and other processes fairly effectively for raising my white blood cell counts between infusion sessions.

There are many online videos for tapping to achieve a variety of results. Look for one associated with your issue. EFT practitioners recommended to me include Rebecca Marina and Margaret Lynch, both of whom have YouTube videos showing their techniques. I took one of Lynch's EFT videos and adapted the wording to suit my particular need. Create your own dialogue, using their patterns, for an effective self-treatment.

To find a certified EFT practitioner, visit www.EFTUniverse.com. EFT can be done by phone.

~~~

Fear of Dying

But when this perishable will have put on the imperishable, and this mortal will have put on immortality, then will come about the saying that is written, "Death is swallowed up in victory. O death, where is your victory? O death, where is your sting?"
—I Corinthians 15:54-55, New American Standard Bible

Fears about dying take many forms, yet probably the most terrifying sting is for single mothers of young children. Practically no woman wants to leave her children orphaned. Who could do a better job of lovingly raising them?

I found it helpful to remember that my children really aren't mine. The Divine has a purpose in everything, including my children, even if I'm not part of the plan.

After my mother's cancer diagnosis, her greatest fear was that her youngest child would not remember her. Fortunately, he was sixteen when she passed.

When I received my first bad scan results, I had to face my fear of leaving my children bereft. Everything seemed surreal as I walked around the house, thinking I could soon be gone. What was there to stop the process? The rebel cells were still alive and kicking me, despite everyone's best efforts. I experienced feelings of hopelessness and my thinking dropped me into alternating moods of resignation and desperation.

In my urge to do something, I remembered I could live in the moment. So I did what I could—I took a walk. I cried, admired flowers, listened to birds, noticed the play of sunlight. A sense of gratitude welled up. I was still alive, right here, right now.

Ken Wilber, in his book *Grace and Grit*, wrote, "[I]t is only in accepting death that real life is found."

Staring me in the face was the opportunity of a lifetime: to re-member who I am and to truly live.

My psychotherapist said dread is simply an emotion. This reminded me to follow the Map of Emotions© by sitting with the fear and excluding the thinking that goes with it, especially the storyline I was telling myself. The terror always dissolved.

My friend Fay Gano encouraged me to relinquish my experience to the Spirit, letting go of the need to control. She reminded me of Julian of Norwich (1342–ca. 1416), a Catholic saint in England who understood the feminine side of the Divine to the level of her bones. When she laid deathly ill, the message she received from the motherly omniscient presence was, "All will be well, and all will be well, and all manner of thing will be well." She recovered and wrote about her sixteen visions in *Revelations of Divine Love*.

Her awareness, I believe, can be applied to everyone, whether we live or die. All will be well, for all lies in the hands of a profoundly loving, all-knowing Being who chooses not to control us, but to love us into relationship.

Perhaps I could become more relaxed about death like the Native American chief in the 1970 movie "Little Big Man" who said, "Today is a good day to die." He got on his scaffolding and waited for death...until it started raining in his face. He got up and continued living.

The Bible proclaims that death has no sting and no victory. We are immortal, imperishable. I believe that when it's our time, we will drop our bodies, and our souls will journey onward.

Thriver Soup Ingredient:

With your journal in your lap, sit with your spine straight. Take a few long, slow, deep breaths. Then ask yourself, "In what ways am I afraid to die?" If no answers seem to come, try writing with your non-dominant hand. If nothing comes then, check in to see if you feel fear in your body. If so, stay with the fear and allow it to be, to intensify, to move, and to dissipate. Then try again. If nothing comes for you, simply do a little more deep breathing and wait for another time to try again.

~~~

Fear of Living

He it is Who created You from clay, and then Decreed a stated term (For you).

—Qur'an 6:2a

According to the Qur'an, I have a designated term. I didn't need to be so afraid of dying. Yet ironically, my fear of dying turned into a fear of living. I didn't notice my fear of living until I watched a travel program about places to visit. The storyline followed a couple as they journeyed from country to country, doing all kinds of activities. It slowly dawned on me how much unconscious dread I have lived with all my life. Fear of falling, fear of not being nice, fear of alcohol. Funny, I willingly jumped out of an airplane and rode some decent roller coasters during my college years, yet soon afterward became terrified of the falling sensation. I hadn't realized how far my fears had advanced.

About nine months after the diagnosis, I wrote a list in my journal. In what ways was I afraid to live? I was afraid to express my needs. I was afraid to stand up to others. I was afraid of more pain, possibly even more cancer. I was afraid of losing control over what I little I could control in my life.

What were my greatest fears about giving control over to the Divine? The Spirit might decide it was time for me to die. The Spirit might ask me to leave my marriage when I had children at home and needed health insurance and income.

Dread had constricted me, batting down my life-force energy. After the diagnosis, it seemed fear might be eating up my body. It was becoming a soul-killer. Then a new tumor festered near my heart, threatening to hammer the coffin shut.

I realized all these fears were fears of fully living—and that they were rooted in a terror of death. Unconsciously, I was afraid that if I expressed my needs in my marriage and stood up to my then-husband, he would abandon me. Then I would be homeless, jobless, and without medical insurance, a form of a death sentence.

It helped for me to understand that if my appointed term on earth wasn't over, I won't die. I will live! I'm not entirely in control of that aspect of existence, according the Qur'an. The Spirit has that responsibility.

I learned to acknowledge and face many of my deepest terrors and advance toward the lesser fears that have dominated my life. It feels much better to face what I am afraid of than to live with the unconscious anxiety that had strangled me for years. I don't know how much dread might have contributed to the start or growth of the cancer. I do know that confronting death has, by itself, removed many terrors. What a gift! I have caught a glimpse, a fleeting glimpse of the soaring joy of the soul when it is no longer shackled by fear.

Thriver Soup Ingredient:

If you are working with a mental health professional, discuss this process with him or her. If you agree it's a useful tool, try this exercise. Spend a little time sitting quietly with a straight spine, breathing deeply. When you are relaxed, pose this question in your journal: In what ways am I afraid to live? If nothing arises for you, shift the pen or pencil to your non-dominant hand and see if you start writing something. Move slowly and be gentle with yourself. Becoming aware of any fears is the first step in letting them go.

Gratitude Attitude

Is not the cup of thanksgiving for which we give thanks a participation in the blood of Christ? And is not the bread that we break a participation in the body of Christ?
—1 Corinthians 10:16, Christian Bible, NIV

In a first-century letter from the Christian Apostle Paul to a church in the city of Corinth, Greece, he identified the Eucharistic meal as an invitation to give thanks for the dying—not the life—of Jesus. The Eucharist was instituted during Jesus' "last supper" before he was crucified. The Greek word *eucharisteo*, from which the word Eucharist is derived, means thanksgiving. Centrally located within *eucharisteo* is the word *charis*, which means gift or grace. *Charis* is closely related to the Greek word *chara*, or joy.

Eucharist embraces joy, grace, and thanksgiving, and the apostle took it the final step—joining all of this with the death of Jesus.

If one can give thanks for the horrific, agonizing death of an innocent man, one can give thanks for anything. And Paul tells the Christians: Give thanks in everything.

Everything.

This is not pie in the sky, nor a pious platitude only within reach of an enlightened spiritual master. This is blissful gratitude that can gush forth from an ordinary human being when the tears have dried. My friend Clark Echols wrote that after his wife—a homeschooling mother, at the time, for their preteen daughter—gave up control over her cancer, her experience of gratitude was hugely magnified and gave her great joy. "It was the freedom from want, need, and control that made this pervasive gratitude possible," he said. "I was daily struck deeply by her expressions of gratitude for simply what I was, and for who I was. Very powerful. And it deepened her relationship with God, which I would not have thought could have been made any deeper or broader than it had already become!"

I cannot grasp the depth of her graceful, joyful thanksgiving, even while she lay completely broken and approaching death. She embodied the Eucharist.

Although I haven't arrived at this level of grace, I can attempt to infuse an attitude of gratitude into life, giving thanks even in the little daily deaths that occur to my ego.

I got to practice during one of my hospital stays, when all I could do was lie in bed. Coincidentally, it happened to be Easter week, a time when Christians celebrate Jesus' last supper through what is now called the Eucharist.

Rather than rage and moan inside, I spent literally hours daydreaming about something I wanted, going into exquisite detail. I had let go of the need to control, and drifted into gratitude—both for the opportunity to explore my daydream, and for the possibility that it might manifest once I placed it in Divine hands. I experienced deep joy, grace, and thanksgiving.

Thriver Soup Ingredient:

Find little things throughout your day for which you can be grateful, even if it's still having fingernails, or being able to get something into your stomach. At the end of each day, write three of these gratitudes, and if possible, record them in a journal. I have a friend who finishes each day writing her gratitudes on her Facebook feed.

~~~

Growing a Lazy Bone

Be still, and know that I am God.

—Psalm 46:10, Christian Bible, NIV

I had a really hard time being still. Unlike most people, cancer didn't teach me to maximize each moment and to see how precious life is. I'd already done that—to an extreme.

During the eighteen months after my first son was born, I almost never got more than three hours of sleep at a time, or even in one night. One of those nights, I spent three hours lying in bed, too exhausted to get up yet too awake to sleep. The next morning I literally cried on my then-husband's shoulder. All that precious time had been totally lost, wasted, rubbed out. I could never retrieve or use them for something worthwhile.

I didn't realize how my stressing over how I spent every minute of my time probably was eroding whole decades from my life. What irony. My work compulsion, rooted in a fear of death, busily created the thing I most dreaded.

The cancer diagnosis had, actually, become a stress-reliever for me. I no longer believed I was totally responsible for the kids, the household, or providing income. In my blurred, drug-induced haze, I couldn't have managed them even if I'd tried. I found genuine relief in letting a lot of it slide. While my time still was precious to me, during my chemotherapy weeks I often found myself sitting in a stupor for hours. At least I wasn't churning thoughts through my head.

My friend Laura Dailey shared with me a story about a woman with cancer who was given only a few weeks to live. This mother went to San Francisco to say goodbye to her two sons. She spent ten days staring at the ocean. At the end of the ten days, she was cured.

How many years had I missed spring because I was too busy sitting at my desk trying to meet deadlines? Perhaps a decade, perhaps two. Far too long.

My compulsion to do something all the time presented me with an ideal spiritual practice: setting aside time to do nothing. I experienced somatic tension when I "wasted time." I found it excruciating to simply sit for hours, especially when it meant others had to do my work for me. Every time I felt a twinge of guilt or the urge to get up and do something "useful," I reminded myself that the most useful thing I could do was relax and get well. This directly challenged my fears about not completing all my projects, which actually was a fear of death.

I soon dreamt I was visiting a wise old healer. All he said was, "Slow down."

I was starting to get the message.

Maria Paglialungo suggested that every time the urge to accomplish came on, to simply breathe. "Patience is having faith in Goddess's time, not yours," she said.

Despite the anxiety, I persisted in the discipline. Gradually the fears lifted, and I began to find great pleasure in simply sitting in our back yard. Sometimes I would drop completely into the gastronomic sensations of a luscious peach or a mellow chocolate truffle. I figured since I won't have taste buds in heaven, I might as well enjoy them here. Why rush the transition? Heaven could wait for my entry.

I knew the shift had finally happened when one of my sons was invited to play at a home that was a thirty-minute drive away. I checked with my son—yes, pick him up at nine. At the appointed time, I drove to the house to fetch him. No one answered the door. After ten minutes I called the boy's mother, and she was about to drop my son off at my house. My son hadn't thought to call and tell me not to pick him up.

Ordinarily, such a situation would have set me simmering for a while. What! Wasting an hour and a half driving and waiting in the cold for nothing! I could have used that time to do this, catch up on that, read this chapter, make those calls, write another entry…. Much to my surprise, however, I found the situation humorous and I peacefully drove home.

My friend Kathryn Martin Ossege has been doing the same spiritual practice—learning to relax, to play, to waste time. She has grown a lazy bone. I think mine's coming along nicely. As a side benefit, I sense it has deepened my awareness of the Spirit pervading everything, even me.

Thriver Soup Ingredient:

If you are driven, like me, try the spiritual discipline of growing a lazy bone. Set aside five minutes daily to sit outside or in a comfortable chair and do nothing. Don't meditate, don't eat, don't think. Just sit. Any time you feel driven to get something done, notice what is going on in your body. Do you feel tension? If so, where is it? Pay attention to it and see if it intensifies, shifts, or dissipates. Go ahead, make your day. Waste a little time. Your body will thank you for it.

∼∼∼

Healing the Shame that Blinds You

ADONAI, don't let me be put to shame, for I have called on you….
                                        —Psalm 31:18a, Complete Jewish Bible

Shame is an emotion, an experience of energy in our bodies. It is not something we can control, nor does it need to control us. It is not good or bad; it simply is. During many of our childhoods, adults used our natural emotion of shame to control us. This produced moods of self-disgust or resignation that now amble along underneath the veneer of our lives. Our Western culture trains us to experience emotions of shame and humiliation, especially about our bodies.

I didn't realize the depth of my own sense of shame until my then-husband held my face in his hands. I was surprised to hear myself say, "Don't look at my face." I revealed to both of us deep humiliation about my pruney-looking skin, induced by decades of worry and topped by chemotherapy and the loss of my ovaries. I became more deeply aware of my feelings about not being loved, wanted, or even seen; of not being "good enough." It tied right into my sense that "I don't deserve." This drove my behavior to please others at my own expense and to defer to others' needs before paying any attention to my own needs.

Part of me wanted to hide the ravages etched onto my face. Part of me wanted to claim my wrinkles as well-earned markers of the strength of will it took to live through my trials.

I needed to own my shame, and I'd been handed the opportunity. I learned the best way to heal shame was to experience its rawness on a somatic level, and then to get my feelings out in the open so they could no longer hide. Talking about them helped bring healing. As I accepted my shame for what it was, it began to lift. I also found that by sharing my experience with others, I became more open and vulnerable to hurt; yet I also enabled others to feel safe sharing their own vulnerabilities with me. This helped create a sense of intimacy and heart connection, which I found deeply satisfying.

I shared my shame on my semi-private CaringBridge.com blog and with my family and friends, and found others could both relate to my sense of shame and offer compassion. I felt restored.

According to my psychotherapist, shame has to be lifted by a spiritual power greater than us. I realized I could come to believe I am good enough, and have enough to finish everything I came into this life to do, including that I am good enough to experience a cure. It was time for me to allow myself to open up my hands and let go of the shame, and to call out to the Divine for assistance with receiving grace.

Thriver Soup Ingredient:

Grab a hand mirror and sit comfortably in a lounge chair. Hold the mirror up to your face and look deeply into your eyes. See what arises for you in your body. What urges come up? What sensations do you feel? Where are they? Journal about your experiences.

∾∾∾

I Want to Live

O Isis, Great of Magic, Heal Me, Release me from all things bad and evil.
—Therapeutic Spell, Ebers papyrus

According to ancient Egyptian myths, the goddess Isis resurrected her brother-husband Osiris after he was murdered by their brother Set. She also cured her son Horus from a lethal scorpion sting. Because of her magical abilities, a prayer to Isis for a cure was recorded in an ancient medical text called the Ebers papyrus.

I took notice of her curing her son of a scorpion sting because, according to myth, a scorpion that feels trapped with no hope of escape will sting itself to death. Someone told me I was vulnerable to this possibility since I had developed cancer—I had stung myself to get out of my misery.

I had been in denial about my mood of resignation before the diagnosis. As one friend put it, there was no sparkle in my eyes. I had already nearly died on the emotional level, and it was possible my body was trying to follow suit by manifesting cancer.

Somewhere, somehow, I needed to resurrect the desire to live.

Anyaa McAndrew, who facilitated my women's circle, sent us a link to a talk show series called "Women on the Edge of Evolution." I bookmarked the web site, but didn't get past the first recording because I was too focused on getting through chemotherapy.

Then my friend Maria Paglialungo urged me to listen specifically to the talk with Melissa Etheridge, a singer and breast cancer survivor. She had a new song out called "Fearless Love." She sings, "I am what I am, and I am what I am afraid of....I need a fearless love, Don't need to fear the end....I want to live my life, Pursuing all my happiness. I want a fearless love. I won't settle for anything less."

I found the song online and listened to it, heartened. I listened to more of the recorded talks, and they raised again my yearning to contribute something meaningful to others' lives through my writing. Dying would take what I have learned to the grave with me. Of what use then was what I worked so hard to gain?

I rose up to the challenge, wanting to be healed and released from all things bad and evil. I decided I wanted to drop the excess baggage that held me in the dirt. I wanted to be healed. I wanted to live. I wanted to live courageously.

Thriver Soup Ingredient:

If you are feeling discouraged and want to give up the fight to live, listen to the song "I Want to Live" by John Denver:

"I want to live, I want to grow

"I want to see, I want to know

"I want to share what I can give

"I want to be, I want to live."

～～～

Journaling: Writing Down to Your Bones

Truthful words are not beautiful, Beautiful words are not truthful.

—Tao Te Ching, 81

The Tao Te Ching speaks to the need for clarity, brevity, and authenticity in our words. This is most possible, for me, through a journal. I have written in blank books since I was eight years old and now have boxes of filled journals. Paper and pen have always been my friends, been there for me, listened to me, reflected like a mirror for me, held my pain and projections, shared my joys and my insights. They have been my most intimate companions on my life's journey.

Soon after the diagnosis, my siblings and I met with Michael Fisch, MD, who worked in the integrative medicine program at the MD Anderson Cancer Center in Houston. I don't recall much from the meeting because I was still reeling in shock after the diagnosis. The one thing I remembered him saying, though, was that cancer patients who wrote about their feelings experienced better outcomes. That sounded easy enough.

Yet I found writing about my emotions more challenging than I expected. I was used to writing down my nightly dreams as well as insights about them; recording events and my thoughts about them; and including ideas and things I was learning. But what exactly was I feeling? Often, nothing. At least nothing of which I was aware. Sure, I'd vented in my journal many times, but I didn't write about my feelings on a daily basis.

I had to learn in psychotherapy that an emotion can be experienced simply as a sensation in my body. It could be a tightened abdomen, a heavy feeling around my heart, or a wrinkled brow. I didn't need to know what the emotion was; I simply needed to give the sensation a little attention without giving it any thought.

My psychotherapist, Sheryl Cohen, encouraged me to start every journal entry with, "Right now I'm feeling..." This was hard for me. In fact, I rarely ever remembered to do it, which demonstrated how resistant I was. When I did remember, I usually had nothing to write.

This practice got harder as chemotherapy progressed. My interest in writing dimmed, and became especially dull during my final regimen in 2011. My mind had become flighty, foggy, and unstable. Neuropathy made holding a pen difficult and painful after writing only a sentence or two.

Gradually, over the years, I did learn to stop and take stock of sensations in my body, and later I frequently wrote about them in my journal. I began having dreams about melting snows and rushing rivers, symbols of thawing and moving emotions. I made progress, and felt grateful for it. I dug deeper and deeper, excavating my feelings, moving toward the level of my bones.

My journal writing now usually has the added dimension of a feeling tone, which gives it more richness and depth. I have gotten better about writing down truthful words. One thing I love about writing in my journal is that I can be authentic, sincere, and completely myself. It frees me to explore exactly what is going on for me, to get it out of my head, and later to have access to my experiences for reference.

Thriver Soup Ingredient:

Try to write in your journal every day, starting with "Right now I'm feeling..." Include whatever emotions come up. The purpose is to help sensations move out of your body and onto the paper, so feel free to ignore writing conventions. The goal is to tell your truth, not create beautiful prose. Include both emotions and your thoughts about those feelings.

~~~

Joy: Predictor of Survival

Homage to perfect joy, to her whose sparkling tiara spreads garlands of light, who with great laughter and tuttara *subjugates demons and their worlds.*

—Stanza 10, "Praise of the Twenty-one-fold Homage"

This stanza pays homage to Tara, a female Buddhist deity known as the mother of liberation. She uses laughter and a mantra to free others from suffering, fear, and disease. Her body, depicted in various colors, provides all beings with perfect joy.

Joy is the most infallible sign of the awareness of the presence of God, according to Pierre Teilhard de Chardin SJ (1881–1955), a French philosopher and Jesuit priest.

If joy heralds the presence of the Divine, then it stands to reason that joy could become an indicator of cancer survival. A study by Sandra Levy showed the psychological factors affecting survival of thirty-six women with advanced metastatic breast cancer. While it's a small study, I think it sheds some light, like the garlands streaming from Tara's tiara:

"After seven years, 24 of the 36 women had died. To her surprise, Sandra Levy found that, after the first year, anger made no difference in survival. The only psychological factor that mattered for survival within seven years seemed to be a sense of joy in life.

"The primary factor that predicted survival, she found, was already well established in oncology: the length of time the patients remained disease-free after first being treated.... But the second strongest factor was having a high score on 'joy' on a standard paper-and-pencil test measuring mood. Test evidence of joy was statistically more significant as a predictor of survival than was the number of sites of metastases once the cancer spread. That a joyous state of mind should be so powerful a predictor of survival was completely unexpected."

My psychotherapist told me early in our process to drop the list of must-do's and only do what I wanted to do—things that brought me pleasure and joy. Even though many supporters cheered me on, I didn't find it easy. I had to give this a lot of thought, and I slowly developed a list: Getting my books published and knowing they are helping others; seeing my children accomplish things; riding a racehorse; watching a beautiful Arabian horse run; and painting spirit horses.

Someone urged me to read trashy novels for fun. No, that didn't interest me in the least. I did, however, decide it was time to reread *Gaudenzia*, by Marguerite Henry. I loved this horse story as a child, and purchased it a few years ago yet never reread it. Carl Jung, father of analytical psychology, said the stories we loved as children tend to carry weight for how our lives go as adults. I found much symbolism in *Gaudenzia* for my current life situation. The mare got injured and was almost put down, but her life was resurrected by two people. She was renamed "joy in living" and eventually won an Italian horserace, called the Palio, several times. The symbolism for me was obvious.

Vince Lasorso reminded me that every beat of my heart sends fresh chemicals through my body. My best chance of surviving is for this rush of moment-to-moment molecules to be happy, joyful, and loving, encouraging my body to regain balance and return to a state of health.

That matches well with what Chardin said. When I experience joy, I experience the Divine within my body; that can only bring about greater good.

So Vince gave me a prescription: Cut out all possible stress, paint my horse figurines, and write my books.

When my then-husband and I took a cruise to Alaska, I wrote on my online blog that I was having too much fun to do any of the healing work I normally did. Vince responded, "Thought you'd enjoy some fun healing." My joy and laughter were subjugating the cancer demons and sparkling outward like garlands of light from a tiara.

Thriver Soup Ingredient:

Bernie Siegel, MD, suggests his patients make "choices based on what would feel right if they knew they were going to die in a day, a week, or a year." This focus gives people an immediate awareness of how they feel and reveals their inner conflicts, which Siegel called the most important job facing the patient. "When the outer choices match the inner desires, energy formerly tied up in contradictions becomes available for healing," he said.

~~~

Living in My Body

Do you not know that your bodies are temples of the Holy Spirit, who is in you, whom you have received from God?

—1 Corinthians 6:19, Christian Bible, NIV

As temples of the Spirit, we are physical containers for the Divine and therefore are holy. When we are present within our own skins, we embody sacred experience, according to Anyaa McAndrew, who led my women's circle during 2009. Our bodies are our home bases, and everything we do starts with our physical responses. If we aren't experiencing our own flesh and blood, we can't feel truly powerful.

I wasn't dwelling in my body, my base of operations. I possessed a shell that I carried around, rather than a home in which I lived. I strongly suspect one of the main purposes of the diagnosis was to help me return to my body. I needed to develop and value my voice, my physical presence, and my personal self. My first task was to become more aware of emotions as energy within my physical form, and then learn to express them in healthy ways.

My psychotherapist helped me realize that while growing up, especially during high school, I felt impotent rage and dread. Those feelings carried over into my adult life and infected my marriage. I had dealt with the feelings by numbing out, living inside my head, and dissociating from my body. I had abandoned myself.

After the diagnosis I learned to be centered, in my own beingness, in my Divine temple, for me. My therapist taught me the Map of Emotions© as a tool for learning to stay in my body. She suggested I take yoga or tai chi as another method of keeping in touch with my internal sensations. And since I tried to take daily walks, she suggested that as I walk, I focus on feeling my feet inside my shoes. Sometimes I switched to watching my breathing or my belly.

While doing these physical activities, I found it relatively easy to stay in my body. Now, staying present to my physical sensations while interacting with someone else? I found that quite the challenge.

I began to notice that when I was in my head, parts of my body would tense up. Ah, I had made a little progress. My therapist reminded me that when I felt physical sensations, I needed to ask myself if I was willing to let the feeling intensify. At first I had thoughts like, "this emotion sure is taking a long time to shift." I had run back into my mind at that point, and needed to drop the thinking and sink back down into my body.

Even after two years, whenever I felt overwhelmed, I would escape back into my head rather than take care of myself.

After three years, those old, life-long habits persisted. My therapist said I needed to set my intention for staying in my body. It actually was an intention to become more fully aware of the Divine within my temple, a way to connect more deeply with the Spirit and awaken more to my own sacredness.

Thriver Soup Ingredient:

Staying in one's body is a challenge when faced with cancer treatment. This attention, however, can be just the ticket for moving into a healthier space. Select a situation each day in which you can focus on physical sensations. It can be while taking a walk, while eating, or while lying in bed. Allow the sensations to be what they are; have compassion for yourself and befriend them, even if they are painful.

$\approx\!\approx\!\approx$

Looking Fear in the Face

And what is the matter with them, that they turn away from the reminder, as if they were frightened donkeys fleeing a lion?

—Qur'an 74:49-51, Cleary translation

My greatest fears, after processing the news of the cancer diagnosis, were not of death. Instead, I dreaded not learning what my soul came into this lifetime to learn, and of the process cancer patients experience while dying—the physical agony combined with complete loss of control. Some days I felt like a frightened donkey.

We can deal with our fears in a variety of ways. One unhelpful method is to ignore the feelings of terror that normally are brought on by a disturbing prognosis. Denial is not a healthy option, and doesn't tend to work for long. My experiences with denial cause me to agree—this approach is ineffective and can be dangerous.

Second, we can try to live with the doubts, worries, anxieties, and even panic that fear promotes when we fall into thinking about what we dread. That doesn't sound like fun. I know—I'm an expert in this technique.

There is a healthier option. My psychotherapist taught me not to be afraid of experiencing the emotion of terror inside my body. For me, it shows up primarily as muscle tension. Experiencing fear doesn't mean we have to live with dread the rest of our lives. Quite the opposite. By allowing fears to be what they are—energy within our bodies—we can feel them within, watch them move around to different areas, dissipate, and transform our lives, through a technique that uses the Map of Emotions©.

The map provided a physical angle on the same lesson I had learned through working with my nighttime dreams using active imagination—the best way to deal with my fears is to face them. Fears can show up in dreams as enemies who chase us. I had plenty of dreams in which my feet felt encased in glue as I tried to escape. Those seeming demons, however, were simply the unconscious parts of myself trying to get my attention. After a few years I learned to face the demon images during active imagination, and then within the dream state. Invariably, the demon transformed into something benign, or even brought a sense of freedom and control. I was discovering gold in the mysterious depths of my mind.

After the diagnosis, I found myself moving into a new level of facing my fears when I had the following dream:

A Doberman pinscher grabs my left hand and bites. It's a firm, but not painful, grip. I feel dread, but remember that dogs who sense fear attack. I release the tension in my body and the terror ebbs. The dog releases my hand.

I had not only faced my terror, I had also learned to experience the emotion of dread in my body while dreaming. I handled the fear by consciously accepting the tension and helping my body dissipate it.

I no longer felt like a frightened donkey fleeing a lion. Nor did I want to run away from reminders to stay steadily focused on the Divine. I had learned to face the lion of my fears and allow transformation to occur.

Thriver Soup Ingredient:

A favorite children's book of mine is *The Red Lion: A Tale of Ancient Persia*. You can read in story form what happens when we run from and then turn to face our fears.

Love YourSelf

Some behold the soul in amazement. Similarly, others describe it as marvelous. Still others listen about the soul as wondrous.

—*God Talks with Arjuna: The Bhagavad Gita*, 2.29a

Widely known speaker Peggy O'Neill describes beholding her Self as a diamond radiating light. She experienced the Divine within her being as amazing and wondrous, and it forever changed her life. She learned to love and accept herself as she was, and to walk tall, even from a height of three feet, eight inches. She is changing others' lives with her message of Self-love.

As a young adult, I had been trained by Christians to be a humble servant to others. Somehow I didn't quite fully absorb the message that we are to love our neighbors as we love ourselves. I did a decent job of it, yet fell far short of the mark. I couldn't very well love others as much as I wanted to if I didn't first have that love within myself.

The diagnosis provoked a wake-up call. It was time to give myself what I had been trying to give others—love. A love that in a twisted way I had hoped to get back for what I gave. I had it backward. First I had to fill myself with love, then I could truly give love to others.

This is not being selfish. This is loving the Divine within one's self. Others will see your light shine and be inspired.

About the time I started treatment, I took a long look in a mirror and was a little astonished to see how beautiful my face is. Full of love and wisdom, a homey, wholesome, comforting face. So I gave myself lovely affirmations about who I am—and the good things coming my way. I felt deeply satisfied.

While sometimes I still feel shame, the majority of the time I grew in Self-love. Gradually I learned to treat the shame as any other emotion: to allow it to be, to intensify, to move, and to dissipate. Then I rose into the experiences of no-thingness, neutrality, or compassion for myself.

I want to increase this Self-love, not as an ego trip, but as a way to honor my higher Self, my inner observer, my soul, strengthening my connection with All That Is. As I deepen my connection with the Divine, perhaps someday I, too, will behold my amazing, marvelous, wondrous soul.

Thriver Soup Ingredient:

Loving your body is essential, one friend told me. Befriend it like you would a sad, wounded child. Find ways to nurture yourself daily. Perhaps you can rub nice lotion on your skin and sing yourself lullabies. Tell your body how much you love and honor it and express gratitude for what it has done for you.

≈≈≈

Map of Emotions©: Let it Be

The gentle and yielding is the disciple of life.

—Tao Te Ching, 76

Those who are yielding and receptive to the sensations of emotions in their bodies are disciples of life, in harmony both within their bodies and with those around them. In contrast are those without flexibility, stiff and unbending. Like a dry twig, they are easily broken.

As humans, part of yielding and being gentle is having full access to our feelings. Emotions are simply energy in motion. For most of my life, many of my emotions had not been moving. They were stuck. Soon after starting with my psychotherapist, she taught me the Map of Emotions©, a guide for experiencing my feelings so I wouldn't repress them anymore.

I found this map incredibly useful for working with the sensations in my body. It involves recognizing an emotion as energy in my body, like tension, and giving it my full attention. By not thinking about the reaction, I could allow the energy to move around, intensify, and dissipate. Ironically, by not attempting to control my feelings, and by not rationalizing them, yet allowing them to be and giving them attention, I felt a deeper sense of control over a disease that had stripped away almost all of my ability to manage my life.

I worked hard on the process. Within two months I found myself trying to experience my feelings for long periods of time, and found this frustrating. My therapist helped me see that I had not been sitting with only my emotions. I also was reflecting on them. Even "this is taking a long time" was splitting into thinking. She compared it to the "Wizard of Oz" movie scene where Dorothy was in the inner sanctuary for the second time and the Wizard said, "Pay no attention to the man behind the curtain." The man, in this case, was the lure of my own thoughts. Instead, I needed to stay in the body, in the feeling, in the moment, in my inner sanctuary. If I stayed with the emotion, it would pass in about ninety seconds.

It took six months for me to notice that when I was focused on thinking, parts of my body would grow tense. I had accomplished round one. Yet instead of moving into part two—going into the tension—I consciously relaxed my muscles. Ah, more work to do.

Later, when I felt depressed, someone called and reminded me that both of our mothers had stuffed their feelings and died of breast cancer. I didn't want to stuff my feelings anymore, yet found myself unable to cry. After we hung up, I prayed for help opening the vault of my emotions so I could feel them more. I soon found myself bawling for about forty-five minutes, experiencing a sadness too deep for words. I had not cried like that for many years.

When I told my therapist about this incident, she reminded me that I can honor and fully experience my feelings in a healthy way without ever crying. The word sadness does not show up on the Map—it's the specific aspects of sadness that appear in various ways, such as hurt, grief, loss, and emptiness. What's important is to feel the emotion in the body and name it, allow it to grow more intense, and allow it to shift and leave. She noted I was judging myself too harshly for not being able to readily cry, saying some of her clients weep profusely as a way to overdramatize while avoiding the actual experience of their feelings.

The key, she reminded me again, is to feel the emotion in the body.

A few months later, during a conversation with another person, I experienced my abdomen clench a slight amount. I immediately asked the other person to rephrase what was said, and I got the response I needed. When I told my therapist about the incident, she got excited because I had successfully gone through a complex process. First I recognized the clench, then I realized I wanted something to shift, and I requested this shift immediately and not in an offensive way. I told her, with sarcastic humor, "Well, it only took me a year." Then I laughed and said, "Okay, now I'm judging myself." She laughed and said, as a way of congratulating me, that I can now conduct the therapy sessions while she watches. Of course, I had many more things to work on, but this indicated a lot of progress.

Nearly two years into therapy, I realized how the Map is actually a mindfulness technique because it moves one deeply into the present moment.

At about the same time, I reached the point where whenever I noticed tension in my body, I stopped what I was doing and processed the emotions. I allowed myself to experience terror, rage, powerlessness, and despair, and they moved out of my body. To my surprise, I even did some crying.

I had become yielding and receptive to my emotions, which enabled me to come more in harmony with my body and with living.

Thriver Soup Ingredient:

If you are looking for a psychotherapist, and struggle with experiencing or expressing your feelings, look around for a therapist trained in the Map of Emotions©. I found it an excellent way for learning how to deal with my emotions in a healthy manner.

~~~

Memory or Imagination: Childhood Sexual Abuse

The enemy is finished, in ruins forever; you destroyed their cities; all memory of them is lost.
—Psalm 9:6, Complete Jewish Bible

Just as ancient cities can be destroyed and lost to history, our personal memories can easily be lost or replaced by false recollections. Our memories are fickle. I got a glimpse of this when, a few years ago, my dad told a story about something that happened when he was younger. Later he reread about that event in his diary, and realized he had remembered the incident incorrectly. This surprised me, since he was an intellectual who always strove for honesty in all his dealings.

Yet this malleability of memory is part of the human condition. It affected me deeply after the diagnosis. Since the cancer occurred in a reproductive organ, I was told by a psychologist that such a cancer likely stemmed from childhood sexual abuse. My stomach felt queasy. I had no memory of any such event. How could this be? Was I one of those individuals who hid the abuse deep in the subconscious mind so I never had to deal with it consciously? Had it really happened, and if so, by whom, and when?

Earlier, when cases of repressed sexual memories showed up in sensational court cases, I had explored these questions. Then I had a night of lucid dreaming and asked if I had been a victim of sexual abuse. I got a "no." Yet maybe this was just my subconscious mind's way of protecting me from the truth until I was ready to deal with it.

I asked a family member, who had worked through therapy for twelve years, if any such thing ever occurred in my family of origin. No, I was told.

Still, after the diagnosis I was encouraged by others to explore the possibility. One person even said she knew it had happened to me because of the tightness in my body.

I went into active imagination, asked for a dream, and meditated. A vague impression came. I explored it, meditated on it, and did active imagination with it. I tried to accept it as evidence of abuse when I was a toddler in a misguided, unconscious attempt to please others. Yet the alleged abuse didn't seem like a real experience. I wrote this unreality off as simply my inability to recall the event because it occurred before my conscious memories began forming around age four.

Then I read "The Memory Wars," an article by Elizabeth Loftus in the magazine *science&spirit*. Her research revealed that biased questions—even changing the word "hit" to "smashed" when asking about a car accident—can lead to false recall. "Our memory systems are capable of creating in unsuspecting minds whole events that never happened. People even claim to recall experiences that would be virtually impossible," she wrote.

I felt I had been pressured into conceiving and then believing something that never happened. I decided to trust my inner sense, my dream response, and my family member. I let go of the need to have a dramatic childhood abuse situation to bolster my sense of being innocent of causing the cancer.

Even if something had happened, it wasn't going to change my current experience. It was time to forget the supposed memory and get on with the work of healing what I did know that needed my attention.

Later, my psychotherapist explained that my body being rigid could simply be the result of a single trauma or the accumulation of internal feelings that I had never witnessed in myself. I didn't need to have a story about it to heal. Healing involved learning to experience emotions in my body, in the present moment, following the Map of Emotions©. Memories of the causes, like memories of a destroyed city, might be lost, yet the healing can still occur. For this I am grateful.

Thriver Soup Ingredient:

If you are sure you have been a victim of sexual abuse during childhood, seek a competent and experienced psychotherapist. The book *The Courage to Heal: A Guide for Women Survivors of Child Sexual Abuse,* by Ellen Bass and Laura Davis, discusses the impact of childhood sexual abuse and how to address it.

~~~

Niceness Dis-ease

Thou preparest a table before me in the presence of mine enemies: thou anointest my head with oil; my cup runneth over. Surely goodness and mercy shall follow me all the days of my life: and I will dwell in the house of the Lord for ever.

—Psalm 23:5-6, King James Version, Christian Bible

This psalm probably was written by David, second king of the United Kingdom of Israel (usually dated about 1040–970 BCE). He expresses trust in the Spirit to provide him with the necessities of life, even in the face of adversity. David's head is anointed with oil, a practice of the ancient Hebrews to recognize kingship, to acknowledge a more powerful connection with the Divine, or to bring healing. David's personal cup of blessings overflowed, possibly spilling into a metaphorical saucer. Whatever filled the cup was for David. Whatever flowed overboard, into the saucer, could then freely be given to another.

The same idea—of giving from the overflow—is spoken every time a commercial airline is about to take off. We're told that if the oxygen masks descend, to put ours on before we help anyone else, including our own children, with theirs. If you don't put yours on, you won't be able to help others.

I understood the concept, yet didn't practice it because I had a bad case of niceness dis-ease.

This illness is based on a fear of the impression I give people, and of not being liked and accepted. The irony is, I probably will be liked more for being authentic than for trying to fit into what I perceive as a role someone else wants for me.

As a child, I lost my trust in unconditional love, so I learned to please others—with nods, smiles, little laughs, and compliance—to my great peril and detriment, taking me to the edge of death.

I gave to the point of exhaustion, and did not replenish myself properly. I had neither the gumption nor the proper boundaries in place to say to my then-husband, "I need to go take care of myself for a while."

I ran near empty for more than a dozen years, and finally my body broke down.

The author of a book on nutrition for cancer wrote about a woman who always ate healthy food, got cancer anyway, and died. He said it might not always be what we're eating that causes cancer—it can be caused by what's eating us. I felt a kinship with that woman, yet wanted to change the dynamic for myself.

While I was in treatment, an acquaintance named Susan gave me a bright, yellow, smiley-face mug and wrote, "See yourself filling that big old smiley cup until it spills over, and THEN you nourish others from the overflow! In fact they just spontaneously get nourished from your fullness."

She had picked up on my inappropriate niceness and knew the antidote. I had posted an apology on my CaringBridge blog for expressing my truth. She probably saw the post and recognized my dis-ease.

I also noticed while watching myself on a camera that I smiled, nodded, and laughed more than normal, another indicator of my unconscious drive to please others at my own expense.

The mug stayed on my personal altar as a daily reminder to fill my own cup first.

I learned that being centered in my innermost being—my Self—isn't selfish. It's sustainable. And it's generous toward others, because if my cup is so full it's spilling over into my saucer, then I automatically have something to give to others.

At the moment, however, my cup was fairly empty. Gini, an acquaintance, reminded me that it was time for me to focus on my deeper Self, to learn to allow life to happen, and to receive from others. It was time for me to speak up for myself and my needs, and to have fun. It was time to replenish myself in the presence of the Divine, and give to others only from the overflow of my cup of Divine grace.

Thriver Soup Ingredient:

If you experience niceness disease, create a daily ritual for being kind to yourself. You can call it High Juice if you like, emulating the British by setting aside time each day to indulge in a lovely drink. Make a list of little pleasures to bask in that will raise your juiciness quotient. Here is a list of possibilities for filling your cup:

Try a new type of tea. Maybe splurge and get a special brand.

Try a new type of dark chocolate, and don't chew. Allow it to slowly melt in your mouth.

Try a new type of fruit. Check out international markets for intriguing possibilities.

Lie down on a patch of grass and watch the clouds float by.

Walk barefoot in grass.

Sit outside and spend time simply listening.

Select a book for pleasure and read a chapter each day.

Buy a flower or bouquet to display on your dining table.

Take a bath with flower petals floating around you.

Old Griefs

O Destroyer of pain, Bestower of Mercy, Fascinating Lord, Destroyer of sorrow and strife, I have come to Your Sanctuary...

—"Raag Bihaagra," Shri Guru Granth Sahib

When we come into our inner sanctuary and experience a deep connection with the Spirit, our pain, sadness, and strife can lift. I needed help with my sorrows to move forward emotionally. The diagnosis frightened me into working on my old griefs to make room for the blessing of rising internal healing energies.

I found this poem by Jalāl ad-Dīn Muḥammad Rūmī, a 13th-century Sufi mystic, encouraging:

Learn from God's Messenger this alchemy:

Be satisfied with what He gives to you.

And when the envoy "Grief" comes to your house,

Then take him to your breast like an old friend!

When I was six years old, we had a kitten named Smokey. One day while meditating, I realized I probably had not completely grieved Smokey's passing, which was my first encounter with violence and death. While still a kitten, Smokey had been attacked by someone with a knife. I don't have any memory of seeing his body, nor of any kind of ritual to mark his passing. I don't think there was much discussion, either. He was taken to the vet and euthanized. I realized I needed to properly grieve Smokey and create a ritual around his death—and for the other two cats we lost while I was growing up.

Anyaa McAndrew, who facilitated my women's circle, gave me the confidence to create my own rituals. I lit a couple of candles in front of our fireplace and played Samuel Barber's "Adagio for Strings" (the saddest music I know). I held a stuffed cat I'd kept since childhood. It is quite worn and missing an eye, reminding me of the children's story, *The Velveteen Rabbit*. Then I sat down and thought about Smokey. In my imagination, he came and sat on my lap. For the third time since I came home from the hospital, I had a good cry. I wrote a letter to each cat we had lost, and then burned their pictures, holding my stuffed cat over my heart. When I finished, I felt gratitude for their roles in my life. I can imagine all three in Elysian Fields, Smokey deliriously chasing mice and birds; Sampson pouncing after butterflies; and Puddie Tat lazily soaking up sun on a nearby rock. I felt content.

Seven months later I decided to delve deeper. I sat down with my early childhood photo album. It contains a photo of me pulling at my hair when I was sixteen months old. To get back into my body's experience at that time, I started twirling my hair at the location where I had pulled it out. Oh, how familiar it felt. I sat with it awhile, feeling nothing. Then it dawned on me. I was experiencing anxiety. I had developed this habit as a toddler to comfort myself. Was something going on outside me causing the anxiety? I don't know. I have a friend with a son who exhibited great anxiety since he was a small child, and his brother showed none of it.

At any rate, I looked anxiety up on my Map of Emotions©. It wasn't an emotion—it was a mood, caused by thinking about the feeling of fear. I had already dissociated from my emotions. So I sat, twirling my hair, and waited to see if fear would arise in my body. After several minutes, it showed up. I allowed it to be, momentarily, then I dropped into the mood of anxiety again. I let my body jerk while releasing high-pitched moans. I let it continue until my mouth and legs got too tired. Then I did Tapas Acupressure Technique to let go of anything else my body was ready to release.

I no longer connect emotionally to the habit of twirling my hair, so that particular grief has dissipated. The Destroyer of Pain and Bestower of Mercy had paid me a most welcome visit.

Thriver Soup Ingredient:

I urge you to work with a mental health professional on this ingredient. Such a compassionate witness can be comforting during your process. He or she can assist you with grieving in a healthy way and enabling you to come out on the other side.

Make a list of things to grieve. It might include the loss of an ability to deeply feel, a sense of abandonment, or even sorrow that you have things you must grieve so your body can heal. You might choose to grieve the time and money it takes to heal, the illness, the loss of relationships, or the missed opportunities you saw while in treatment.

Go back to the source of the pain. Enter into your body and feel the grief, using a technique suggested by your mental health professional. Ask your body questions. Comfort yourself in a way that works for you.

~~~

Opening My Heart

In the Name of God, the Compassionate, the Merciful HAVE we not OPENED thine heart for thee? And taken off from thee thy burden, Which galled thy back? And have we not raised thy name for thee? Then verily along with trouble cometh ease. Verily along with trouble cometh ease. But when thou art set at liberty, then prosecute thy toil. And seek thy Lord with fervour.
—Qur'an 94:1-8, Rodwell edition

According to Islamic tradition, the Archangel Gabriel cut open the prophet Muhammad's chest, pulled out his heart, cleansed it, filled it with wisdom, knowledge, mercy, and grace, and then placed it back inside his chest. This might have occurred to him during a time of despair to give him hope and the strength to overcome adversity.

During my time of despair, nine months into chemotherapy that didn't seem to be helping much, my own chest was ripped open in a dream.

My psychotherapist and I had been discussing Marion Woodman's *The Crown of Age*. Woodman, a Jungian psychoanalyst who had cancer herself, called the illness an autoimmune disease, and said all such illnesses were death wishes. My therapist and I discussed what possible death wishes I might have had. All the possibilities we unearthed were rooted in fear.

My therapist, however, encouraged me to see the cancer not so much as a death wish as an invitation to reopen my heart so I could heal my broken emotions. I needed to deeply face my anger, fear, powerlessness, and hurt, thereby reviving my emotional life.

By opening my heart, I also would feel more connected to myself, to others, and to the Spirit.

Soon, I had the following dream:

I'm on a boat full of people. An old woman I know with short, curly, white hair takes me upstairs. Then I see her take a small blackbird, hold his chest toward her, and cut the bird's breast wide open! The bird's eyes are shut tight and it screams in agony. The woman ignores the bird's pain. She doesn't seem to have any good reason for torturing the bird.

My therapist saw the dream representing my process: What opens my heart? The blackbird probably represented my shadow, or unconscious, self. The old woman was my wiser feminine nature. It felt like torture to open my heart.

To gain more comprehension, I acted out the part of the old woman in the dream. In my house I walked up some stairs, holding a little stuffed bird and a small knife. I focused my awareness inside my body. While pretending to be the old woman, was I feeling rage? No. Fear? No. Ah, it's mostly grief. I was reminded of the Mayans cutting open human chests as sacrifices to the gods. Yet she had only opened the bird's breast—she had not taken out the heart. As the old woman, I spontaneously held the bird to my own heart, and instantly felt love and compassion.

Then I switched roles and became the blackbird. Wrapped in blankets, I experienced my chest being cut open. I felt fear, rage, pain, and powerlessness. My body writhed and shook while I screamed, moaned, cried. Finally I ended with an experience of neutrality, of nothingness. The emotions had lifted into textures and the energy moved out of my body.

I had begun reframing the purpose of the illness as an invitation to learn how to open my heart. Could I be like the thirteenth-century Sufi poet Jalāl ad-Dīn Muḥammad Rūmī, who figuratively tore at his own breast to vent his pain?

> From reed-flute hear what tale it tells;
> What plaint it makes of absence' ills:
> "From jungle-bed since me they tore,
> Men's, women's, eyes have wept right sore.
> My breast I tear and rend in twain,
> To give, through sighs, vent to my pain.
> Who's from his home snatched far away,
> Longs to return some future day....
> —"The Reed Flute"

My heart had been like Rūmī's reed, cut off and separated for so long from the cane field that it had closed down and would not even make the shrill noises in response to its pain. It was time for my chest to be torn open so my heart, like the prophet Muhammad's, could be pulled out for cleansing and purification. With an open heart, I could experience my deepest yearnings. One of those is to experience bonding with others, yet the greatest is a longing for a profound connection with the Divine. When the task of conventional medical treatments ended, I could more fervently seek the Spirit.

Thriver Soup Ingredient:

Vince Lasorso explained that when one is in a lot of pain, it's difficult, if not impossible, to meditate. So if you want to meditate but find your mind wandering endlessly, accept that this might not be the right time to fervently seek the Spirit.

As an alternative, Connie Lasorso suggested spending time in your imagination creating a beautiful sanctuary for yourself. Let your mind roam freely and play. Each day you can add a new detail. It will be a lot more fun than stressing or berating yourself over an inability to meditate.

~~~

Paradigm Shift Happens

Yet he knows the way I take; when he has tested me, I will come out like gold.
<div align="right">—Job 23:10, Complete Jewish Bible</div>

I have been tested with the refining fire of one of the worst diagnoses someone can have; and I have emerged like gold. Vince Lasorso, who has worked with cancer patients for about thirty years, calls me his poster child for making the emotional paradigm shift necessary for survival.

The purpose of healing, according to my friend Judy Merritt, PhD, is not to continue going about our lives as if nothing had happened, but "to allow the lessons and their healing wisdom to sink in and do their transformation work...the shedding of old skin, old ways of being and doing."

I felt a lot of confusion about where to begin. Confusion is a great starting point, a friend said, because it means a shift can occur. "You are not in control and doing the same old same old. You are open to knowing another new way."

If I could find the right internal switch, maybe that would help me shift into a new paradigm. Perhaps it involved finding the core emotional wounding that led to the cells rebelling. My psychotherapist had no definitive answers, so I felt I needed to do more exploring in the subconscious realm.

One switch I realized I needed to make was to let go of the workaholic side of my personality. After a few months of psychotherapy, I dreamt I was invited to move into a large, beautiful home. I went back to the office building where I lived, packed all my things, and a man moved all my boxes into the new house.

According to Carl Jung, father of analytical psychology, the place where one lives in dreams represents one's psyche. It makes perfect sense that psychologically, I had been living in an office building. How wonderful to be moving out of a work environment and into a beautiful new home! This pointed to at least one paradigm shift I needed to make to become healthy again.

I began to inspect everything in my life. No stone was left unturned. I worked with each item I unearthed, and made hard choices. Did this serve my goal of being healed and cured? If yes, it stayed in my life. If no, it had to go. The hardest, most painful choice of all was to leave my marriage of twenty-two years. After two years of questioning, I concluded that I needed to live in a peaceful sanctuary, even if it meant no health insurance and the possibility of living in poverty.

Perhaps this was the final switch that needed to be made, because my next scan was—unexpectedly—clean. Vince tells me he sees a great deal of confidence in me now that wasn't there before the diagnosis. I had been tested by the hottest fire and come out as gold.

Thriver Soup Ingredient:

Paradigm shifts are difficult and can feel excruciating. If you are determined to survive, take a good, hard look at everything in your life. Anything that does not serve your goals needs to be eliminated. Anything that pulls at your energy, drags you down, or makes you feel bad, needs to go. This can be the hardest part of healing, yet sometimes it is necessary for survival.

∾∾∾

Power of Powerlessness

But ADONAI—it is he who will go ahead of you. He will be with you. He will neither fail you nor abandon you, so don't be afraid or downhearted.

—Deuteronomy 31:8, Complete Jewish Bible

Fear and dismay have dogged me all my life. Through psychotherapy, using the Map of Emotions©, and energy work, I learned one of my behavior patterns has been to drop into the mental state of resignation. I do this when I feel hopeless about a situation and powerless to change it. After one therapy session, something clicked into place for me. Perhaps the word "resignation" didn't have quite as negative an overtone for me as the word "victim," another mood I dropped into so I could numb out my hurt.

Feeling newly empowered, I encountered another opportunity that day to experience the feelings of powerlessness in my body. I did not. Following the familiar rut in my brain, I stayed in my mind and fell into the mood of resignation. As soon as the episode was over, however, I recognized at a deeper level than before what I had done to myself. I had given up what I wanted on a mental level without checking in with my body.

I returned to the individual, feeling tension in my abdomen, neck, and jaw. I was able to stay more conscious of my inner experience. I expressed my needs, and did not back down until I got them met. Rather than finishing with the usual moods of resignation and resentment, I walked away with a surge of energy and a sense of satisfaction—a far more pleasant experience.

The next morning I dreamt that I was putting some outdated books into a bonfire. I think this symbolized an inner transformation of some old beliefs and attitudes that no longer served me—patterns that have held me back. By burning them up, new energy was released.

By allowing myself to feel powerlessness and fear in my body, these emotions lifted. Staying conscious stopped the drop into resignation. I had opened up to Divine help and healing by remaining receptive to my inner experiences. The Spirit faithfully went before me and stayed with me, lifting away my fears.

Thriver Soup Ingredient:

My friend Lois Clement told me her method of prayer. It helps bypass resignation and moves the heart into a sense of allowing, even while experiencing feelings of powerlessness. Calling in her spiritual guides, she spends a lot of time expressing gratitude. This is followed by imagining herself filled and overflowing with divine light. She asks to be open to divine guidance and asks how she can be of service. This type of practice can deepen one's experience of gratitude and peace.

$$\sim\sim\sim$$

Rock the Block: Warming the Heart of Stone

Freya married Odur.... One day, however, Odur went away, and she knew not where to find him. She wept in sadness, tears falling from her sorrowful eyes and splashing upon the rocks of the earth. The hard rocks became soft and allowed the warm tears to reach their very centres and there they solidified to become fine pieces of the purest gold. Other tears fell into the sea and became amber of the most beautiful quality.

—"Freya and Odur," *The Viking Gods: Pagan Myths of Nordic Peoples*

The power of feminine warmth and love to restore, uplift, and bring healing shows up in many myths. In the tale of Freya and Odur, I especially like how Freya's tears softened hard rocks. It reminds me of the girl Gerda whose tears saved her friend Kai in one of my favorite fairy tales, "The Snow Queen," by Hans Christian Anderson.

One day, while lying around in a post-chemotherapy daze, I watched a similar motif play out in the children's video, "Sylvester and the Magic Pebble." I had never come across this story among the thousands I had read to my children when they were young. In the tale, a mule named Sylvester finds a magic stone that he soon discovers has the power to fulfill his wishes. On his way home, he encounters a lion and, in terror, wishes he were a boulder so the lion could not gobble him up. Instantly, the pebble grants his wish.

For months, his parents desperately search for him, yet find no trace. Reconciled to the fact that their son is gone forever, they one day prepare a picnic lunch and go into the countryside. Sylvester's mother unknowingly sits on the boulder that had been her son. Her motherly warmth stirs his heart of stone, helps him revive, and he is able to return to his true self. The family is joyfully reunited.

At the same time I had been reading Dawna Markova's book, *I Will Not Die an Unlived Life*. Dawna said when our minds are still like water in a calm pond (a goal of meditation), we can look into the depths and see all our mental and emotional junk lying at the bottom—stuff we avoid noticing when we are busily stirring the waters with ceaseless thinking.

That night, just before falling asleep, I saw a spontaneous image of myself shoving a huge stone into the pond of my mind. That boulder sat in the pool, taking up space, weighing down my psyche, and blocking my view. The metaphors of the rock in the pond combined with the story of the mule and his pebble, for me, became apparent. As a young child, I allowed fear to turn parts of my heart to stone—a measure of self-protection I no longer needed. The boulder still sat in the pond of my mind. It took a life-threatening illness to awaken my awareness to its presence.

The image of the big rock sitting in my mind's pool remained so vivid I felt compelled to draw a picture of it.

Later, when discussing these events with my psychotherapist, she said the boulder I saw prior to drifting off to sleep could have been placed in my mind from either a combination of experiences or a single event. Regardless of its origin, it did not require a personal story to be removed. I could allow the rock to marinate in the pond without forcing it to break up, shrink, or move. I could mentally sit atop the stone and meditate on its purpose. I could bring warmth and love to the rock, just as Divine Mother, expressed through Freya's tears, could continue to warm my heart.

Gradually, the boulder softened and shrank as I meditated and let go of a variety of fears. By opening to the process, and to the warmth of the Divine Feminine, my heart of stone became more pliable, and I awakened more from my unconscious slumber.

Thriver Soup Ingredient:

Consider reading the children's book *Sylvester and the Magic Pebble*, by William Steig, or watching it on the "Storybook Treasures" DVD titled "Strega Nona and More Stories About Magic" from Scholastic. Amberwood Entertainment has a nice DVD version of "The Snow Queen," based on Hans Christian Andersen's fairy tale. Imagine yourself warming to the feminine aspect of the Divine and receiving motherly comfort and compassion.

~~~

Rock Unblocked: Amber Transmutations

I saw what looked like gleaming, amber-colored fire radiating from what appeared to be his waist upward.... This was how the appearance of the glory of ADONAI looked....
—Ezekiel 1:27-28, Complete Jewish Bible

The glory and presence of the Divine can be imagined in the beauty of amber (fossilized tree sap), rendered translucent when light pours through it. Amber showed up for me in mediation not long after a spontaneous image had arisen of a huge boulder sitting in the middle of the pond of my mind. The rock blocked my view and the free flow of water.

Symbolically, my new clothes dryer quit at the same time, indicating I was stuck somewhere in my process of taking on a new persona. (Apparently I was not progressing toward the newly cleaned clothes, which symbolizes a fresh way of being in the world.)

The appliance repairman said the dryer's heating element burned out because the exhaust pipe was clogged with lint. What a perfect symbol for the blockage in my psyche. The repairman explained that I needed to purchase a duct cleaner and do a little roto-rooting in the venting tube to remove the obstruction. I followed his directions, with assistance from my sons, and soon had a clean pipe.

Later, as I was meditating on the rock in my mental pool, I experienced a spontaneous image of a couple of people heaving a large round piece of amber over the stone.

A little more than a year later, at my fiftieth birthday party, my long-time friend Julia Lynch blessed me with a gleaming amber bracelet. It sits on my altar, reminding me of the presence and glory of the Spirit.

Thriver Soup Ingredient:

Place some amber, or a picture of amber, on an altar as a reminder of your ability to transmute cancer into healthy tissue through the presence of Divine light in each of your cells.

≈≈≈

Shadow Work: Dark Night Rises

When she entered the seventh gate, from her body the royal robe was removed. Inanna asked, "What is this?" She was told: "Quiet, Inanna, the ways of the underworld are perfect. They may not be questioned." Naked and bowed low, Inanna entered the throne room. Ereshkigal rose from her throne. Inanna started toward the throne. The Annuna, the judges of the underworld, surrounded her. They passed judgment against her. Then Ereshkigal fastened on Inanna the eye of death. She spoke against her the word of wrath. She uttered against her the cry of guilt. She struck her. Inanna was turned into a corpse, a piece of rotting meat, and was hung from a hook on the wall.

—*The Descent of Inanna*

Inanna was the queen of heaven for the ancient Sumerians in Mesopotamia. She decided to visit the Underworld to attend the funeral rites of her sister's husband. Her sister, Ereshkigal, was queen of the underworld. To enter into her sister's domain, Inanna was forced to give up everything. Ereshkigal represented Inanna's shadow-self, her neglected side, her deep wounds that she had repressed, all the split-off parts of herself she had denied and cut off to achieve her earthly accomplishments. Judges in the underworld saw this, and condemned her for it. Ereshkigal struck her dead.

When we resist or ignore our shadow sides, the cut-off and ignored parts of ourselves, we lose our creativity, vitality, and sexual energy. We sink lower and lower, losing pieces of ourselves bit by bit, and can eventually become ill.

Splitting starts for us in childhood. Kids hide behaviors from adults, then start policing their own thoughts. To be accepted, children create false selves. Their true selves are separated out and sink into their unconscious minds. As adults, we might view parts of our shadows, such as being stubborn, as something positive, such as being determined, to defend ourselves against others' judgments. Women often use their false senses of themselves to get what they need. They might act seductively or overly dependent in attempts to gain attention, love, power, or freedom.

These unwanted parts of ourselves don't disappear. They lurk, unsuspected, in the unconscious parts of our minds. The more light we present to the world, the deeper the darkness that waits patiently in the unconscious for the right opportunity to spring out and get our attention.

I spent some time exploring these repressed aspects of my personality, using active imagination. I discovered a stereotypical, old-fashioned, prudish, nasty inner judge. He wore a big, curly white wig and dark robes and wielded a gavel. I gave him an assignment: list ten things he likes about me. He did it.

I also discovered my inner critic: a man wearing black leather, with black and white spiky stripes on his face and head, and little sharp knives poking out of his knuckles. He was really angry, ready to rip things to shreds. He hungered for more attention.

These aspects of myself needed to be integrated back into my personality, because they were contributing to my illness. "Anything that is repressed causes destruction, a breakdown," wrote Dean Ornish in *Love and Survival: The Scientific Basis for the Healing Power of Intimacy*. "It is the real self, the undefended self, that is always fine, happy, light."

When we become aware of our shadowy aspects and work with them, we relieve our bodies from the burden of having to carry them. This is when the spiritual sides of ourselves come to the rescue. Inanna's servant, Ninshubur, represented Inanna's spiritual self. Ninshubur eventually managed to rescue Inanna. We, too, can be rescued from unconscious parts of ourselves that turn venomous if we do the inner work to bring our internal darkness into the light.

Thriver Soup Ingredient:

Robert Johnson, in his book, *Owning Your Own Shadow*, explains the importance of balancing the good with the bad. This can be done through rituals such as burning, writing, drawing, sculpting, dancing, or burying. One practice I did for several months after the diagnosis was to write angry, nasty letters to people about my true feelings concerning their behaviors. Then I created a little ceremony and burned the letters as a way to let go of the resentments.

≈≈≈

Spiral Staircase

A waterpot becomes full by the constant falling of drops of water. Similarly, the wise man, little by little, fills himself with good.

— *The Dhammapada*, 9:123

The contents of the unconscious mind are just that—unconscious. The wise unconscious mind normally will not allow itself to flood our impetuous yet unprepared egos with its contents. Little by little, our unconscious minds provide new content for our conscious minds to assimilate. I found this acutely frustrating because I felt I needed to resolve my emotional issues quickly to survive.

In my pushiness, I got ahead of the game—and my unconscious mind said, "Stop. Come back where you belong and move forward only when you have what you need." This showed up in a dream after a visit with Gary Matthews, a shamanic counselor.

In the dream I saw two staircases leading to a party at the top of a bridge; one spiraled and the other moved upward at right angles. (To me, they represented the masculine and feminine pathways of energy traveling up and down the spine. The party at the top, I believe, is spiritual bliss.) I had climbed nearly to the top of the stairs with many other people before realizing all the people were carrying trays of food. I had none. I asked a girl, "Where did you get the food?"

"Down at the bottom," she told me.

Deeply disappointed, I trudged back down to the bottom and waited in line to get provisions for the journey back up—food, which represented self-nourishment of whatever kind I needed.

My dream clearly communicated that I wasn't ready to climb to a new level. I had unwittingly tried cheating by not doing the required "work" at the base, and so was sent back down to start over.

Yet all was not lost. A couple of days later I dreamt I met a woman who had come into her power. She represented this aspect of myself rising into more awareness, and I gained more resolution of a second-chakra issue: outgrowing the whiny kid who gave away her power and played victim.

Just as some physical injuries can fester, some emotional wounds might never fully heal. Our lives are like spiral staircases. As we ascend, we revisit the same injuries over and over, just at different levels. The lions waiting at the gates of these wounds get fiercer each time we cycle around the helix. Gary admonished me to face these beasts: "Stand up to life with grace and power!"

Also like the curved staircase, I usually need to hear important messages over and over until I finally am ready to receive them. Friends might find this infuriating—I know some of mine have. Yet with love, they have consistently dripped their precious pearls of wisdom into my water pot, filling it a little more each time.

Likewise, by filling our own water pots bit by bit, we eventually can reach greater consciousness by patiently and persistently plodding up our spiral paths. When we reach an appropriate level of growth, the unconscious usually rewards us with expanded awareness.

Thriver Soup Ingredient:

Make a spiral wind catcher to remind you of the tendency humans follow in their growth—winding around, ever-upward, returning to the same lessons—yet at a higher level than before so the teaching moves more deeply into us.

What you will need:

A hard, flat surface you can get messy, such as newspaper on a table top

Two pieces of 12x12 cardstock of two colors and/or designs, one representing feminine energy and one representing masculine energy

Glue stick

Large, flat, circular object, such as a plate or lid

Pencil or pen

Scissors

Hole punch

Yarn or string for hanging

Lightweight decorative items, like ribbons, stickers, and glitter that can be used to represent your cancer journey.

Lay one piece of cardstock face down on your work surface. Cover the back side with glue. Carefully lay the back side of your second piece of card stock directly on the glued side of the first piece of paper. When done, you should have the feminine and masculine sides facing outward.

Take your large, flat, circular object and place it on your paper. Trace around it with a pen or pencil.

Cut out the circle. Continue cutting into the circle in a spiral direction. After the initial inch or so of cutting, keep your cutting width as consistent as you can. Keep cutting around until you reach the center.

Lift up the spiral from the center, and use the hole punch to place a hole in the center. Tie your piece of yarn or string through the hole. Then decorate the spiral with your lightweight symbols. Hang it in an indoor location where it can be caught by an air vent, or outside where it can catch a breeze yet won't get wet.

Whenever you look at it, offer a prayer of gratitude for how far along the spiral you have moved.

~~~

Tapas Acupressure Technique: The Deed Hunter

"Therefore I tell you, whatever you ask for in prayer, believe that you have received it, and it will be yours. And when you stand praying, if you hold anything against anyone, forgive him, so that your Father in heaven may forgive you your sins."

—Mark 11:24-25, Christian Bible, NIV

I discovered, soon after the diagnosis, that I was a resentment holdout from childhood. It was time for me to reach a place of forgiveness. For this, I turned to the Tapas Acupressure Technique, a method created to help a person ease stress and let go of painful issues from the past. The technique involves focusing on a group of statements while touching acupressure points on the back of your head and on your face.

As with the Emotional Freedom Technique, I would rate the temperature of the ruptured feelings from ten to one, with ten being the most intense to one being almost gone.

My first use of TAT involved a painful experience from the time I was six, and it ranked a ten on the emotional scale. I worked with TAT for about thirty minutes, and got the intensity down to a two. Then I looked at my third eye, on the inside of the middle of my forehead, and saw a gorgeous blue circle. Then I heard a "good work" in my mind. What a beautiful affirmation.

Every few months I had another TAT session. I realized the puffy red sties on my eyelids and infected boils on my arms that erupted when I was a girl mirrored my unconscious rage. At the time I got sties, I also learned not to cry, being given the verbal threat, "If you don't stop crying, I'll give you something to cry about." By this time, chemotherapy had dried out my eyes, so I was putting cream into my eyes again, reminiscent of the creams I put in my eyes while dealing with childhood sties.

My days of being a good girl were over. That ingrained way of operating was my sure path to the gravesite. I learned through TAT to say phrases such as, "It's over now. I can relax now and let it go. I can breathe. I can forgive now."

Through TAT I accepted and moved through the rage, sometimes allowing my body to shake violently in my chair for up to ten minutes. Eventually I moved into forgiving others and forgiving myself. This clearing opened up a wider channel between the Spirit and me, enabling more Divine love to flow into my body.

Thriver Soup Ingredient:

If there are emotional issues from the past that still plague you, and you think TAT might be of some assistance, visit www.tatlife.com/ to find out more.

∿∿∿

Visiting the World of Shadows

Hades did not disobey but spoke to his reluctant wife of what would be hers when she was with him.... Then, when she leapt up with joy to begin the long trip back to her mother, he secretly slipped her a pomegranate seed. Unwittingly, she ate it, thus ensuring her return to the underworld.

—Homeric Hymn to Demeter

The Greek god Hades rules the place of the dead, also known as the underworld. Psychologically, it is a place of darkness, despair, or depression, an experience into which many cancer patients fall.

This underground area does not, however, have to devour us—it can be mined for gold through the use of imagination. Energy intuitive Maria Paglialungo worked with me several times to go deeper into Hades to learn pieces of my emotional puzzle so I could heal and bring more conscious awareness into daily life.

When pretending mentally to venture down, I always went with the guidance of a fellow underworld traveler. I asked for and received the presence of my animal totems and spiritual guides to protect and assist me. I found myself descending through a spiral stairwell, similar to that of old stone castles in Europe. The first several times I saw tiled images of angels lining the walls. After enough visits, those mosaics became actual angel figures walking down the stairs with me.

The next stage was leaving the stairs to walk in pitch black, not knowing where I was going or what lay ahead. Dread made forging ahead difficult, yet I felt encouraged by all the spiritual assistance I was receiving.

I kept walking until I came to a dimly lit cavern. There I would meet individual characters from my past. Sometimes they would transform into vicious animals, and parts of my body would ache.

A variety of emotions surfaced—among them shock, rage, and shame. Frequently, my body shook. Sometimes I screamed into a pillow.

I would not have done such deep work on or about myself if my life literally had not been hanging on the line. Maria provided trusted guidance on my inner journey.

After one particularly intense session, I felt regal, like a queen, leaving Hades and returning to ordinary consciousness. Only later did I learn my process mirrored Persephone's mythic journeys into the depths. By negotiating with the Divine, I was able to return to normal waking life with greater wisdom, insight, and love.

Thriver Soup Ingredient:

If you are working with a mental health professional and have the energy and strength, ask this person if she or he is competent at, experienced in, and willing to guide you through a journey of your imagination into the underworld. Much gold might be hidden there, yet care must be taken to ensure your safe return to normal waking consciousness.

D. Mending the Mind

Introduction to Mending the Mind: Entering Peace Like an Arrow

> *Your worst enemy cannot harm you as much as your own thoughts, unguarded. But once mastered, no one can help you as much, not even your father or your mother.*
>
> —Dhammapada 3:43

Our minds—our thoughts, our pointless ruminations on trivialities, the stories we tell ourselves about our lives—can be the worst type of enemy. They can keep us stuck for decades in resentment or guilt or anxiety that eats away at our health. They can even drive us mad.

After a cancer diagnosis, unguarded thoughts can lead us down one empty rabbit hole after another. It's easy to slip into one and not have the strength to crawl back up to the surface. This can lead to more unnecessary misery. Who needs that?

Fortunately, we have an alternative. The practice of mindfulness is about training and then mastering the mind so we are freed from its vagaries. One Buddhist nun wrote long ago, "I, a nun, trained and self-composed, established mindfulness and entered peace like an arrow. The elements of body and mind grew still, happiness came." When we guard our thoughts diligently, we have the ability to calm ourselves and experience peace.

My mindfulness training came in the form of learning to stay conscious of my body and my thoughts, no matter my circumstances. This involved paying attention to what I was thinking from one moment to the next. I began watching the chatter of thoughts whizzing around in my brain. I found this easiest in the morning between the time I woke up and the time I got out of bed. Often I discovered my mind reviewing the same script over and over, like a bad newsreel. What a silly waste of time and energy, especially when I had one foot in the grave. I realized I had better things to do with my brain.

My psychotherapist taught me that the minute I recognize I'm falling into an old mental rut, I can divert my attention toward feeling my feet in my shoes or focusing on my breath. The more I practiced, the easier it became. This practice also helped me fall asleep at night, as long as my brain wasn't churning too much and I already felt tired.

I began to identify less with the mental gyrations and more with the part of me able to witness the rehashing. According to author Ken Wilber, this is the one Witness existing within each of us; the Divine looking out through my eyes, which is the same Spirit that's looking out through each person's eyes. And it is my true Self, the same true Self that exists in each person.

I was learning how to be more mindful by living in the now rather than regurgitating the past or running mental movies about the future; it involved experiencing each moment as it arose, without labeling, judging, or creating stories around something.

I also began to more fully understand the incredible power of the mind. For example, I have heard several times that the mind can instantly alter the body's chemistry. It has been documented that people with multiple-personality disorders can have medical conditions that only appear with one of their personalities. Conditions such as diabetes might instantly appear when one of the multiple personalities is present and disappear completely when that personality recedes. I joked that perhaps I should develop this disorder and adopt a personality that didn't have cancer. On a more serious note, I recognized that if someone can do that, then training my mind and awareness can have great benefits in every area of life.

I am able to tame my mind for brief bursts when I am aware enough to notice during the day. I'm not master of my mind yet; it still runs the show during the vast majority of my waking hours. Yet when I am paying enough attention, I can jump off the merry-go-round and re-enter my body so I can find some peace. And along with the peace comes a growing ability to hear my intuition, which will prove to be of more help to me than my parents ever could provide.

Thriver Soup Ingredient:

Try paying more attention to your moment-to-moment thoughts. Perhaps if you notice a script running through your head, write it down to get it out, to free up some space so you can be more present in your life. The more you observe your thoughts, the more power you will have over them, and the more peace you probably will experience in your life. If being in the present moment involves planning for the future, try to do your scheduling with full body awareness to keep grounded in the now.

A Reason to Live

I will not die; no, I will live and proclaim the great deeds of Yah!
—Psalm 118:17, Complete Jewish Bible

About a month after my diagnosis, energy intuitive Maria Paglialungo wanted me to come up with a reason to live. Of course, I said "to eat chocolate." Truly, though, it couldn't be for my children or for anyone else. It had to be for me. To live my life so I could tell others about the deeds of the Divine in my healing.

One friend had faced the same question. Did she want to live or not? If yes, why? She decided her answer was yes—because she wanted to experience the Divine within her body. She sought enlightenment, and oriented her life around that objective. Health returned to her body.

I learned I don't need a specific reason to live. I only need the drive to live.

So, what could resurrect that drive in my life, the urge to thrive that had receded decades earlier? I returned to the original question and my half-joking answer:

To taste chocolate,

To smell roses,

To witness more sunsets,

To ride horses again, and

To write more books, my preferred vehicle for sharing what I have learned.

Tai chi master Vince Lasorso reminded me to focus on the goal without strain, because stress damages the immune system. Bypassing the tension enables joy to emerge from these activities. The ultimate joy is experiencing the Spirit expressed through one human form.

More than a year into treatment, I suddenly felt a deep assurance that all of this—the marriage, the cancer, the end of the marriage and my cure—were part of a process to bring about my healing so I could be of service to humanity on a larger scale—something I could not have done without either experience. I sensed something big and good waiting for me when the preparations have been completed. I shall live, and I shall tell the deeds of the Divine in my life, edifying and assisting others on their journeys deeper into the Spirit.

Thriver Soup Ingredient:

Ask yourself the question, "Do I really want to live? If so, for what reason?" If you have no answer, choose today to live for something. Maybe it's to eat a chocolate truffle you've been saving, or to call someone you haven't spoken to in a while. Then tomorrow, have another reason to live that day. Gradually come up with a list of reasons to live, and access the drive to survive.

≈≈≈

Affirmations: Great Expectations

All that we are is the result of what we have thought: it is founded on our thoughts, it is made up of our thoughts. If a man speaks or acts with a pure thought, happiness follows him, like a shadow that never leaves him.

—*The Dhammapada*, 1:2

The importance of my mind's role in my life came to light one summer while working at a conference center. I stayed in an apartment with a lovely woman, Fay Gano. Soon after moving in, I walked out onto the old wooden balcony. My foot fell through the floor.

I went to the center's nurse, who told me I'd end up with a scar on my shin. My roommate, however, disagreed. She told me about affirmations, and suggested the following adapted from one taught by Emile Coué (French psychologist and pharmacist, 1857–1926): "Every day, in every way, with God's help, I'm getting better and better." It's beautifully open-ended and positive. It also is something your mind can believe, so it will resonate with your heart and emotions.

Every day that summer, during the thirty-minute walk to and from my office, I said that affirmation and visualized a clear shin. To the nurse's amazement, my skin healed beautifully.

After the 2009 diagnosis, my brother, Jim Bright, taught me to write out each of my affirmations five times every day. Author Louise Hay suggested in one of her books to hold your throat and speak the affirmations out loud. My psychotherapist pointed out that we have to deal with our emotions about issues before we can expect affirmations to be effective. It's a matter of aligning the mind, which can be fooled, with the heart, which speaks its own truth. I also learned it is the emotions, not the words, that the cells in our bodies pick up. So speak words you truly believe in with deep feeling.

Your mind is powerful. Use it to the fullest extent possible. Clear out as much negativity as you can—including from the unconscious mind—and allow happiness to become like a shadow that never departs.

Thriver Soup Ingredient:

Create your own powerful affirmation. Here are a few I like; perhaps you might find something useful among them:

Divine healing love, energy, and light now saturate every cell in my body.

My body now heals itself naturally, easily, and quickly.

The Spirit continually flows through me, bringing healing energy into my body, mind, spirit, and life.

I am successful.

Find a blank notebook. If you are able, write your affirmation in the present tense, usually with the word "now." This tells your body you are ready to receive it. Avoid all negative words like "no" and "not" and negative prefixes and suffixes such as "un" and "less." Instead, craft your words into exactly what you desire. Make sure it is something with which both your mind and your heart can agree.

For a bonus, try setting your affirmation to a familiar tune, such as "Jingle Bells" or "Happy Birthday to You." Then you can sing it while cooking, taking a shower, or walking to keep your mind occupied with what you are moving toward.

Jim suggested writing an affirmation by hand five times each day (this is why one sentence is most useful—it is far easier to maintain the practice when it takes five minutes or less). As you are writing the affirmation the first time, say it loudly; as you are writing the affirmation a second time, speak it in a normal voice; for the third, talk softly; the fourth time, whisper; and the fifth time say it silently to yourself.

As you write, hold your other hand to your voice box so you feel the vibrations created by the words.

During the whole process, allow yourself to emotionally experience what your life will be like when this affirmation becomes a reality. Add some sort of visual to your affirmation to include yet another of your five senses, further engaging your mind in a positive experience.

When you are done writing and saying your affirmation, close with a sense of gratitude, even if it is simply for the ability to speak or think an affirmation.

∽∽∽

Anxiety Pills

Do not be anxious about anything, but in every situation, by prayer and petition, with thanksgiving, present your requests to God. And the peace of God, which transcends all understanding, will guard your hearts and your minds in Christ Jesus. Finally, brothers and sisters, whatever is true, whatever is noble, whatever is right, whatever is pure, whatever is lovely, whatever is admirable—if anything is excellent or praiseworthy—think about such things.

—Philippians 4:6-8, Christian Bible, NIV

If I wasn't too much of a worry-wart before the diagnosis, I was after. For a cancer patient, anxiety is almost a given, nearly as insidious as the disease itself. "Oh, no! What if I can't control the nausea on the next type of chemotherapy? What if my scan shows a new nodule? What if I die during surgery?"

The what-if's can crowd out everything else, even to the point of making you throw up. It can overwhelm at almost any stage of the process, including when treatment is over and someone is considered cured.

My psychotherapist pointed out that anxiety starts with the emotion of fear in the body. For me, the fear usually showed up in my tense face and gut. Then my brain kicked in, producing anxiety. I had "so many bad thinks," as Vince Lasorso pointed out.

The key to letting go of the anxiety and the bad thinks was to refocus my attention on the sensations in my body. I realized my thinking about my dread was my way of escaping the actual emotion, which showed up as uncomfortable sensations in my body.

Through practice, I was able to identify the fear in my body, to allow it to be what it was, and to stop my bad thinks. While learning this technique, it helped me to refocus my mind on things that were beautiful, admirable, and true—the reflection of sunlight on pine needles, the sweet scent of cinnamon, the vibration of a dulcimer. Another prescription for anxiety that helped was to pray. Bringing my fears to the Spirit and asking for assistance helped me let go of some bad thinks. A third method was refocusing on anything for which I could feel grateful. Even a small thing, like "Today I opened my eyes again."

With practice, the need for anxiety pills—if you take them—might lessen. Maybe you can, after discussion with your doctor, ditch them. You can create a new prescription—one that relies on your focused attention and reduces the chemical burden on your body.

Thriver Soup Ingredient:

When you feel anxious, check in with how your body feels. Are you tense in your face? Does your chest tighten? Does your stomach contract? Try to let go of your thoughts and simply focus on the sensation in your body. Allow it to be what it is. Allow it to move around; allow it to get intense; and allow it to dissolve. And if your brain still insists on thinking, try to redirect your thoughts to the Divine or practice offering gratitude—even if only for a moment.

~~~

Be Self-full

In a deep-dug pit a man buries a treasure with this thought: "In time of need 'twill be a help to me, or if the rajah speak ill of me, if by a robber I am plundered, or to pay my debts, or when food is hard to get, or when ill-luck befalls." Such are the reasons in this world for burying a treasure. Yet all this treasure thus well concealed in its deep hiding-place—It profits the owner not at all.

—"The Hidden Treasure," *Khuddaka-Patha*

My inner treasures had been buried most of my life. I had not been authentic with others because of an unconscious desire to please. My behavior, I later realized, was rooted in fear of abandonment.

Cancer opened the lid of my internal treasure box and I slowly began to regain my true Self. Vince Lasorso encouraged me from the beginning to be selfish—not in a narcissistic way, but in an authentic, rich, Self-full, Self-focused way. My therapist added that one of my spiritual lessons was to pay attention to my needs first.

My acquaintance Susan explained that caring for others before ourselves leaves us without inner selves and only leads to resentment and rage. "We gotta find our true inner power and live from the place that Barbara Marx Hubbard referred to as 'vocational arousal'—juicy with our passion and life purpose, bringing forth the brand or individual ray of the collective light and spirit that only we each can offer to the world."

I learned that being self-full involved honoring who I truly am, remembering that my eternal soul simply is experiencing human conditions, and realizing the Spirit is living and experiencing the world through my life. As a being created from light and love, I deserved the loving attention only I could give myself.

Bernie Siegel, MD, wrote, "An unreserved, positive self-adoration remains the essence of health, the most important asset a patient must gain." Such a standpoint can even reverse illness, "almost as if the individual is reborn and rejects the old self and its disease, thereby becoming able to identify the tumor as something distinct and separate from the new self."

Gradually I opened to this new way of viewing life. When my hair started falling out, I donned a turban and dubbed myself Turbanator. My sense of Self-fullness grew. It felt wonderful, like walking out of a murky, slippery slough of despondency and up onto firm, dry land.

I began to understand that my authentic Self—my truest treasure—is my greatest gift to myself and others. It was unprofitable while hidden deep inside, yet offers riches untold when finally brought into the light of awareness.

Thriver Soup Ingredient:

Find an enchanting piece of stationary and a beautiful pen. Write a love letter to yourself on it, describing all the beauty within your soul and all the kind things you have done for yourself and others. Take your time, and dress up your prose with juicy, lush, rich adjectives. When you are finished, offer up gratitude to the Divine for these gifts, and cherish them within yourself.

∾∾∾

Blame Games

As he went along, he saw a man blind from birth. His disciples asked him, "Rabbi, who sinned, this man or his parents, that he was born blind?" "Neither this man nor his parents sinned," said Jesus, "but this happened so that the works of God might be displayed in him."

—John 9:1-3, Christian Bible, NIV

In this Gospel story, Jesus' disciples wanted to blame the blind man or his parents for the blindness. My questions along the sarcoma journey were similar because of the shame I experienced about the diagnosis. What did I do wrong to bring about the cancer in my body? How could I have let this happen? What flaws in my character or way of thinking or methods of dealing with life brought this on?

Even Marion Woodman, widely known Jungian psychoanalyst, listed six reasons why she might have contracted uterine cancer, and all of them were based in her psyche. She clearly saw a connection between mind and body.

I probably could have come up with at least a dozen quite valid reasons for why I had the diagnosis. All of them led to a sense of guilt, which was counter-productive anger turned in upon myself.

Treya and Ken Wilber exposed their tussle with this issue throughout their book *Grace and Grit*, and Ken wrote more about it online. For five years, others gave them opinions on what she had done spiritually wrong, yet none of the theories were the same. The individuals who spoke did, however, share the "arrogant assumption that they knew what was really moving Treya, or their own fears projected onto Treya and read back to her as the cause of her cancer."

Fortunately, this took place during the 1980s. There seems to be more acceptance of cancer now since it is widespread, so I didn't face much in the way of others' blame. I manufactured enough for myself.

Self-blame is self-defeating because it creates negative thoughts that interfere with the body's attempts to heal itself. It would be more beneficial to practice forgiving myself for anything I might have done that contributed to the illness.

It helped me to know that Woodman, who spent decades healing her own psyche, and Sri Ramakrishna, an enlightened spiritual master, still ended up getting cancer; yet billions of people don't get cancer, even if they are sleepwalking through their lives, never dealing with their issues. Even many whose lives exhibit evil don't get cancer.

Of course there are emotional, mental, and spiritual factors that can come to play in an illness. I wanted to understand all those factors affecting my situation in my attempt to control the cancer. I figured if I could comprehend how it originated, then I could diminish its effects on my life. And maybe even be cured.

Yet I have learned that our egos do not control or create our realities. The Divine is not a great vending machine in the sky we can use to dispense whatever goodies we want if we insert a prayer, nor is the Spirit a vengeful being who punishes us.

Do our egos influence reality? Sure they do. I live within a complex mystery, which opens up space for me to make choices that affect what occurs in my life. This relieves me of the need to blame myself when things head south, or the ego trip that comes when life seems to be going well. It opens doorways into gratitude and self-acceptance.

A more helpful stance that moved me beyond self-blame was to consider how to maximize the cancer encounter to bring about healing, or even a cure. This is what Treya did during her five-year cancer journey. Cancer can be viewed as an initiation into a more profound manifestation of inner wisdom. What I have experienced is an alchemical process resulting in inner gold more valuable to me than anything. I would, however, like to live long enough to manifest this new wisdom in such a way that others will benefit.

Another important direction could involve probing how I might mine the occurrence for more precious insights. The diagnosis could refocus my attention on living inside of and loving my body, rather than treating it as a shell I carried around out of necessity. As Vince Lasorso suggested, it could expand into questions such as, "Who do I want this new Heidi to be? What qualities do I want to possess?"

The best attitude is what my psychotherapist urged me to adopt: to simply accept cancer for what it is and move forward. Drop the self-blame and ask how I can best use this experience. To judge myself as flawed for contracting an illness was to potentially miss the point. After all, the enlightened master Jesus said the blind man and his parents were blameless. The purpose of the blindness was simply to glorify the Divine. Perhaps that is the purpose behind your cancer as well.

Thriver Soup Ingredient:
Ponder this poem by Jalāl ad-Dīn Muḥammad Rūmī, a 13th-century Sufi mystic:
When my soul soared
To that blessed sphere
I was free of the tyranny
Of "why?" and "how?"
At last
The thousand veils lifted
And I could behold
The hidden secret.

∾∾∾

Bucket List: As You Like It

I died regretful of three things. What were they? I never had enough of beholding the Exalted One. I died regretting it. I never had enough of hearing the good Norm. I died regretting it. I never had enough of serving the Order of Brethren. I died regretting it.

—"After Death," *Anguttara Nikaya*

No one wants to die with regrets.

Not even the two men from opposite ends of the economic spectrum who meet in a cancer hospital in the 2008 comedy-drama "The Bucket List." They form an unlikely friendship and make lists of the last things they want to do with their lives before they "kick the bucket" (die).

The bucket list included simple things like "laugh 'till I cry" and "help a complete stranger for the good," along with a catalog of world travel destinations.

My then-husband and I laughed heartily through the movie when it came out. After the cancer diagnosis, he encouraged me to write my own bucket list. Naturally it included things like watching my kids graduate from high school and college, attending their weddings, and holding their children in my arms. I didn't have any control over those events, so I decided to use a visual to help make them a reality. Using click art, I printed out two images of graduation caps and taped them onto the glass front of a family portrait so it looked like both sons were graduating. It looked tacky, yet conveyed the right message.

Otherwise, I felt I had already done most of what I wanted to do, so my list of what I could control was quite short—see the northern lights in Norway, take a cruise to Alaska and see Denali, and spend Christmas in Heidelberg and Rottenburg, Germany.

I cheated on the first item—I found a video on YouTube.com showing a night of northern lights above Norway.

Couldn't cheat so easily on the trip to Alaska. My then-husband planned a wonderful vacation the following summer, and my ankhologist helped us plan around the three-week event. Even while living with chemo side effects, our vacation fulfilled everything I'd hoped for and more. We witnessed glaciers calving in Glacier Bay; watched the midnight sun at 2 a.m.; and basked in awe at the sheer immensity of Denali Peak.

As I moved through my process, my bucket list grew. I found that when I was experiencing down time in the hospital, I could still fill my mind with wonderful fantasies. I recalled Viktor Frankl's 1946 book *Man's Search for Meaning,* in which he explored his experiences as a Nazi concentration camp inmate. He found that prisoners who tended to survive were those who could envision themselves doing what they loved in the future.

Even if I don't physically live out my fantasies, I will have relished living them in my mind. Not everyone is lucky enough to reach remission with its open door to fulfill a bucket list, but the imagination can almost always be accessed.

I want to feel I lived an abundant, joyful life, experiencing as many of my dreams as possible. I want to avoid a mind clouded with regrets when I pass. Having a list of items guides me as I move toward greater internal fulfillment.

Thriver Soup Ingredient:

Using your journal, make out your own bucket list. There is no limit. Be expansive, and go for the really important and joyous items. What do you really want to do with your life? What unfinished business do you have—to experience, to give, to heal, to learn? List at least ten items and prioritize them. Then commit to finishing them, and ask the Divine to grant you the time and the means to complete your list. As you cross each item off your list, add another for fun and see how far you can get.

~~~

Cause of Cancer: Checkmate

Surely this present life is only a play, and pastime! but if ye believe, fear God; He will give you your rewards.

—Qur'an 47:36, Rodwell edition

The Islamic prophet Muhammad had perspective on this game we call life. If what he wrote is true, life is but a chess tournament, cancer sits across the playing board, and we've been check-mated. I didn't really understand the rules of this game, much less know how to respond to the threat of losing this round.

I thought that by learning the rules, I could control the outcome of the game. At first I subscribed to the belief that my emotions were the seedbed from which my illness grew, making me responsible for my illness. There's nothing quite so guilt-producing and emotionally damaging as self-blame.

As time went on, I learned that dinosaurs and wild animals have died from cancer. My psychotherapist told me about a theory that it might take ten generations for changes in brain structure to produce schizophrenia. Perhaps the sarcoma had been generations in the making.

My friend Mica Renes pointed out that some New Age adherents expect us to be able to create happy, healthy lives, but—like Muhammad said—that's not why we are here. We chose these bodies and our parents for specific lessons. Life is messy. Giving up control is part of the lesson.

My vista opened up.

One friend suggested viewing cancer not as a disease but as a survival mechanism. This could make looking at the underlying cause more possible because this perspective would reduce the sense of shame that often accompanies the illness.

I found assistance from Ken Wilber's book, *Grace and Grit*. His wife Treya, who had cancer for five years, believed cancer had many causes, including one's genes, the environment, choices in life-style, and personality. To believe that only one's personality brought on the illness overlooks the fact that thinking we are in control of everything in our lives is a destructive illusion.

I could feel my body let go of tension, especially in my abdomen. I didn't have to blame myself so much anymore. I didn't have to pretend to be in control or impress others with how hard I worked at resolving old issues. I didn't have to struggle so insanely hard to do everything "right" to survive.

That didn't leave me free of responsibility. Ken explained the importance of determining if the disease originated on the physical, emotional, mental, or spiritual level. Then, it's best to treat the illness primarily from that level. For example, if the cause of cancer is smoking, the first approach to treatment is to stop smoking. If there is a mixture of causes behind the cancer, then use a corresponding mixture of responses. I also would recommend addressing the illness on all levels, at least to some extent, to increase your chances of survival: physical, emotional, mental, social, and spiritual. Because of the deadliness of the diagnosis I was given, I knew I needed to treat each aspect of my life if I was going to survive.

If you're not sure about which arena in your life gave rise to cancer, then start with possible physical causes before moving to the emotional, and make sure those bases are covered before moving to the mental, and so on. I chose to work 100 percent on each of these aspects to maximize my chances for survival.

I suspected numerous contributions to the diagnosis. On a physical level, my mother had passed from cancer and my father caught cancer early, indicating a genetic predisposition. During my first pregnancy, the embryo planted itself too low in my uterus, which I have since heard can be a precursor to cancer. I later had fertility treatments for a couple of years. On the emotional level there were multiple potential contributors, especially stuck and unconscious feelings.

I don't know if any or all of them had caused the cancer, and it eventually had little impact on my journey. Even if I had been told the illness was simply a natural phenomenon, I still would have followed the journey I made because I felt called to do so. I felt compelled to be 100 percent active in addressing any possible physical, emotional, mental, spiritual, and social causes.

Whatever its root cause, a cancer diagnosis is a checkmate, a time to pay more attention to the game of life. Explore your options for survival. Along the way, you might find the process an initiation into profound grace.

That sounds like the perfect prize to me.

Thriver Soup Ingredient:

Here are some questions to play with and explore. Perhaps something useful might show up for you as you journal about them.

If I had a pet that was diagnosed with cancer, would I blame the pet?

Is it possible I contributed to the cause of this cancer? If so, in what ways? For me, the answers fell into the emotional range: stuffing feelings, working too much, not paying enough attention to my body. Even while exploring these, I continued addressing the cancer in the realms of the body, mind, spirit, and social interaction. I wanted all my bases covered.

Is it possible I was allowing the cancer to continue? If so, in what ways? For me, I eventually discovered that by staying in my marriage, I wasn't providing my emotional aspect with the space to heal. I needed to remove myself from the stress caused by the relationship before my body could relax enough to rebalance itself and get well.

How can I change my life to remove these obstacles to my cure? For me, I had to move out of the house and make a separate life for myself. I needed to learn to take care of my needs first and to enjoy my life.

≈≈≈

Cherishing My Gifts: Bringing *Hidden Voices* into the Light

Do not neglect your gift...

—1 Timothy 4:14, Christian Bible, NIV

Part of my journey through cancer involved learning to deeply accept, develop, and use my many gifts.

In 1998, soon after my youngest son was born, I gave birth to my first traditionally published book: *Hidden Voices: Biblical Women and Our Christian Heritage*. Because I had an infant and a preschooler to care for, I didn't devote the time to promoting the book that it deserved; when my time began to open up, I became ill.

Fortunately, the book sold well on its own.

In April 2010, I found out the nodule in my lung was regrowing, and my then-husband had said he wanted out of the marriage. I had a long talk with a friend about how I could have financial security on my own, with no job, when I was in treatment for stage IV cancer. He told me maybe it was time for me to write a best-seller.

And then came the most amazing, auspicious coincidence. After searching amazon.com for another book, I decided to check on *Hidden Voices* just for fun. I noticed it no longer was available, yet seven new copies were being offered through other sellers. For the first time, I looked at this page and was shocked to see the price of my book ranged from $28 to $2,499!

I was fairly certain the final price is a misprint. However, for such a price to show up when it did—while I was starting my second type of chemotherapy treatment, fearing for my life and my marriage—indicated several things to me. First, I needed to recognize that my financial supply ultimately comes from the Divine, not from an organization or from other human beings. Second, I needed to recognize that I am a valuable human being, with important gifts to offer to others. Third, I needed to continue seeing the importance of *Hidden Voices* in helping Christian women see their own value. Fourth, I needed to get busy writing my other books because of the value they would give to others.

A psychotherapist and friend, Judy Merritt, PhD, found even more value in my online find: "Perhaps that price is the Universe's subtle way of telling you something about your voice... something about the Divine healing energy that lives in your body...something about how outrageously valuable your body, your voice, your spirit are to the world...so valuable, that no real price can be set, and the value is no mistake...like the women in the Bible, whose roles and voices you took 5 years to unearth, you are one of them."

Nearly a year and a half later, just for fun, I rechecked *Hidden Voices* on the amazon.com website. Much to my surprise, a new copy was on sale for $248.49. Unlike the $2,499.99 price, this did not appear to be a typo. The next highest was priced at $139.02, and the next at $127.69, all from different sellers. I realized, once again, the Divine was telling me to go out and talk about the issues raised in my book.

My brother, Walter Bright, explained these hilarious and odd book prices: "The selling prices are often not set by a person. They're set by a computer program set up by the seller to 'scrape' other prices for the same item from Amazon's web site, and use that to set their own price. They do this because they are putting thousands of books up for sale.

"Those programs use various algorithms; some set a price a percentage higher than any of the others, some a percentage lower. They'll often check the other prices regularly and reset theirs."

Despite this news, I again did a search for *Hidden Voices* to see how it was doing at the local library, and stumbled across a second traditionally published book written by me. I had created some church curriculum material that the denomination had turned into a book. Being deeply involved in treatment when it was published, that knowledge had somehow escaped me. I was thrilled.

Even after a year into my remission, an online copy of *Hidden Voices* was being offered for $999.00. The Divine still wouldn't let me off the hook. I needed to cherish and use my gifts, which meant it was time get out and talk about my book. To honor the guidance I received, I joined Toastmasters International to become a better speaker, with an eye toward creating speaking engagements on themes presented in my books.

Thriver Soup Ingredient:

Pay close attention to seeming coincidences. They might hold messages for you. For greater clarity around synchronicities in life, read *The Three "Only" Things: Tapping the Power of Dreams, Coincidence and Imagination* by Robert Moss. Moss created a practice called "active dreaming," an original synthesis of dream work and shamanism.

Disease is Evil: A Farewell to Harms

Protect her, moreover, from every affliction and ailment, from all pain and sickness, and from what-soever may be abhorrent unto Thee.

—"CXLVI," Prayers and Meditations

Pain and sickness are abhorrent to the Spirit. Twentieth century spiritual leader Bruno Gröning taught that illness is evil and not within the will of the Divine.

I had the tendency to think that I would only be cured if it was the will of the Divine. After much reading, I came to understand that the Spirit is not the author of sickness and confusion, but the bringer of joy, bliss, love, and good health. In Matthew 8:16-17 of the Christian Bible, Jesus was reported to have healed all who were sick, not just a select group.

During my journey, I thought about Randy Pausch, PhD, who wrote *The Last Lecture* and died of pancreatic cancer in 2008. He believed he would die of the disease because that's what he was told by those whom one of my friends had called "the high priests of health."

And he did.

Did he have to? Perhaps. Perhaps that was his specific purpose, to learn from the experience and to teach others how to live. Thousands gained wisdom from his book. As it says in the Christian New Testament, "where sin abounded, grace did much more abound." I'm not saying Pausch sinned. I'm saying where there is evil, as was the illness he died from, grace can enter in and bring about much goodness. Certainly his wisdom has richly blessed many others' lives.

Many people, however, are living for several years with pancreatic cancer, especially through the care of Nicholas Gonzales, MD. Part of the alternative doctor's program involves patients consuming large quantities of pancreatic enzymes each day.

Our bodies do break down because we live in a broken world and within bodies that are susceptible to illness. That doesn't make us or our behavior evil for experiencing an illness. Rather, the disease itself is evil, the opposite of the goodness of health. While I do not believe illness is caused by the Divine, I do think the Spirit allows disease to strike and death to occur simply because it is a part of our human condition. Yogananda wrote, "There can be no images of light without contrasting shadows. Unless evil had been created, man would not know the opposite, good." Beyond that, I believe the Spirit can use a disease, and even death, to bring about greater good, as I think happened with Pausch. In addition, I believe the Divine can cure anything, if that serves a higher purpose. Those surviving for years with pancreatic cancer are providing hope for thousands of people expected to die in a matter of months.

A few months after my treatment ended, someone told me about a cancer patient who was told to "get her affairs in order." While the bearer of bad news might have thought he or she was being honest about a given situation, such a phrase can steal hope like a child letting the air out of a balloon. I reacted to the story with a sudden rush of fury. I said, "You know what I think of people who say that?" and held up my finger. This was not my old style by any stretch. It reflected a "take your prognosis and shove it" attitude that raises life force energy in the body. One friend had said many times it's the women who get angry who get well.

Following a cancer diagnosis, feeling rage about the abhorrent dis-ease that grips our bodies can bring up vital life-force energy that promotes healing. Understanding that the Divine wants health and healing for us can strengthen us to find ways to live longer. Or it can lead to grace that cures without our doing anything. Or even if we try everything and work as hard as we can to live, we still might not. It is mystery. So even if the Divine allows us to pass into the next life, the evil of cancer in our bodies will still be eliminated. It loses no matter what we do—or don't do.

Thriver Soup Ingredient:

Ask for protection from the evil disease cancer. Demand your Divine right to a cure. As you talk to the Spirit, see if you can feel your life force energy rise and give you strength. We can always hope that we are among those who will live longer. Yet, like Randy Pausch, some of us won't make it, no matter what we do or believe. Perhaps the Divine has an inscrutable reason for this. Whatever the outcome, however, at least we will know we gave it our best—and possibly helped others live better lives as a result.

≈≈≈

Exercising the Will: How to Tame Your Dragon

Now when the Blessed One had thus entered upon the rainy season, there fell upon him a dire sickness, and sharp pains came upon him, even unto death. But the Blessed One, mindful and self-possessed, bore them without complaint. Then this thought occurred to the Blessed One, 'It would not be right for me to pass away from existence without addressing the disciples, without taking leave of the order. Let me now, by a strong effort of the will, bend this sickness down again, and keep my hold on life till the allotted time be come.' And the Blessed One, by a strong effort of the will, bent that sickness down again, and kept his hold on life till the time he fixed upon should come. And the sickness abated upon him.

—"The Book of that Great Decease," *Buddhist Suttas*

Buddha had incredible willpower, and used it to bend sickness to his need. Kenneth Pelletier, MD, studied the psychology of numerous patients who recovered from illness despite great odds, wrote Bernie Siegel, MD. Their five characteristics held in common included:

1. Deep internal shifts that occurred through spiritual practices.
2. Improved interpersonal relationships.
3. Choosing a diet offering optimal nutrition.
4. A deepened sense of both the spiritual and material aspects of life.
5. A felt sense that they regained health as a result of their own difficult struggles.

Like the Buddha, these people used strong determination to bend their illnesses so they could recover. They apparently took nothing for granted: they took control of whatever they could and worked with whatever they had to elicit healing responses in their bodies.

I didn't come across this list for more than two years, yet felt I had followed each of the points. The clean scans certainly came after "a long, hard struggle." And I feel I did the other four items.

I think in my case, the clean scans were a matter of Divine grace, others' prayers, and my hard work.

When I look at what I have done and hear others' stories, I am amazed at how much more I have done to help myself. Surely if what I have done is not enough, there is nothing more I could have done or not done that would have helped. Others have done far less and been cured. I threw my whole being into this process. For me, healing was more than a full-time job.

One practice that came out of the process was learning more fully to select my thoughts at every moment, just as I pick out my clothes for each day. That is all I can control. Yet those thoughts, applied with force of will, lead to discipline that can bring desired results.

Thriver Soup Ingredient:

Take the ideas presented in *Thriver Soup* that you find useful, and others you find appealing, and apply them to your life with intense willpower. Acknowledge the grace to grow and change that comes from the Spirit.

∿∿∿

Family Patterns: Repetition Compulsion

But he said to me, "My grace is sufficient for you, for my power is made perfect in weakness." Therefore I will boast all the more gladly about my weaknesses, so that Christ's power may rest on me.
—2 Corinthians 12:9, Christian Bible, NIV

The Christian Apostle Paul had a "thorn in the flesh" (no one's sure what that was), and when he asked in prayer for it to be removed, he was told that the Spirit's power was made perfect in his weakness.

One weakness many people share, that can highlight the grace and power of the Divine, is a repetition compulsion. Alberto Villoldo, PhD, in his book *Shaman, Healer, Sage*, explained it well: "We gravitate to people and situations that will allow us to relive the circumstances of the original wounding in an attempt to heal it."

In my life, the compulsion took the form of an unconscious drive to recreate and repeat unhealthy behaviors I experienced during childhood. This weakness was necessary for me to wake up and see the patterns. I couldn't hope to change my unconscious proclivities until I saw them. Herein lay the perfection of my weaknesses.

Two years after the diagnosis, Vince Lasorso was doing energy work on my body. He asked me what was going on when my mother, who'd had breast cancer, went into remission. As I thought about his question, I began to see a connection between her situation and my own. As recognition of my compulsion to repeat her pattern dawned, Vince said he felt my body let go of a lot of energy. Then he asked what was going on in her life when the cancer returned. Again, when I connected her situation with my own, he said he felt my body let go of a lot of energy. I realized I needed to break those unhealthy patterns.

The next day I met with Hari Sharma, MD, my Ayurvedic physician. He said my Ayurvedic pulse and other indicators showed that I was quite healthy, my blood was clean, and there was no need to detox. This was not a great surprise, yet I was pleased with his confirmation. He expressed surprise that I'd developed a lung nodule a few months before and was recovering from its surgical removal. After telling Dr. Sharma about my experience with Vince the day before, we both agreed the issue for me was stress. I needed to remove the significant sources of stress from my life. He made several recommendations, including an Ayurvedic formula for easing the effects of stress on my body.

By recognizing my pattern, which was a repeat of my mother's experiences, I was able to make changes that led to my entering and staying in remission. My weakness had led to insight and greater opportunity for the Spirit to manifest power in my life.

Thriver Soup Ingredient:

If you had another family member with a serious illness, take a look at the circumstances surrounding the person's age and life situation. See if you can find a parallel with your situation. If so, ask yourself what you can change to alter the pattern in your own life. Discussing this with a mental health professional might bring greater clarity.

～～～

Forgiveness: Stairway to Heaven

I forgive all beings, may all beings forgive me. I have friendship toward all, malice toward none.
—Jain salutation

Forgiving all beings, including ourselves, is a tall order, yet an extremely important goal—especially for cancer patients. When we harbor resentments, play victim or martyr, or feel disgust, the one against whom we experience these moods isn't damaged by them. Instead, we are. These mental constructs, if left untended, can wreak havoc on our immune systems at a time when we need these disease-fighting abilities the most.

I am not diminishing the pain done to us. Sometimes the agony inflicted is unbelievable. Yet I came to understand the importance of forgiveness when I looked at the broad range of my existence. I think it is possible that my inability to forgive in previous existences has led me to the great pain in my current life. For me to prevent more pain in my future existences, I believe I need to reach a place where I can forgive myself and all other beings—including the Divine—for everything.

By harboring resentments toward others, I was creating mental stories and living in the past instead of experiencing my life in the now. Every time my mind replayed the old painful sagas, my body responded by dumping toxins into my bloodstream. That was the last thing I needed.

The cancer experience invites us to make amends with others, ourselves, and the Divine. This includes being able to forgive everyone for everything. It is a gift we can give ourselves in the midst of our physical trials.

All humans suffer. When some suffer, they lash out at others in a misguided attempt to ease their own pain. When I was profoundly hurt by someone decades earlier, I was encouraged to forgive. I tried, yet eventually realized I simply wasn't ready. I needed to do some healing before I could authentically and completely forgive. It took seven years, yet when I did, I physically experienced a weight lift off me. It was I who benefitted from my finally being able to forgive. I felt so much better.

I also came to realize that by not forgiving others, I was trying to insist they become who I wanted or expected them to be, not who they were. I wanted to remake them into my image. It was a declaration of basic inequality between them and me. That ego-based position needed to go.

When we forgive ourselves, we let go of guilt and self-criticism, learning to accept the parts of ourselves that have caused distress. By experiencing and accepting these forbidden, seemingly unacceptable, or forgotten elements of our personalities, we can become more whole. This frees up energy for physical healing. The Spirit forgives us as well. I like what the Qur'an says in Sura 4:106: "But seek the forgiveness Of God; for God is Oft-forgiving, Most Merciful."

Forgiving the Divine for our circumstances enables us to open to the possibility that the Spirit really does know what's best for our growth. I don't think we are limited to this finite human experience. I believe we have eternal souls that entered into human bodies to learn and grow, and what we gain will be ours forever.

Practicing forgiveness is a spiritual discipline, because each incident for which we can forgive provides an opportunity to heal something within ourselves. Forgiveness is best practiced on an ongoing basis. We have the choice of being enslaved to our pain and self-defensive egos or becoming free within our souls. It might take several attempts at letting go before we are released from our resentments, blaming behavior, victim or martyr status, self-pity, anxiety, desperation, resignation, or disgust around a particular event or circumstance. It's human, and it's okay. We can forgive ourselves for not fully forgiving; and we can always be willing to be willing to be willing to forgive. Then we can live what members of the Jain religion teach, which is to wish no harm on any being and to practice forgiveness as long as we inhabit human bodies.

Thriver Soup Ingredient:

Obtain a bowl or cup for your home altar. Some people might want to use a Tibetan singing bowl.

Whenever you feel the need, intentionally fill the bowl with your negative thoughts and emotions around the need to forgive yourself or others. When the bowl is filled, raise it up in front of you and ask the Divine to take it. Then ask the Spirit to fill your bowl with blessings and love. Lower it back down and emotionally receive the goodness that flows from the Divine. Close with thanksgiving.

~ ~ ~

Gift Nobody Wants

How resplendent the luminaries of knowledge that shine in an atom, and how vast the oceans of wisdom that surge within a drop! To a supreme degree is this true of man, who, among all created things, has been invested with the robe of such gifts, and hath been singled out for the glory of such distinction. For in him are potentially revealed all the attributes and names of God to a degree that no other created being hath excelled or surpassed. All these names and attributes are applicable to him. Even as He hath said: "Man is My mystery, and I am his mystery."

—Bahá'u'lláh, *The Book of Certitude*

Bahá'u'lláh (1817–1892), founder of the Bahá'í Faith, saw humans as invested with vast gifts that potentially can reveal all the attributes of the Divine.

I heard many people say cancer was a gift to them because it changed their lives for the better. When the illness shows up, however, it's generally not seen as a gift.

My family quickly saw the gift of cancer show up in my life. They expressed surprise that I seemed happier and more relaxed than I had been for decades. They wondered at first if I was putting on a show, but they eventually saw it as genuine. My neighbor also commented on how much more relaxed I was. What a nice affirmation of the changes I made in my life.

A few months after the diagnosis, I had begun feeling quite content about my situation. I saw myself on an accelerated path of growth and insight, healing areas of my life I didn't even know needed it. Growth felt good. I was filled and surrounded by love and support. I usually was free of pain. I began truly enjoying my life, doing things I never allowed myself to do before, and starting projects I had put off my entire adult life. I smiled as I thought about how this learning process helped me become an even better writer, a prospect I found extremely fulfilling.

Then I received an email from a relative who said, "I really think you are going to beat this cancer. You have a sparkle in your eyes that I haven't seen since your childhood photos."

I nearly cried.

I wasn't done receiving the many gifts of cancer. After nearly two years of chemotherapy, when another regimen was about to exact its toll, I looked in the mirror. A wrinkled-up, freckled old face fronted my growing bald patches. My marriage was over; my life had been stripped; my body felt weak, exposed, and vulnerable. I felt like a kitten tossed into a rapidly roiling stream, drowning in terror. Heaviness, like a millstone, settled in my gut.

At the same time, I acknowledged that my inner light shone forth more powerfully than ever, and will continue to do so. It's like being a sealed clay pot full of gold coins; the jar has to be broken before the coins can spill out and be of use.

Would I trade what I have gained? No, I believe this was meant to be, exactly as it happened. As I write each entry in this book, a deep sense of purpose and fulfillment fills me with satisfaction. I received a multitude of gifts from cancer; others have gifted me with love, support, prayers, and presents; and now I am preparing this book, my gift for others, revealing attributes that make cancer survivors reflections of Divine attributes.

So, in a way, I was glad I was on my final attempt at chemotherapy and there was no drug routine afterward, as sarcoma patients have few options. Before, I had felt jealous of women with other types of cancer—they had many different, helpful drugs to try. My bag of tricks was empty, and I had been fully thrust into the arms of Divine Mother for healing. It was time for me to become that atom resplendent with knowledge, that drop surging with vast oceans of wisdom.

Thriver Soup Ingredient:

Sit in your favorite meditation posture. Take several slow, deep breaths. When you are centered, imagine yourself to be a drop of the ocean. When settled in that image, ask the Divine to infuse you with knowledge and wisdom. Allow it to arrive inside you in whatever form it comes—as a rainbow, a waterfall, or perhaps streams of light. Sit with this experience for a while, basking in the love and joy.

Close with deep gratitude.

∼∼∼

I Will Survive

[H]e who is able to control himself is mighty.

—Tao Te Ching, 33

Prognosis: Time to master myself. And time for miracles.

With the chemotherapy regimen prescribed by my first ankhologist, I was given a seven percent chance for a cure. My brother, Jim Bright, wrote, "I would rather take a risk on an experimental treatment than commit to one with such a low probability, and 7% is just too damn low. So low it makes me wonder, did those folks get better because of some other factor, like the will to survive? Even a broken clock is right twice a day.... How can a treatment be unsuccessful 93% of the time? Sounds to me like the wrong path. Then again, 7% sure beats zero."

We proceeded to find another ankhologist, going to Houston, New York City, and settling on Dr. Larry Copeland at Ohio State University. He didn't give me a percentage cure rate. He expected survival of two to three years—one to two years longer than the other two ankhologists. He also took into consideration that my lungs were fairly clear, rather than full of nodules, as had been expected due to the state of my abdomen when the doctors found the cancer.

So I raised the question on my private blog: Does each of us have a set expiration date? If my expiration date is set, then it doesn't matter if I smoke or eat a gallon of ice cream a day; however, the quality of my life between now and that point will be improved considerably by eating well and taking good care of myself.

I read in one source we have five possible exit points in each lifetime. If this is true, I didn't know how many I'd already blown past. I can think of at least two from childhood and one from young adulthood.

One friend responded, "I agree with your assessment that when it's our time to leave, we go. Whether we devour Twinkies and Big Macs or sip wheat grass tea. I think the healthy choices we make only affect the quality of our life, not the quantity."

Another provided a different perspective. "It could be that your expiration date isn't yet set. Really, it's not. And you are right that eating well and taking good care of yourself is important to you and to your children."

Whichever theory is true, one friend wrote about how she balances living life while preparing for death. "I regularly ask myself: if I only had one day, week, month to live, would I do anything differently? If the answer is yes, I do it. If the answer is no, I give thanks. It works for me."

It's a good practice. And I still felt there was an order to the universe, that all will be well in the end—whatever that entails.

In the meantime, it's not over 'til it's over. Anita Moorjani battled cancer for four years, lay in a coma with her organs shutting down, and had a near-death experience. A few weeks later she walked, nearly cancer-free, out of the hospital. She had been told it wasn't her time yet. She wrote about her experiences in *Dying To Be Me: My Journey from Cancer, to Near Death, to True Healing*. "My body is only a reflection of my internal state," she wrote. "If my inner self were aware of its greatness and connection with All-that-is, my body would soon reflect that and heal rapidly."

I also heard the story of a woman told she was supposed to die of cancer at age forty-two. When the time came, she begged the Divine for a reprieve, and it was granted. I don't know how much longer she lived, but she zipped past that particular checkout point.

I have since heard that the statistics doctors tell us are for information, not condemnation. That made the most sense to me.

So maybe survival is part self-mastery, part Divine will, part internal healing, part timing, and part who-knows-what. And maybe it's different for everyone, as we all have our own individual paths.

Whatever it is for me, I want that will to survive, and I want to learn self-mastery.

Thriver Soup Ingredient:

Listen to the refrain in the song "I Will Survive" by Gloria Gaynor, and imagine that the one not welcome anymore is the cancer. Sing the refrain and visualize the cancer as something ugly in your house and you are kicking it out into the street.

Image Cycling: The Bengston Technique

All of them look to you to give them their food when they need it. When you give it to them, they gather it; when you open your hand, they are well satisfied.

—Psalm 104:27-28, Complete Jewish Bible

The opening hand is a gesture of giving. As we open our hands to give, we also receive. This became clearer to me when I learned about the healing technique taught by William Bengston. I'd never heard of the Bengston technique until I met John Hill through a mutual friend. He explained that Bengston did a study on mice injected with a type of cancer guaranteed to kill them within twenty-seven days. He created a list of twenty things he wanted for himself, then put a visual with each desire. He turned those visuals into a mental movie he played over and over while holding his hands around a cage of infected mice, one hour each day. He also visualized energy looping from one hand, around his shoulders, through his head, down to the other hand, and jumping across to the first hand (so the energy ran through the cage of mice). The mice all got cancer—and all were cured.

Bengston followed this experience by teaching groups of volunteers the same technique. New groups of mice were cured by the volunteers.

Bengston turned his technique of image cycling into a course called "Hands-on Healing." The six CDs include background on the technique and detailed instructions for the exercises.

The basic idea involves selecting at least twenty specific things we want (such as a celebration party for entering into remission, rather than a generalized idea, such as being cured), creating a visual image for each item, and stringing the pictures together into a mental movie clip. The training involves learning to run through these images so quickly they flash by at incredible speeds. It seems to me the technique somehow gets one's ego out of the way so deeper healing energies can be accessed.

Although John warned me it's hard for most people to come up with twenty items, I quickly came up with about thirty. The threat of death hanging over one's head brings clarity, no doubt. Then I searched online for images to match the top twenty items. I practiced visualizing each item, in order, while running the energy from hand to hand, then through my body, in a constant cycle.

I was opening my hands to both give to and receive from myself so I could be sated with more goodness from the Divine.

Thriver Soup Ingredient:

Make a list of twenty specific things you would like to experience or manifest in your life, like a clean scan. Come up with a visual image for each item, such as you giddily holding your clean scan report in an upraised hand.

When you sit in meditation, hold your palms on your lap, open and facing each other, as if you are holding a large ball. Visualize energy looping from one hand, around your shoulders, through your head, down to the other hand, and then jumping across the empty ball-shaped space and into the first hand. I like to start with my left hand and move to the right, as I have been taught that the left side of the body is more receptive and the right side is more active.

While moving the energy loop, start visualizing, in the same order each time, the twenty items you want to manifest in your life. Keep running the images through your mind, like a mental movie, while moving the energy through your body. Repeat as long as it's fun and worthwhile for you. As you practice, move the images more quickly, until they become a blur of emotion while the energy courses through your body.

When you finish, offer gratitude to the Divine.

This exercise will give you some familiarity with the Bengston technique, and then you can decide if it's something you want to pursue.

Inner Patriarch: Dialogue with Self-appointed Judges

"Do not judge, or you too will be judged."

—Matthew 7:1, Christian Bible, NIV

There is a wounded part of me that likes to judge others. It uses up a lot of my energy and makes my body and mind more stiff. I have attempted to drop it for years, and it has persisted.

While attending the women's circle led by Anyaa McAndrew, I became more conscious of that inner judge. Then we did exercises designed to bring us in touch with our inner patriarchs and inner matriarchs. These are two of what psychologists have called archetypes. These aspects of our psyches can influence us without our awareness, and in ways we don't always comprehend. In Western culture, these aspects often are wounded.

The wounding probably evolved and spread during the five generations of witch hunts in Europe, begun by the Spanish Inquisition. Mothers tried to protect their daughters by telling them to be quiet, not be seen, and not do anything outside the norm so they would not be accused of being witches. According to Anyaa, this developed into a wounded inner masculine figure in women's psyches which she called the inner patriarch. It usually shows up in our lives as criticism. We see unhealthy male energy outside ourselves and criticize it, rather than looking toward our own unhealthy inner masculine that wants to be healed.

I had gotten to know some of my other inner archetypes, but I was in for a shock when I did this exercise.

We formed groups of three. Anyaa asked one of us in each group to get into a meditative state. Then a partner would ask the meditator's inner patriarch four questions while the third partner wrote down the verbalized answers. When I meditated, I was horrified by what came out of my mouth. My inner patriarch had a low opinion of women and I let him take all my power.

Anyaa suggested we thank our inner patriarchs for cooperating with us by answering our questions. Then, back in meditation, we were asked to call in our priestess archetype to assign jobs to our inner patriarchs.

I felt a heavy sigh escape when Anyaa said we could continue working with our inner patriarchs, assisting them with transforming into wise old men. Part of the process involved focusing on the different feelings evoked by the inner patriarch and the inner priestess aspects during imaginative discussions with them. I had been merged with and debilitated by my inner patriarch, giving him control. After this exercise, I could ask my priestess self to hold my power.

Next, during a meditative state, we dialogued with our inner matriarchs. Again, I felt stunned by my responses. My inner matriarch had a low opinion of men, yet saw them as more competent than women. She saw me as weak and frightened, and lacking healthy personal limits.

My inner work became clear: go into meditation, act as my priestess-self, and converse with my inner patriarch and matriarch. I needed to give them work to do and set healthy boundaries for them.

These dialogues were followed by a dream in which a masculine figure kissed me, loved me, and wanted to marry me, but I told him the cost would be high. He had to work for it and needed to gather energy. Later still, I dreamt that I had gotten married. I believe this is the inner marriage of my masculine and feminine energies. I had watched for this dream for decades, and finally it arrived. I had thought such as dream was the grand finale, the final stage—the union of heaven and earth, the integration of body and soul. I realized in the dream that it was only another step in a long, long process.

With continued spiritual practices and psychotherapy, I gradually developed my positive masculine qualities—for me, the primary aspect was healthy boundaries and the courage to stand up for my needs. I learned not to judge myself so harshly, which lifted the compulsion to judge others.

Thriver Soup Ingredient:

It's hard for anyone in Western culture to escape having wounded inner masculine and feminine aspects to their personalities. If you are interested in exploring your inner patriarch, a good place to start would probably be the book, *The Shadow King: The Invisible Force That Holds Women Back* by psychotherapist Sidra Stone, PhD.

Internal Conflicts: My Money or My Life

The Blessed Lord said: O Pandava (Arjuna), he who does not abhor the presence of the gunas—illumination, activity, and ignorance—nor deplore their absence; Remaining like one unconcerned, undisturbed by the three modes—realizing that they alone are operating throughout creation; not oscillating in mind but ever Self-centered; Unaffected by joy and sorrow, praise and blame—secure in his divine nature; regarding with an equal eye a clod of clay, a stone, and gold; the same in his attitude toward pleasant or unpleasant (men and experiences); firm-minded; Uninfluenced by respect or insult; treating friend and enemy alike; abandoning all delusions of personal doership—he it is who has transcended the triple qualities!

—*God Talks with Arjuna: The Bhagavad Gita*, 14.22-25

The Hindu Bhagavad Gita outlines the qualities of a liberated soul, free from ordinary human ties. The yogi experiences no attachment to humans or situations and remains ever-tranquil.

Uh, not me. Soon after the diagnosis, I applied for disability benefits and started receiving income from the federal government to cover the income I had been receiving from free-lance work.

An internal conflict over the checks quickly developed. If I got well, the checks would stop. How odd to feel tied to being ill to get my social security money back from the federal government. How strange to prefer, at one level, the money over my health. I clearly needed to let that attachment go.

I realized it more fully while working with certified Emotional Freedom Technique practitioner Mim Grace Gieser. She asked, "What is keeping you from fully accepting healing?" I felt shame around my answer—as long as I was ill, the checks would continue.

As we talked, however, I came to realize the issue for me wasn't the money because I enjoyed working from home and running my own small business. No, it was about time. When the disability checks stopped, I would probably need to return to full-time work. I wanted, instead, to continue working from home and writing books.

Mim took me through a long tapping session and my number representing the internal conflict crept down from a five (out of ten) down to a four. Apparently this conflict had deeply entrenched itself. It took many tapping sessions on my own to reduce the conflict.

Gradually the issue resolved itself, especially after my treatments ended and my energy started to return. I felt more amenable to the idea of going back to work one day.

I still lack the equanimity toward all things that a yogi experiences. And that's okay. Maybe someday, as I continue trundling along my path, it will happen.

Thriver Soup Ingredient:

In your journal, write down the question, "What is keeping me from fully accepting healing?"

Then meditate for about twenty minutes. When you are done meditating, return to the question. See if anything arises for you that can be recorded.

If so, begin working with whatever this barrier is, using whatever technique you find useful.

Lamp unto My Feet

Thy word is a lamp unto my feet, and a light unto my path.
                                        —Psalm 119:105, King James Version, Christian Bible

The writer of this psalm compared the word of the Divine to a lamp that could only light one's way, one step at a time, through the dark of night. At the time the psalm was written, there would only have been access to Iron-Age oil lamps, used in the Middle East from 1200 to 536 BCE. These small clay saucers were pinched around the edges with a spout at one end for the wick. One little flame would be all the light it could produce.

The writer had light for his path, meager as it was. Well, where was my lamp? Why wasn't anyone able to light my wick? I felt abandoned by the Divine, drowning in the dark, unable to see the next step with any clarity. How easy it would have been to take a misstep, fall down a rabbit hole, and lose my chances for survival.

Instead of basing decisions on clear evidence—there wasn't much research on this orphan cancer—we relied on guesswork. Any signposts were hard to spot, and knowing the best direction to take was difficult at best. Groping in the shadows of my life, I turned to consultations with others, meditation, and prayer for guidance.

After my second type of chemotherapy had stopped working, we had a conference with my ankhologist, known as "The Wiz." His final option was a drug that would involve spending five days in the hospital every three weeks. Originally I had no intention of continuing with this type of chemotherapy. Why bother? What good would it do? The Wiz had known fewer than half a dozen people in thirty years who got rid of their nodules with such a regimen.

I didn't think my wick would ever light up.

Then the Divine spoke words through my then-husband, igniting my lamp. He asked about possibly removing the nodules by surgery and then doing the chemo. This way we could have the nodule cells sent for analysis to determine which drug to combine with ifosfamide for the greatest possible effectiveness. He also felt this was a good path because I still had only two nodules. As he and The Wiz talked, I felt my body flood with a wave of positive energy, the way it does when I finally realize what a dream symbol means. My then-husband later told me he felt the same way.

So it was decided—lung resections followed by the final chemosabe.

By staying present in my body, I was able to notice when the positive rush of energy washed through me, like the wick of a lamp suddenly igniting and spilling light out around me. The Spirit had provided holy words through my then-husband so we could more clearly see the next step of my journey.

Thriver Soup Ingredient

Christian singer Amy Grant uses this Bible verse as the springboard for a song called "Thy Word." A search on the internet should bring it up so you can listen to it.

~~~

Leaving the Land of Confusion

For God is not a God of confusion but of peace.

—I Corinthians 14:33, New American Standard Bible

So much confusion, so little peace.

After sixteen chemotherapy treatments, I expected a clean scan. Instead, two nodules were growing in my lungs.

First I went into shock. Then I went numb as a way of protecting myself against the emotional pain. About an hour after the news, I couldn't stand the idea of being in the house where I had spent so much energy and time on healing work. In despair, I drove to a local nature preserve, took a long walk, and had a good cry.

How could I have felt so sure I was done with the whole cancer scene when I so obviously wasn't? At least I had been right about one thing—I no longer needed the chemo I'd been given. Gemcitabine and docetaxel had run their course and were spent.

My mind gyrated with confusion. When I returned home, I looked at my Map of Emotions©. I realized confusion is not an emotion. Rather, it's a mood—an indication that I was swimming in my head, dissociating from my body. Once again I had fallen back into my tendency to hide in my mind, attempting to understand, dissect, and analyze my situation so I could avoid feeling emotional pain. Usually I come out feeling better, giving myself the illusion that the more I understood, the more I could control a given situation. Even with my new awareness about my behavior, I allowed this familiar pattern to continue yet again, with the knowledge that I was consciously choosing this coping mechanism.

Confusion, as a mood, is what I fall into when I am avoiding the emotion of despair in my body. That emotion was exactly what I felt. Prior to the scan results, I experienced genuine confidence, an upbeat, positive attitude. My dreams and others around me indicated I was moving toward remission. I had done everything humanly possible to bring it about.

And there I sat, with the sht regrowing in my lungs.

Part of me wanted to fall into my familiar mood of resignation, to give up the fight, to stop trying so hard to live. Yet the emotions of dread about the pain that cancer can create, along with the terror of suffocating to death, drove me back into wanting to do all I could to stave off the perceived end as long as possible.

One thing I hadn't done—with gentle reminders from others—was to let go of the need to control my situation and to hand it all over to the Ultimate Healer. It wasn't up to me whether I got well or not, although I could greatly influence the process and its outcome.

I also knew no matter what the scan said, I was going to continue with my healing practices. I needed to continue with the same intensity—not as a means for controlling but as a way of making my life more tolerable for myself and my family. I needed to live in the moment, to breathe, and to be grateful for the many wonderful blessings I had.

Thriver Soup Ingredient

If you fall into confusion, remember it's all in your head. Confusion might be the result of thinking about your feelings of powerlessness, emptiness, despair, hopelessness, or shame. Stop the thinking. Exit your head and take your awareness into your body. Notice your physical sensations without labeling, judging, or fixing. If you follow the Map of Emotions©, the energy eventually will lift into a texture like compassionate gratitude or possibly a simple sense of witnessing yourself.

∽∽∽

Lucky or Unlucky? God only Knows

Misery, alas! rests upon happiness. Happiness, alas! underlies misery.
—Tao Te Ching, 58

Is getting a cancer diagnosis miserable misfortune or happiness-inducing good luck for us? Or is luck even a part of the equation?

There is an ancient story about the luck—both miserable and happy—of a father and his son. One day their only horse escapes. The neighbor comes over to sympathize. The father says, "Maybe it's bad luck, maybe it's good. Who knows?"

The next day, the horse shows up with a whole herd of mares. Now the father is rich. The neighbor comes over to celebrate. The father says, "Maybe it's good luck, maybe it's bad. Who knows?"

The next day a horse kicks the son and breaks the young man's leg. The neighbor comes over to sympathize. The father says, "Maybe it's bad luck, maybe it's good. Who knows?"

The next day the military comes to recruit soldiers, and the son can't join because his leg is broken. And so the story continues.

The Tao Te Ching says it succinctly: Bad luck hides within good things, and good things can come out of what appears to be bad luck.

For me, while I felt quite unlucky to have the diagnosis, many good things came out of it: fabulous support from family and friends, new friendships, a cruise to Alaska, and a whole new life for me. Sometimes it takes a crisis before we can see life more clearly and make better decisions.

Our vision is limited; we don't know the future. If you feel unlucky and miserable for getting a cancer diagnosis, know that happiness and good fortune might lurk within it, if we only have the eyes to see.

Thriver Soup Ingredient:

Always look for the good hiding in seeming misfortune.

One way is to make a list in your journal of all the good things that have come out of your cancer diagnosis. Are your friends pitching in to help? Are you closer to your family members? Are you making more time to take care of yourself? Are you eating more nutritious foods? All of these changes, and many others, might be cause to celebrate.

∽∽∽

Making Decisions: An Answer is Blowing in the Wind

For wisdom is better than pearls; nothing you want can compare with her.
—Proverbs 8:11, Complete Jewish Bible

The natural pearl has long been known as the queen of gems because it was so rare and valuable. The biblical writer who said wisdom was better than pearls selected, for comparison, the most valuable item known to humans at the time.

Wisdom comes with experience, usually through making decisions and witnessing the consequences. I preferred to lean on others' wisdom rather than gaining or trusting my own. Doubts—based in my unprocessed emotion of fear—plagued me. I had a long history of giving away my power. My psychotherapist kept reminding me to find ways to strengthen myself and honor what I knew rather than listening to and depending upon others for all of my major decisions.

My fear-based behavior of giving others more credence than myself continued. Week in and week out, my therapist pointed out to me where I had choices, could be empowered and could act assertively in family life. My insecurities about my own wisdom and insight continued. It probably stemmed from my childhood, during which I felt invisible and my emotions were devalued. It took me decades to understand that I was a sensitive child. I had grown up in an intellectual environment where instincts and intuition were given little intrinsic value.

It was time to reclaim those lost parts of myself.

I created an Emotional Freedom Technique session for developing my personal power and removing emotional blockages.

With growing intention, I gradually learned to keep my feet underneath me and decide what I wanted, when I wanted it, and how to influence my life's course. I slowly grew in my ability to listen to my instincts and intuition. I gained the strength to avoid agreeing to anything unless I felt sure it was what I wanted. Like a strand of pearls, orb by orb, I began to try on more wisdom. I liked how it felt.

Thriver Soup Ingredient:

When you have difficult choices to make, sit quietly and try on each decision and see how your body responds. Be receptive to inner promptings that stir your soul. These might provide you with a clue for which direction to take.

～～～

Medical Intuition

"For my thoughts are not your thoughts, and your ways are not my ways," says ADONAI.
—Isaiah 55:8, Complete Jewish Bible

We cannot truly know or understand the mind or activities of the Divine unless we become enlightened. Since there aren't a lot of fully awakened beings around, the vast majority of us are muddling around in the dark.

During March 2010, I talked with a woman diagnosed with stage IV cancer who had undergone chemotherapy. She said she felt clean and several medical intuitives said they sensed no cancer in her body. Yet a couple of weeks later she had a scan that showed a tumor. She headed into more intense chemotherapy.

After our conversation I felt anxious, vulnerable, and doubtful about my experiences. What if I was completely wrong about a dream that seemed to indicate my cancer was gone? What if the medical intuitive who said she sensed no cancer in my body was wrong? I felt shame around appearing stupid and being "wrong" about my perceptions.

I brought my anxiety and fears about my upcoming scan into a conversation with a Self-Realization Fellowship nun. How does one reconcile feeling clean and medical intuitives saying one is clean with scans that show more tumors?

The nun had talked with many women who had cancer, and recalled one medical intuitive saying the woman's spiritual body—a subtle, second body that corresponds to one's physical body yet cannot by perceived by one's physical senses—was clear. When the spiritual, or astral, body is clear, the physical body tends to follow this pattern. Perhaps those intuitives had picked up on the astral body's condition of my friend. Her scan showed what was current, not what was to come—a clean body. Perhaps she just had to endure one more chemo routine to achieve the total health for which she and so many others had visualized and prayed. Time is a relative phenomenon, and the Spirit's work is not limited by our perceptions. The Divine way of thinking and doing can be far different from ours.

As it turned out, my acquaintance never went into remission, and I had more nodules growing in my lungs. No medical intuitive is ever 100 percent correct. Relying on others to intuit our circumstances can lead to false expectations. Instead, a medical diagnostic test can verify your personal situation.

The mind of the Divine is beyond anything we—including medical intuitives—can understand. We often cannot make sense of why things happen as they do, nor do we always comprehend the Spirit's intentions behind our circumstances. Life is a mystery. Acceptance of this parameter can prevent some anguish that might result from unmet expectations.

Thriver Soup Ingredient:

Avoid asking medical intuitives about your situation. They are not machines that can record with pinpoint accuracy what is living in your body. Neither do they possess a clear channel to what the Divine is thinking, planning, or doing. They are human and therefore unable to be 100 percent objective. If what they tell you is correct, it wasn't necessary to ask them—the scan will show the truth as far as it is able. If the intuitives are wrong, their words can have a devastating effect on your emotions. Let the medical diagnosis tell you what you need to know at that time about the situation for your physical body.

≈≈≈

No Coincidences: The Wizard of Odds

From a distance ADONAI appeared to me, [saying,] "I love you with an everlasting love; this is why in my grace I draw you to me. Once again, I will build you; you will be rebuilt, virgin of Isra'el. Once again, equipped with your tambourines, you will go out and dance with the merrymakers."
—Jeremiah 31:3-4, Complete Jewish Bible

I believe everything happens for a reason, even if we don't comprehend it. We are loved with an everlasting love. Whatever happens, we will, at some point, dance with joy—even if it's in heaven.

After my first lung resection and soon after starting my third chemotherapy regimen, I received my first book from the American Cancer Society, *You are Not Alone.* (St. Elizabeth Healthcare, in Edgewood, Kentucky, the hospital where I was to receive the chemotherapy infusions, apparently was the only treatment place to order the book for me.) It contained pages specifically about uterine sarcomas. I was struck by one sentence after its discussion of stage IV: "Sarcoma often comes back and spreads to the lungs. If there are only 1 or 2 small tumors, these may be able to be removed with surgery. Some patients have been cured by this treatment."

Cured! I wanted to dance with excitement that the ACS could say something so bold about this illness—especially when the Memorial Sloan-Kettering Cancer Center physician pretty much said it couldn't happen. I had been a great candidate for surgery because I only had the same two nodules for more than half a year, possibly longer.

On the same day, I received a forwarded email showing a photo of a truck beside a highway. At seventy-five miles per hour, the pickup had slammed through a guard rail, flipped over a huge concrete culvert, and sat facing the opposite direction, right on the edge of a deep chasm. If the truck had landed a few more inches to the side, the two occupants would have been plunged to their deaths. Instead, they were unharmed except for a few bruises. Whether the photo and story were true or not, it gave me the message: if it's not your time, it's not your time.

Later that day, I met with a woman who told me I still had important things to do with my life—don't waste it on trivialities.

My friend Charley had just called me a sponge. I'd been a sponge for knowledge all my life. Soon I would be giving my sponge another big squeeze so new contents could gush out to assist others on their journeys.

These events reinforced for me the belief that there are no coincidences. Seemingly disconnected events in my life occurred during a brief span of time to display a common thread. Father of psychoanalysis Carl Jung would call these synchronicities. I realized, by paying attention to them, that there still are important things I am supposed to do with my life that will be of service to others. This knowledge filled me with deep gratitude and joy. I knew that I, too, would one day be dancing with the merrymakers.

Thriver Soup Ingredient:

See if you can spot some synchronicities in your life. When they appear, offer gratitude to the Divine for ordering your life and providing hope for the day of dancing.

≈≈≈

Questioning Faith

Then the Lord answered Job out of the whirlwind: "Who is this who darkens counsel with words without knowledge? Get ready for a difficult task like a man; I will question you and you will inform me! "Where were you when I laid the foundation of the earth? Tell me, if you possess understanding!"
—Job 38:1-4, Christian Bible, NET

Job was a man described as "sincere and upright, God-fearing and shunning evil." He subsequently lost everything, including his health. He and his friends struggled to figure out answers to the perennial question, "Why?"

Sometimes I felt like Job. Cancer claimed my health, and with its demise went my marriage and financial stability. I walked away from a large suburban home and moved with my younger son into a cottage that was smaller than the living room and kitchen of the marital home. I went into debt and struggled to pay my divorce lawyer and the relentless monthly medical bills.

"Why?" It was a question I struggled with for years. Why did the Divine allow cancer to exist? Why did it viciously visit me in early middle-age? Why was I thrown into a situation where I needed a loan to pay my bills?

I had tried all my life to do what was right and take care of my health. My situation felt outrageously unfair. Hadn't I been good enough to deserve better? Was I being punished for some unknown sin? Was this bad karma?

Fortunately, I didn't have it as bad as Job. My children lived through the crisis, I had modern medical and complementary care, and I had the invaluable love, assistance, and support of family and friends.

My psychotherapist helped guide me through these questions. Did I believe the Divine was a judge and punisher? Or did I believe the Divine was a comforter, redeemer, healer, and one who could cure?

I would not, could not believe in a Divine punisher. The universe was too stunning to be created by a big meanie in the sky.

I sank back down into my Western religious roots: "God is love," says the Christian Bible. "With everlasting love have I loved you; therefore have I drawn you to Me with loving-kindness," says the Jewish Bible. "But I cast (the garment Of) love over thee from Me," says the Qur'an.

Whatever the cause, whatever the reason, I landed, like Job, on the side of mystery.

Where were you when I founded the earth?

I do not understand the "Why?" or the "Why me?" and decided that was okay. How could I—with my puny brain, living on a planet that is nothing but a dot in an outlying solar system that is hardly a speck in the universe—understand the workings of the Divine, who created all there is? And who still loves—*loves*—me?

I do not comprehend this love. It is, however, a love I feel deep within my body. It is a love I hear when I listen to the roar of silence. And it is a love I see in the snowflake, in the sunrise, and on the faces of my family and friends.

I am satisfied.

Thriver Soup Ingredient:

Sit quietly in a chair and place your elbows in front of you on a table or desk. Use the index fingers of each hand to close your ears. Listen carefully. Ignore the sounds made by your body. Listen more deeply. You might hear a hum or a roar. If you think you've identified the sound, take your fingers away from your ears and see if you can identify the sound again. This sound is called om, aum, amen, amin, and hum. It is said to be the sound of creation, the vibration of the universe. When I become distressed, I tune in to this roar to remind myself of the love of the Divine surrounding and filling me at all times, no matter the outer circumstances in which I might be embroiled. I find peace and comfort in this sound of silence.

~~~

Re-member

"Therefore you are to be perfect, as your heavenly Father is perfect."
—Matthew 5:48, Christian Bible, New American Standard Bible

In this verse, Jesus encourages his disciples to be "perfect," from the Greek word *telios*. I think *telios* probably is better translated as whole, complete, or mature. I liked the idea of being whole. I wanted to piece back together my wholeness, my holiness, the original messages of my cells lost in layers of life. My friend Judy Merritt reminded me that these cellular messages are messages of love, health, and wholeness. Energy intuitive Maria Paglialungo encouraged me to relax more and deeply meditate to re-experience myself as a soul living in a physical body. My essential nature is light and love, and deeply experiencing that nature could automatically bring health.

Jon Kabat-Zinn, PhD, mindfulness meditation teacher, would concur. He said healing comes from a sense of already being completely whole. When we taste that wholeness, our bodies respond by restoring themselves to the deepest homeostatic balance to which they are capable of moving. Such a perspective was quite different from the evangelical Christian mindset I had been taught, including the belief in original sin. It took years of study before I realized this doctrine is not supported by the Hebrew Bible or the gospels of Jesus. It started with the Apostle Paul and was later developed by the early Church fathers to counter other Christian beliefs that cropped up in the ancient world.

Gradually, I came to think more in terms of original wholeness. While perhaps we don't all come into this world as perfect little beings, we usually do start out with more wholeness than where we end up by the time we become adults. As we grow, our tendency is to separate ourselves from others and even from parts of ourselves, rejecting aspects of our personalities that we experience as negative. The personal ego sees itself as distinct from other human beings.

I had come to see split-off, rejected aspects of my personality as separate. They sank down into the shadowy realms of my unconscious. I projected those characteristics onto others: She's too nice. He's too angry. She talks too much. He's too overbearing.

The cancer cells, reflecting my psyche, were parts of myself that probably rebelled and split themselves off from the whole to lead their own, parasitic lives.

It was time to turn within to see myself as whole, to see my cells as whole, and to re-member my parts into the wholeness that I truly am.

Thriver Soup Ingredient:

As you deal with cancer, re-member all the parts of yourself and think in terms of your wholeness. As Vince Lasorso told me, "Think global!" Recruit the power of your whole system to transform your entire body, not just individual battlefields. Allow the grace of life to permeate you. Let go of thoughts such as "kill the cancer." Instead, affirm, "Balance and harmony are my body's natural states of being."

~∼∼

Recognizing Scams: Buyer Beware

...be ye therefore wise as serpents....

—Matthew 10:16, King James Bible

Whom does one trust when it comes to finding complementary cancer treatments? Patients often are frightened, vulnerable, and desperate, making us ripe for trusting scammers who peddle false hope and useless, expensive wares. We need to be wise as serpents when considering our options.

This is where having a large support community can be beneficial. I came across plenty of miracle cures, asked my supporters for advice, and avoided blowing my wad on useless sht.

Often a rip-off artist will have a website filled with mysterious lures, overstated half-truths, a multitude of adjectives and descriptions, and boatloads of seemingly powerful testimonials. The way I figure it, if what the scammer is trying to sell really works, all that hype is unnecessary. I'd suggest skipping the product.

If the item seems greatly overpriced, it's probably worthless.

If a person suggests something is a cure for cancer, skip it. If it truly cured cancer, everyone would know about it quickly enough. I find it hard to believe the product would be kept a secret because nearly everyone knows someone with cancer and would want to give it a try if it really worked.

Even websites claiming to have scientific backing for their products need to be carefully perused.

If you come across a product you think is promising, do an internet search, including the word "scam." Read and weigh what pops up. Some scam reports clearly are unreliable, while others probably are legitimate. Be persistent. Go deeply into your internet search. Sometimes I had to search through ten pages of online results to find good information about a particular product.

Use your best radar: your own instincts, a gift from the Divine. If you have trouble accessing your inner guidance system, find someone with a gift for intuitive understanding and ask for assistance. Be wise as a serpent to avoid costly traps and scams.

Thriver Soup Ingredient:

One way to find an answer to any questions about whether to try a product or not is to ask your body a yes-or-no question about it. Meditate for about twenty minutes. Ask again, and see how your body feels. If your body feels good, you can probably give the product a try. If you experience a little discomfort, it might be best to pass.

≈≈≈

Resentment: Raging Bull

Get rid of all bitterness, rage and anger, brawling and slander, along with every form of malice.
—Ephesians 4:31, Christian Bible, NIV

Bitterness and rage might feel satisfying in the moment, yet over the long haul it is we who are damaged, not the offending party. Resentment and bitterness, in particular, are poisons that can fester until they explode into disease.

I had read in Louise Hay's book, *You Can Heal Your Life*, that cancer is probably caused by profound hurt or long-term resentment. It also could arise from the pain caused by a secret or grief that has eaten away at one's self. Arthritis, she wrote, was caused by one feeling unloved, along with criticism and resentment.

Ah, the word resentment showed up in both. While I can't speak for anyone else, I knew these emotional issues were true for me. Cancer was my clarion call to bring any such self-righteous feelings into awareness and then let them go.

My psychotherapist confirmed this for me when she commented one day that I was dripping with resentment, and when I am resentful, I become passively aggressive. Even though I had not been fully aware of this mood within myself, I knew she was right.

It was time to face my pain and work through it. It became especially critical because I learned that resentment, blame, and contempt (moods I experience when I start thinking about the emotion of anger in my body) lower white blood cell counts. Sure enough, when I had episodes of rage, my white cell counts dropped even lower.

I went home that day and wrote up several lists of different areas where I experienced resentment during my life. The number of items I wrote astonished me, and I knew it was far from complete. I experienced impotent rage at how I had been hurt by various people during the previous five decades. Creating the list gave me a broom for sweeping out my psyche's basement.

When I did active imagination one day, I decided to dialogue with the cancer. I imagined getting small enough to enter into my own lungs. Asking for the support of my spiritual guides, I journeyed to a lung nodule. The lump appeared to be a black mass on pink tissue. I explained to the mass that it either must transform into healthy cells or it will die—I will kill it or my body will expire, which also will end its existence. I asked what brought it to me. It responded: rage and resentment.

Again, I knew it was time to flush out all my bitterness.

Five decades of resentment is a heavy load to unleash, and I knew I needed help. I went to see my Emotional Freedom Technique practitioner, Mim Grace Gieser. She suggested I tap my thighs as I talked about the situations that created some early anger. I shuddered and spasmed with rage as we did EFT. By feeling my anger inside my body and in the moment, I gradually let go of the bigger resentments in a healthy manner that caused damage to no one. I could feel a shift in my body, and a sense of peacefulness arose. Some of the psychic poison had dropped away.

I drove to Whatever Works Wellness Center to have a little healing ritual in their labyrinth. Having planned ahead, I had packed my costume butterfly wings, representing the rising of my new self. I walked the grove's path and stopped at the Mother Mary alcove. I prayed, burned the paper listing my resentments, and offered a little butterfly gift.

My therapist later said the cost of giving up my resentment is becoming open and frightened. That can feel like a high cost, and yet it is minor compared to the cost of festering resentment that poisons the body. By feeling anger in the moment, rather than allowing it to turn into a resentful mood, we can manage our feelings in a way that leads to greater health, which benefits everyone.

Thriver Soup Ingredient:

The *Co-Dependents Anonymous* book contains a terrific and thorough section on how to work through resentments as step four of its twelve-step program. If you have the time and energy, consider finding a meeting and asking someone in the organization to assist you with working through the exercises. Otherwise, do what you are able on your own. Any resentments you can drop will be helpful, and your body will appreciate it.

≈≈≈

Self-acceptance

Therefore the sufficiency of contentment is an enduring and unchanging sufficiency.
—Tao Te Ching, 46

We are enough. Really, we are. Even when we don't feel or act like it. We don't need more of anything to be sufficient in the eyes of the Divine.

Women in Western societies are acculturated to appear perfect in every way. This posture is both rigid and self-abusive, especially because each of us carries our own image of what perfection is supposed to be. When we come from this programmed stance, it is easy to blame ourselves or others for our shortcomings. This can lead to a variety of outcomes, including jealousy of others, cruelty toward ourselves and others, or passive-aggressive behavior.

I have a friend whose cat demonstrated this for me one day. Her cat attacks its own tail. I laughed with abandon the first time I saw it happen. The feline pounced on her tail several times, hissing angrily. This cat had not recognized her own tail; seeing it twitching was unacceptable to her. She projected fear and anger onto her own body part and assaulted it.

Humans behave in similar ways. We possess personal features that feel unacceptable. When they are unacknowledged and projected out onto others, then we want to attack. When we accept the dark sides of ourselves as part of who we are, then they no longer create negative emotions. I want to become more like a cat that accepts its own tail for what it is.

After working with my psychotherapist, I gradually found this happening with my judgmental thoughts. In the past, I used to be so unaware of my negative, nasty thoughts that I would repress them immediately as they started to arise. I pushed them back down because I wanted to be a "nice" person and did not want to see myself as judgmental.

Now when they arise, they are not immediately shoved away. Instead, I see them as what they are—negative, nasty, judgmental thoughts, yet still only thoughts, completely harmless by themselves. I don't need to berate myself for having them; they are simply part of the human condition, just as a cat's tail is part of a cat. This knowledge frees me to do what the Buddhists teach people to do during meditation—simply notice my thoughts and let them float away. No need to hold onto, think about, or act upon them.

I am sufficient, in and of myself. I am enough in the eyes of the Divine. I am learning to accept myself for who I am, even cherishing formerly unacceptable parts of myself. It feels lovely.

Thriver Soup Ingredient:
The following visualization can assist with enhancing self-acceptance.

Sit comfortably in a chair with your back straight and palms turned up in your lap. Take a few slow, deep breaths. Then imagine yourself surrounded by beings who love you—real or imagined. Breathe their love in through every pore of your body. When you feel sufficiently self-accepting in the moment, come back to your everyday life. Try to hold that feeling and attentiveness with you as you move through your day, your week. If you realize in the moment that this perception of self-care isn't present, simply pause and turn your thoughtfulness to reconnecting with a feeling of self-acceptance.

≈≈≈

Setback: Possible Prelude to a Cure

Trust in ADONAI with all your heart; do not rely on your own understanding.
—Proverbs 3:5, Complete Jewish Bible

I did not understand, and I did not feel trust in the Divine with even one millimeter of my heart. After two years of chemotherapy and a lung resection, a PET/CT scan showed the sht was back. A fifteen-by-fifteen millimeter nodule sat in my lower left lobe, taking up room in a depression right next to my heart.

For the first twenty-four hours I took refuge in my head, conscious that I was avoiding feeling any emotions in my body.

The next day I finally started to allow bits of emotion into my awareness. My psychotherapist asked me why I consciously avoided doing the Map of Emotions©. It's so simple to do. I didn't have an answer except I was afraid of being aware of my body's responses, afraid of touching vast emotional trauma: anger, fear, grief, loss, powerlessness, despair.... I am grateful that even while in shock, I was able to maintain enough consciousness to be aware that I was avoiding my emotions.

The following day I saw my ankhologist and fell into overwhelm. Dr. Pavelka showed the spot on the scan. It was about half an inch around and sat right next to a major pulmonary vein, like a stubborn person with its arms crossed. We couldn't see anything between the nodule and the vein. The doctor said it was highly unlikely the nodule had invaded the vein. However, its position made surgery tricky. Radiation probably would cause too much damage to nearby tissues.

We all felt fairly certain there wasn't much point in doing more chemo. We had used up all the known options for endometrial sarcoma. That part brought relief, yet also raised more fears for me.

Another surgery loomed.

And then I remembered the little green inchworm I'd watched climbing up a large stone behind a statue of Mother Mary in the Whatever Works Wellness Center's labyrinth. The creature got close to the stone's peak, paused, rose up onto its back legs, and slowly veered off to the right side. I felt disappointed that it did not climb all the way up, thinking the little garden show I was witnessing might be one of those coincidental signs from the universe.

I sat and waited, watching the worm slowly sense its way across the rock face. Then it stopped, rose up again onto its back legs, turned, and crawled its way to the top. It showed me I would climb my own mountain, inch by inch, even if I veered off track for a while.

Sure enough, after the second lung resection, I had clean scans. My own understanding, in which I had trusted, proved false; the Divine came through, and I felt deep gratitude.

Thriver Soup Ingredient:

According to the teachings of German healer Bruno Gröning, one's body might undergo a healing crisis in which one feels more pain or experiences worse symptoms for a while. This is later followed by a cure. Reports from the Circle of Friends in their newsletter repeatedly show this phenomenon. A setback, therefore, might actually be the prelude to a cure.

Songs Bubble Up

We laud you with delightful songs for you are the Mistress of joy, the Mistress of music, the Queen of harp-playing, the Lady of the Dance.
—Song of praise for the Egyptian goddess Hathor

Hathor was an ancient Egyptian goddess of music, joy, and dance, among other personifications. I like her because sometimes songs will bubble up into my conscious mind and play repeatedly in my head. When a song seems to come from nowhere, I don't consider it a coincidence. I happen to think it's the universe giving me a message, trying to get my attention.

A song can be prophetic, though we can't always know until we have hindsight.

Nine months into treatment, the refrain "I'm clean, clean, clean" from the song "Clean" kept running through my mind. Actually, two spots had been cleaned up, and only one remained. While it took another eighteen months to manifest, this song did provide me with hope I desperately needed.

One month later, while I was involved in my second chemotherapy regimen, I woke up with the song "I Can See Clearly Now" playing loud and clear in my mind.

This song seemed to tell me that I would receive exactly what I was requesting, and it might have been related to my emotional work in psychotherapy. My therapist pointed out that my maiden name, "Bright," was a repetitive phrase in this song. She also noted how the phrase "bright, sun-shiny" also pointed to the "bright smiley face" symbol I used to remind myself and others to see my body shining brightly with Divine healing energy.

After my first lung resection, the phrase, "I seek to cure what's deep inside" from Toto's song "Africa" kept playing in my head, so I felt a physical cure might be in process and my emotional healing was continuing.

Even if these lively songs were not telling forth the future for me, they still enlivened my days and gave me hope. These happy feelings could only serve to enhance my health, so I belted out the songs whenever I could, without disturbing others: in the car, at home alone, or wherever.

If I felt up to it, I danced with the music. I think the Hathor aspect of the Divine also found pleasure in my joy.

Thriver Soup Ingredient:

Pay attention to any songs that spontaneously arise in your mind or heart. Sing them out loud if you can. You can try an internet search for a performance of the music, then play it and learn the lyrics. Dance to it, if you can, to jiggle those happy feelings into your cells.

～～～

Spirit Helps Those who Help Themselves

Verily never Will God change the condition Of a people until they Change it themselves (With their own souls).

—Qur'an 13:11b

While the phrase "God helps those who help themselves" is sometimes quoted as a Bible verse, it actually doesn't appear in the Bible. The Sura quoted above, from the Qur'an, comes closest to this idea. The concept already had been developed through ancient Greek tragedies more than a thousand years before the Islamic prophet Muhammad was born. The Bible does pick up on the concept in the Book of Hebrews (6:11-12, Christian Bible), which says, "We want each of you to show this same diligence to the very end, so that what you hope for may be fully realized. We do not want you to become lazy, but to imitate those who through faith and patience inherit what has been promised."

As the Qur'an and the Bible say, our getting well might need to involve our putting forth diligent effort to change ourselves. If we are diagnosed with lung cancer and keep smoking anyway, then we aren't doing our part to get better. Sitting back and waiting for a miracle is probably ineffective for the vast majority of humans. It's like the joke about the man who prayed faithfully for years to win the lottery, yet didn't win it, until finally he hears a Voice say, "You'll have to buy a ticket first."

I'm not saying a miracle cure can't happen. It just might be someone's fortune in life to have that blessing. Or someone might simply experience a profound internal shift that changes the body's chemistry and brings about a cure. These, however, are not the norm.

After talking with other cancer patients, I came to realize how much I have done to save my life—it seems to be far more than the majority of others with a cancer diagnosis. Surely if what I had done was not enough, there was nothing more I could have done or not done that would have helped. Others have done far less and been cured.

Oddly, about eighteen months into treatment, I awoke up from a nap with a message—I'm not going to get well from all my work. Apparently I had been trying too hard. There is diligence, and there is overkill. There are delicious soup recipes, and there are unsavory smorgasbords. I needed to step back, relax, and allow. It was time to strike a healthier balance between diligence and simply being. I also smiled when I realized that perhaps, if I dawdle and delay working on what I feel the Spirit has asked me to do with my life, I might get to live longer.

Thriver Soup Ingredient:

I found that people responded quite well to me when I worked hard to help myself get better. They tended to be more supportive, perhaps because they knew that their assistance, combined with my efforts, would produce a better outcome. Helping yourself by taking responsibility for every choice takes one out of victim mentality and into an "I can do this" mode of operating. This sends positive messages to one's cells, which will help the body as it works to heal itself.

∽∽∽

Using Cancer: Don't Waste Your Sorrows

Brethren, be earnest, mindful, virtuous, and steadfast in your aim. Guard ye your thoughts.
—"It is Time for Me to Go," *Pali Canon*

Our thoughts hold great power. They shape and influence our experiences of life. And of cancer. By guarding our perceptions, as the Buddha taught his followers to do, we can turn our thinking around. We can shift from viewing ourselves as victims of disease to exploiting the cancer as a means for achieving our highest personal objectives.

At some point during my illness, I made it my aim to steadfastly use the cancer for my own purposes. I didn't want to waste my sorrows—I wanted to use them as instigators of change. I found physical pain and the threat of death to be especially great motivators. If I could avoid some suffering by taking better care of myself and doing my psychological work, with earnestness, mindfulness, and steadfastness, then I would—with the added benefit of changing my life in positive ways. I had to work hard to protect my thoughts from victim or failure mentalities, and to spur myself onward so I could change everything in my life that I wanted to transform anyway.

Treya Wilber, in the book *Grace and Grit*, described using breast cancer to grow in every area of her life. She chose to look at death, along with the meaning and purpose of her life, more closely. She wanted to find and follow a contemplative path. She sought greater self-kindness and self-love, desiring to more easily express her anger and be more open to intimacy. On a physical level, she decided to exercise and eat well. "And most of all," she wrote, she wanted "to be gentle with myself about meeting or not meeting those goals."

My earnest aims also involved several areas of my life: socially, to improve my relationships and be of service to others; physically, to improve my food choices even more; emotionally, to really dig deep through psychotherapy so I could heal old wounds; mentally, to learn better concentration; and spiritually, to deepen my connection with the Divine. Along the way I hoped to learn more about my life's purpose and follow it.

I love how it all turned out. My steadfastness in bringing earnest mindfulness to my processes brought broad and deep rewards. I had used cancer, instead of letting cancer use me. I am grateful.

Thriver Soup Ingredient:

May you take this quote from the movie "The Curious Case of Benjamin Button" to heart: "It's never too late to be whoever you want to be.... I hope you live a life you're proud of. If you find that you're not, I hope you have the strength to start all over again."

It Takes a Village 277

E. It Takes a Village

Introduction to It Takes a Village: Sharing the Moment...Sharing Life

When Jesus had entered Capernaum, a centurion came to him, asking for help. "Lord," he said, "my servant lies at home paralyzed, suffering terribly." Jesus said to him, "Shall I come and heal him?" The centurion replied, "Lord, I do not deserve to have you come under my roof. But just say the word, and my servant will be healed. For I myself am a man under authority, with soldiers under me. I tell this one, 'Go,' and he goes; and that one, 'Come,' and he comes. I say to my servant, 'Do this,' and he does it." When Jesus heard this, he was amazed and said to those following him, "Truly I tell you, I have not found anyone in Israel with such great faith. I say to you that many will come from the east and the west, and will take their places at the feast with Abraham, Isaac and Jacob in the kingdom of heaven. But the subjects of the kingdom will be thrown outside, into the darkness, where there will be weeping and gnashing of teeth." Then Jesus said to the centurion, "Go! Let it be done just as you believed it would." And his servant was healed at that moment.
—Matthew 8:5-13, Christian Bible, NIV

The centurion in this story was willing to forgo his status and pride to advocate for his servant. His love for this man and his faith in Jesus moved the Christ to extend healing to the servant.

The love and faith of my family and friends buoyed me through years of treatments. I felt continually amazed by the kindness and generosity of so many people—many who never met me and others whom I had not heard from in years.

While recovering from my first surgery, dear friends surrounded my hospital bed and spent an hour praying over and for me. Later, women encircled me with chants and laid hands on me while praying. My body, relishing this attention, shook with energy moving up my spine.

One friend said, "Do you see how much you inspire others? It's false humility not to accept this. And it's not about you. It's about bringing people together in love and joy, making community."

Jesus and Bruno Gröning encouraged people to gather in community and pray together because this increases our ability to access healing energy. My community of loving people was pivotal in my recovery, especially because one of my primary issues and needs has been to emotionally connect with others. Dean Ornish, in his book *Love and Survival,* cites study after study demonstrating that people who are emotionally and physically supported through illnesses have much higher rates of survival than those who go it alone.

Even better results can arise for the patients who find others with whom they can share true feelings on a daily basis. This simple, yet difficult, practice sends positive messages to the body that encourage healing.

I found that when I had a specific need, I thought about who might be the most interested in assisting me. Setting aside my ego, I made my request. Roselie and Jim, can you help me find people to stay with when I travel to other cancer centers? Paula and Cathy, can you drive me to and from Columbus for my lung surgery? Debbie and Cynthia, can you take turns changing my surgical bandages once I get home? I found my family and friends more than happy to help, and I felt deep gratitude for their love and faithfulness. I think the centurion would have been proud of me.

Thriver Soup Ingredient:

Gather together a group of your friends who know each other. Form a circle. Select one person to move into the middle and who is to remain silent.

Those forming the circle of friends then say only words of affirmation and encouragement to the person in the center.

When it is your turn in the center, receive the loving words into your heart. Write them down later in your journal, and express gratitude for this gift.

∾∾∾

Bright Smiley Faces

Dear children, let us not love with words or speech but with actions and in truth.
—1 John 3:18, Christian Bible, NIV

My family and friends expressed their love for me not only with words but with action. Soon after the diagnosis, my sister purchased a bag of bright yellow smiley-face pins that we wore as reminders to pray and think positive thoughts.

A week later, I met Charley, a fellow writer whose work I'd read several times in a local publication, *Infinity*. As we talked, I said I had stopped writing for the local holistic magazine *Whole Living Journal* because of my new medical condition.

A month later, I came across a deeply moving and delightful column Charley had written about my situation for *Infinity*. He intuitively knew the symbol for my journey was bright yellow smiley faces. His article encouraged others to place smiley faces where they could see them as a reminder to pray for me.

Images of bright yellow smiley faces started arriving on notes and cards, lifting my spirits. I purchased about 100 smiley-face buttons and gave them away, requesting prayers in the process. I began visualizing my body as a big, happy face, filled with individual cells that beamed their smiles with heavenly light.

Many people would later tell me they kept their buttons in visible locations and would pray for me whenever they looked at them. I saw those yellow smiley faces in several retail shops I frequented. Seeing this symbol bolstered my confidence in my outcome.

Soon, Maria Paglialungo got out a treasure map she had made years earlier. On the bright yellow paper sat the word "Enlightenment" with a yellow smiley face used as the dot over the letter "i." Later Maria added eyes and glitter, transforming the whole poster into a big smiley face and taping it to her refrigerator. I copied her image and her choice of location so it could be a constant reminder of my purpose and her love.

More yellow smiley faces showed up during my treatment. My brother, Jim Bright, and his wife, Janet, sent a bouquet of sunny flowers in a round pattern with dark green pipe cleaners used as eyes and a mouth. Later, they sent a whole package of yellow smiley-faced goodies, including window clings, measuring spoons, a towel, and a cup with a lid and straw that I use every day at my desk. Susan Smith-Sargent and Brecka Burton-Platt gave me large mugs with bright yellow smiley faces on them. Judy Peace gave me some old-style-clasp smiley-face buttons that I wear on my clothing.

I am surrounded by tangible expressions of others' love in action, represented for me by a symbol of healing. My joyful surroundings promote healing, and I feel sunny with delight.

Thriver Soup Ingredient:

Come up with a simple symbol that represents what you want for this journey. Angels, butterflies, dragonflies, roses, or ribbons are just a few ideas. Buy these images as stickers or pins and hand them out to people while asking them to pray for you.

∾∾∾

Cancer Support Community

[B]etter a neighbor nearby than a brother far away.
—Proverbs 27:10b, Complete Jewish Bible

When the cancer disaster strikes, support is critical. For many people, there is no family around to help out. That's where a close neighbor, in the form of the global network of Cancer Support Communities, can be of tremendous service.

This non-profit organization provides free support groups, counseling, education, and healthy lifestyle programs for people affected by cancer. The CSC even offers participants personal web pages and blogs to extend patients' support systems.

My local Blue Ash, Ohio, CSC is housed in a beautiful, spacious building. A volunteer always greets people with a warm smile and does what it takes to find answers to questions; a gorgeous outdoor courtyard provides a peaceful setting for quiet time alone or visits with friends; a wonderful library is filled with helpful resources; a lovely living area provides comfortable sitting for educational programs or group meetings; individual rooms lined with couches covered with blankets offer a safe setting for support groups; a modern kitchen enables chefs to present cooking classes and groups to meet for potlucks; and an art room is filled with fun and useful supplies. During occasional Ladies' Night Out gatherings, we've eaten delicious dinners and been entertained with interesting and fun programs.

I've enjoyed a variety of classes, from art to yoga. Everyone there has been touched by cancer, so an immediate connection of understanding forms among participants. There's no need for pretense or hiding the illness, as everyone has been in a similar boat. I've made friends with some of the women, and have supported many in prayer. Many, in turn, have prayed for me.

I am grateful for the CSC, a close neighbor with understanding, along with caring support that is there for me on a daily basis.

Thriver Soup Ingredient:

To find a Cancer Support Community near you, go to www.cancersupportcommunity. org/Default.aspx and look under the "Cancer Support" tab to find a community near you. All programs are offered free to those affected by cancer.

〜〜〜

CaringBridge: An Interactive Blog

Dear friends, let us love one another, for love comes from God. Everyone who loves has been born of God and knows God.

—1 John 4:7a, Christian Bible, NIV

I had no idea how much I was loved until my family and friends spread the word about the cancer.

Years earlier, I had a friend on the website www.CaringBridge.org, a personal health social network with an interactive blog. I was amazed by the support she received. I fantasized that if I ever ended up needing such a website, I might have support from maybe half a dozen people at best.

Well, I was in for a fabulous surprise. As soon as my friend Kathryn Martin Ossege got the news about the illness, she set me up on CaringBridge with a somewhat private blog. She and my then-husband contacted everyone they knew who might be interested in providing support. She later said she wanted to create one spot where she could provide daily reports for friends and family about my condition and progress. She updated everyone until either my then-husband or I could post. She only used my first name and two initials so the blog would not be found by anyone who was not personally invited. She chose a setting that required people to log in each time they visited. This felt safe to me, so I decided to participate.

During the three-year life of the blog, I posted nearly 800 times. There were nearly 15,000 visits and 800 guest posts—some from people I never had and probably never will meet. I cannot imagine the vast amounts of prayer on my behalf, and am deeply grateful for this wonderful, supportive community.

Maria Paglialungo suggested at one point that I place an intention statement on the blog so everyone could pray the same way. I liked her idea because I believed if everyone prayed the same way or offered the same intention, then the likelihood of our having a positive outcome was greatly increased.

I also took my laptop when I went in for surgery, and was able to give my supporters quick info bites so they could pray specifically as I went through recovery. I found their responsiveness extremely comforting, allowing me to let go of some of the muscle tension in my body. I knew people were praying for me in my hours of greatest need.

My heart feels warm as I remember how my dear friends and family loved me in the most instantaneous manner possible through online health social networking.

Thriver Soup Ingredient:

You can obtain a free, private, online social health blog to raise support for your situation. Try the Cancer Support Community option at www.cancersupportcommunity.org/MainMenu/ Cancer-Support/My-LifeLineorg.html or www.CaringBridge.org.

$$\approx\approx\approx$$

Dances with Women

Finally, Ama-no Uzume, the goddess of mirth and dance, came forward with a plan. Uzume climbed upon a large upturned tub that resonated like a drum, and began her dance. Her feet drumming, her dancing ecstatic, she removed her undergarments and then, once she had the undivided attention of the eight hundred divinities, she lifted her kimono and exposed her vulva. They laughed, clapped their hands, and shouted.

—"The Myth of Amaterasu," Jean Shinoda Bolen

In this Japanese fairy tale, the sun goddess is hiding in a cave and won't come out. This is dreadful for the community, and they must find some way to lure the sun back out. Using an age-old idea, another goddess plans for and then creates laughter and dance to draw the attention of Amaterasu. The people celebrated, because when the sun goddess returned to her proper place, the people would live.

I wanted to dance myself to celebrate my life, yet could hardly believe it when I gathered my wits and pulled up my sweat pants to attend belly dance lessons.

As I had heard, the class proved fun and provided good exercise. I also felt at ease exercising only with women.

Facing my body shame, I wrote about the experience on my blog. The subject of photos inevitably arose. Uh, no thanks. How ridiculous I'd look in a belly-dance costume, with a large abdomen resembling a road map of downtown Manhattan.

Still, I had a great time.

I learned that belly dancing was developed by women for women, to be done in the presence of women. It met a social need and helped relieve tension during menses. It also can help women learn to relish their bodies.

My friend Norma Wirt, a belly dancer, wrote, "It's hard to feel sad when you hear that mysterious music and see the fluid movements of the women. One of the first things you'll learn is that your arms will follow the 'melody' of the music. Your hips and pelvis will carry the beat of the drums. It took me a while to get my body parts moving the way I was supposed to, but once you let loose and feel the music, your body will respond without much effort from you."

My friend Kathy Nace wrote, "When I decided to take flamenco...I had no idea what else would rear its ugly head! I had somehow learned that my body was totally irrelevant except as a shell for the real me, and I ignore(d) it as much as I could. This was a huge rent in the fabric of my wholeness as a created being. Being in class weekly and having to face ALL myself in the mirror... was so hard. And yet, I celebrate so much that I absorb through my senses, which reside in this body."

A poem by Jalāl ad-Dīn Muḥammad Rūmī, a 13th-century Sufi mystic, came to mind—one which says our bodies are woven from the light of heaven. We literally are composed of stardust.

I learned from psychotherapist Anyaa McAndrew that dance brings vibration into and enlivens the body, making it more present to the woman. A woman can express her gifts through her physical being, and can use dance to convey self-love and self-care. A woman's way of meditation can be movement, which tends the feminine aspect of the Divine within her body.

Lakota medicine man Leonard Crow Dog, before a Native American Ghost Dance, said, "While dancing, your body will be the altar."

So, if you are able, go dance and find your ecstasy within. Allow joy to vibrate through your body, making it an altar for your prayers.

Thriver Soup Ingredient:

If you are physically able to belly dance, find a local class and check it out. Have fun! If there aren't any classes around, do an internet search for belly dance videos. Watch, participate, and maybe even invite a friend to do it with you. Feel joy in movement as you learn the basic steps. Delight in the nuances of muscle use. Dance in front of a mirror, look yourself in the eye, and cheer yourself on as you master this new skill. Perhaps you might find the music of Loreena McKennitt an inspiration, especially the album "An Ancient Muse."

Death and Rebirth Ceremonies

A believer is not terrorized by death's calling.

—*The Japji*, 13

As cancer patients, the specter of death can loom a little too close for comfort. All sorts of terrors can surface and make us miserable. Even a deep faith can sometimes be seriously shaken by the grim prospect of dying from cancer.

Facing this fear can loosen up something old and unwanted that you can then get rid of. A good way to face one's fear is to stage your own death ceremony and explore your emotions as they occur. By getting into our pockets of terror and despair, we can experience some healing and move deeper into the Divine.

My women's group, led by Anyaa McAndrew, conducted death and rebirth ceremonies during 2009 to help us drop some of our fears and live more fully. Rain saturated our Halloween on Saturday, October 31, our day to die. I dressed in all black for the second time in my adult life. We wrote our own obituaries, keeping them light and humorous at Anyaa's suggestion. I wrote mine to the tune of "Ding dong, the witch is dead," from the movie "The Wizard of Oz."

Each of us made a flammable doll to represent the parts of ourselves we were ready to let die. Mine involved an empty paper towel roll that I stuffed with my baseline CAT scan results, a few pictures and several words written on scraps of paper. Since I was fighting so hard to save my life, Anyaa suggested I die to the parts of myself that needed to die so I could be reborn.

As the sun set, we solemnly took turns walking up to a fire pit. There we read our obituaries and tossed our death dolls into the blaze. Each of us had ceremonially died. We returned to our beds in silence.

Sunday brought gorgeous, sunny weather. We processed our death experiences and designed our own rebirthing ceremonies. I wore all pink and asked the women to form a human tunnel for me to pull myself through on my forearms. I gave each of them a word to use as a starting point for encouraging me through this birth canal. I bent forward and began the push through the human portal. By the time I got through, I was quite tired and laid down on my "receiving blanket," an angel throw that the women had saturated with their healing energy. Maria Paglialungo placed a smiley-face button on the blanket. The women showered me with red rose petals and more encouragement, placing their hands on me. I was birthing a new, healthier me. Some of the fear had died, leaving more space for faith and for my mind to soar closer to enlightenment.

Thriver Soup Ingredient:

If you are experiencing some fear around the possibility of death, create your own death and rebirth ceremonies to allay them. First, write your obituary, in a lighthearted way. Then gather flammable things that represent the parts of yourself you want dead. Combine them together somehow and burn them in a carefully tended fire. Spend some time in silence, contemplating your experience. Then create a rebirth day to celebrate what you are birthing in yourself. Use your imagination and move with what feels right and freeing to you. Two songs that might provide a helpful background for rebirthing are Karen Drucker's "You are Healed" and "I will be Gentle with Myself" from the album "The Heart of Healing."

~~~

Faith of Our Family and Friends

Some men came carrying a paralyzed man on a mat and tried to take him into the house to lay him before Jesus. When they could not find a way to do this because of the crowd, they went up on the roof and lowered him on his mat through the tiles into the middle of the crowd, right in front of Jesus. When Jesus saw their faith, he said, "Friend, your sins are forgiven."

—Luke 5:18-20, Christian Bible, NIV

In Luke's account of a divine cure, some men acted on their loving faith to help their paralyzed friend. They did not allow throngs of people, ordinary barriers, or socially acceptable behavior to intimidate them. Determined, they clambered up unto the roof of the overcrowded home where Jesus sat teaching. They hauled up their friend, who lay on a mat, and removed tiles to open up the roof. Persistently seeking access to the divine healing presence, they carefully lowered their friend so he would softly land right in front of Jesus.

Even though I had read the story many times, I had never noticed that Jesus did not say to the paralyzed man, "Your faith has made you well." Instead, Jesus noticed the faith of the man's friends, and then forgave the paralyzed man so he would be cured.

How I needed the love and faith of my family and friends! They rallied around with practical assistance, tenaciously seeking or providing the best treatment for me despite financial barriers and time constraints. They prayed with faith when I had none. Sometimes months went by without my whispering a word of prayer or doing any meditation because I felt too sick, fatigued, overwhelmed, or depressed. My heart swells when I recall how so many of them persistently prayed for me every day—some for nearly three years. Other friends visualized, lit candles, and set positive intentions for a healthy outcome.

I am filled with gratitude for everyone's faith and faithfulness. I feel fortunate to have such wonderful family and friends who cleared a path so I could more deeply encounter the Spirit and move into remission.

Thriver Soup Ingredient:
Let your family and friends know of your appreciation for their faith and faithfulness, and if you are inclined, reference the text above about the friends of the paralyzed man. Sending thank-you cards provides you with the opportunity to open up to more gratitude and lifts the spirits of your recipients.

≈≈≈

Fun with Friends

For where two or three gather in my name, there am I with them.

—Matthew 18:20, Christian Bible, NIV

Several times during my treatment phase, I got together with two or three friends to have fun doing what I had wanted to do for years. I could feel their love warming me, and I knew they represented the love of the Spirit manifesting in human form.

A couple of times Rebecca Woods, Laura Dailey, and I toured some of Cincinnati's churches to view fabulous stained-glass windows. We saw a variety of styles, including a large Tiffany-created image of Archangel Michael. I was struck by the large number of churches and windows dedicated to Mary, the mother of Jesus. All this spectacular art was there for the viewing; all we had to do was figure out where they were and plan our visits. Rebecca outlined our tours, called ahead to ensure our access to the sanctuaries, and off we went to explore. We had a lovely time entering into gorgeous spaces, absorbing their ineffable peace and beauty. For the first time, we entered St. Mary's Cathedral Basilica of the Assumption in nearby Covington, Kentucky. There we viewed the world's largest church stained-glass window, along with an individual window dedicated to St. Agatha, patron saint for those with breast cancer.

Rebecca topped off our visits by giving me a lovely Hallmark stained-glass window holiday tree ornament that was part of a series. "Now I have to stay alive long enough to collect them all!" I wrote. I actually outlived the series—only three types were created. I own one of each.

The ornaments will always remind me of our little gathering of friends in the name of the Spirit, soaking up the sacred as we gawked at great art.

Thriver Soup Ingredient:

Think about a few things you've been wanting to do with friends yet never did. Contact them and ask them to plan a fun outing around those ideas. Then go and have a great time.

≈≈≈

Gratitude's Gifts

And remember! your Lord Caused to be declared (publicly): "If ye are grateful, I will Add more (favours) unto you."

—Qur'an 14:7a

My friend Kathy Nace understands that the real source of abundance in life is found in practicing gratitude for what we already have, small and large. When she came to visit me, her face lit up as she recounted her 500-somethingth experience for which she gave thanks. She had taken up the spiritual practice of looking for, and writing down, 1,000 gifts already in her everyday life, modeled after author Ann Voskamp's discipline which she wrote about in *One Thousand Gifts: A Dare to Live Fully Right Where You Are.*

I thought about Kathy's words and looked at my fingers—how old and worn they looked, a far cry from the beautiful hands of young actresses. And yet, I felt deep gratitude for them. How much they have done for me! How many people they have touched, how many thousands of meals they have prepared, how many millions of words they have typed, how many dozens of blank books they have filled with the outpourings of my soul. How beautifully and wonderfully I am made.

My friend Fay Gano added richness to the practice of living with thanksgiving by suggesting I try to feel gratitude for exactly where I was. Where was I? In the midst of miserable chemotherapy treatments and surgeries, with no job and a husband who wanted out of our marriage. Give thanks? More like give hell.

Fay, however, understood and practiced an ancient truth—to offer thanks, even in the midst of the most discouraging circumstances, even without knowing any answers to desperate questions. Thirteenth-century Persian poet and Sufi mystic Jalāl ad-Dīn Muḥammad Rūmī described how to receive the vicissitudes of life in his poem, "The Guest House." He calls each of us a guest house and encourages us to welcome everything that shows up, whether joy or depression. "Even if they're a crowd of sorrows, who violently sweep your house empty of its furniture, still, treat each guest honorably. He may be clearing you out for some new delight...each has been sent as a guide from beyond."

My life certainly was being cleaned out. I could only hope the Spirit was making room for some new delight. Maria Paglialungo said it more graphically: be grateful for all the sht in our lives, because it's really only fertilizer. When sht happens, plant some seeds in it. Watch what grows.

I'm surprised and quite pleased with what grew out of my sht; I am glad for what was cleared out of my life and delighted by the new. It took time, yet my increase came—in the form of profound gratitude, light-hearted happiness, and deep joy.

Thriver Soup Ingredient:

Even in the midst of chaos, pain, and change, there is much for which we can feel gratitude: the loving concern on a friendly face, the warm caress of sunshine, the sweet fragrance of fresh air, the gentle massage of a shower, or the creamy smoothness of a chocolate truffle. It is through receiving these simple gifts that a divine experience manifests richness and abundance in our lives.

If you are so inclined, challenge yourself to write down 100 things in your journal for which you are grateful. It probably will be easy for you to come up with a few dozen rather quickly. As you move through your day, watch for more items to add to your list. Observe how this level of attention shifts your focus and experience. This might inspire another topic for your journal.

~~~

Laughter: Have a Joke and a Smile

Baubo cheered the goddess with her bawdy humor. Her jests brought a smile, and then when she lifted her skirt and exposed herself, Demeter laughed and was restored.
—*The Metamorphosis of Baubo: Myths of Women's Sexual Energy*

Baubo knew the restorative nature of laughter. While her actions seem odd by today's standards—how could this bawdy action elicit laughter?—ancient Baubo figurines show females with their skirts raised to expose their round bellies and vulvas. Jean Shinoda Bolen, MD, said, "Once the vulva was the entrance to the body of the goddess, and cleft-like cave entrances were painted earth-red in reverence."

Such laughter, which author Winifred Milius Lubell said often is associated with the trickster figure and with fertility, "was often used in sacred and joyful rituals to ease a stressful situation, to set painful matters in perspective, to restore balance."

Baubo used humor to help lift the Greek goddess Demeter's spirits when she could not find her daughter, Persephone.

Laughter gives your diaphragm, abdomen, lungs, chest, and face an enjoyable little workout. It also increases oxygen levels in the blood and tones the whole cardiovascular system. After laughing, all your muscles relax, including your heart. Your blood pressure and pulse rate temporarily drop. You might be able to tolerate pain a little better, and your digestion will improve. Your immune system also functions more optimally.

Laughter has proven to be the best medicine—I have heard stories of people who cured themselves of cancer by watching comedies every day for months.

After the diagnosis, I decided to give laughter yoga with Judi Winall and Pam Hall a try. This practice combines laughter for no reason with yogic breathing. The routine was developed by Madan Kataria, a physician from Mumbai, India. It uses the philosophy "fake it 'till you make it," because the body cannot differentiate between fake and real laughter. Either way, you get the same physiological and psychological benefits. Thousands of social laughter yoga clubs have sprung up around the world. According to the official laughter yoga website, "Laughter is simulated as a body exercise in a group; with eye contact and childlike playfulness, it soon turns into real and contagious laughter."

I attended my first laughter yoga meeting with my friend Laura Dailey. She later wrote, "What a treasure to see and hear you giggling, chuckling, snickering, guffawing, hootin' and hollerin' at laughter yoga! With all your God-given joy, that little tumor doesn't have a chance!"

I've continued attending on occasion. My sister, Roselie Bright, knit a funny little hat for me, which was perfect for laughter yoga. I also wore Willy braids (fake brown braids coming out of a folded red bandana), and Laura wore funny socks. Silliness was the name of the game.

Going as far as Baubo isn't necessary to lift my spirits.

Thriver Soup Ingredient:

Visit laughteryoga.org/ to find a club near you. An internet search can pull up numerous videos of laughter yoga that you can watch and with which you can laugh. Additionally, you can order cartoon and joke books and audio files from your local library, and watch or listen to comedies. It might be helpful to find a way to laugh—or at least smile inside—each day.

≈≈≈

Reiki: Let Your Fingers do the Talking

Their Light will run Forward before them And by their right hands, While they say, "Our Lord! Perfect our Light for us, And grant us Forgiveness: For Thou hast power Over all things."

—Qur'an 66:8b

For light to stream before someone and from the right hand, one must be filled with Divine light. I imagine Jesus had this kind of energy, perhaps not visible to most humans as light, yet powerful enough to cause instantaneous healings by touching others. Many individuals through history have been known to heal people by touch, and even from a distance, without personal contact.

A system of hands-on healing was developed in 1922 by Japanese Buddhist Mikao Usui. It involved the transfer of universal life-force energy through a practitioner's hands into the body of a client. This method was called Reiki.

Brecka Burton-Platt, a Reiki master, got me started on this healing path with training for the first two levels. She gave me an initiation, or attunement, in which the energy centers in my body, known as chakras, were opened so my body could become an effective conduit for the flow of life-force energy. I learned some Japanese words used as healing symbols to do in combination with the practice.

Being my typical self, during my attunements I felt nothing in my body. Nada. I have faithfully practiced nearly every day since my first training. It involves prayer, drawing the symbols on each hand using only fingers from the other hand, and then placing the hands on or above various body parts and asking the universal life force to penetrate and heal. After two years of nearly daily practice, I still felt nothing.

I kept going, however, because soon after learning Reiki, I asked in meditation what practices would be the most transformative on my healing journey. One by one I went through my list. I got little response from most modalities, yet with the Reiki I got a strong "yes." And so I continue, by faith. Sometimes my hands do get a little warm while I practice, which I find encouraging.

I have added a few things to my personal practice to enhance whatever flow is there. I gather energy into my hands by rolling them around each other, as if stretching out a hand muff. I do auditory toning for whatever body part I'm concentrating upon. And I say the words for the Reiki symbols while visualizing light streaming into the crown of my head, down to my hands and into my body.

Does it work for me? While many people report experiencing physical sensations, I didn't for more than three years of almost daily practice. I believed, however, that I, like every human, could be a conduit for Divine healing energy, whether I felt it or not. I will gladly receive all the Divine light my body can stand.

Thriver Soup Ingredient:

If Reiki interests you, ask around to see if you can sit in on a Reiki energy share session to see for yourself what Reiki involves. Then you can make a better decision about whether Reiki is an art you would like to pursue. Read up on the various types of Reiki and select the training that most suits who you are.

~·~·~

Shamanic Breathwork

In their trouble they cried to ADONAI, and he rescued them from their distress.
—Psalm 107:13, Complete Jewish Bible

In the straits of my terror of death I cried out to the Divine, and was provided with a new way to clear out old emotional baggage as a path toward healing: Shamanic Breathwork. A practitioner is someone with access to, and influence in, the spirit world through trance and/or ritual. The Shamanic Breathwork process was developed by Linda Star Wolf, DMin, PhD, as a synthesis of her personal healing experiences with breath work, the wisdom of indigenous people, depth psychology, and addiction recovery models.

Through an induced altered state of consciousness, practitioners can transform and integrate past traumas, develop closer connections with their spirit guides, and receive visions about their sacred purposes in the world.

I had been meeting with a circle of women for a process designed to awaken my inner divine feminine self so I could share it with the world. Part-way through the nine monthly meetings came the diagnosis. I soon understood that to have any chance for a cure, I would need to face my emotional wasteland and heal.

One of our meetings landed on Halloween 2009—a good day to practice dying to the old, and to allow unwanted emotional baggage to rise into conscious awareness and dissipate. Our group of about a dozen women put on blindfolds and lay down on mats in the Half-Moon Temple at Isis Cove near Whittier, North Carolina. Our facilitator, Anyaa McAndrew, explained the process and then played music designed to enhance our experiences and assist us with bringing unconscious material to the surface of our minds. We were instructed to breathe quickly for three minutes while focusing on each of seven chakra, or energy center, locations on our bodies, starting with the root chakra at the base of the spine. Also at each chakra, we were to move our right hands counter-clockwise over the chakra location to release blocked energy, and then to move our hands clockwise to receive positive energy back into the chakra.

I moved into a trance-like state. Because I felt unconditionally accepted and loved by the beautiful circle of women lying near me, I dove completely into my experience. Two or three times, with facilitator Anne McQuinn's help, I sat upright in a birthing posture and screamed with all the force I could muster: "Get this sht out of my body!" I wanted to evict the evil child that had possessed my womb. I wanted to birth it by belting out primal screams. In between bursts, I lay down in the fetal position to regroup and recover.

As the music continued and we moved up to higher chakras in our bodies, I gradually calmed down. Toward the end, my body felt like flowing water—peaceful, at rest.

I don't know if the experience ultimately made any difference in the disease process, yet I felt a letting go of rage and terror and dread. My forcefulness gave other women permission to verbalize their own pain. Together, we made lots of noise—cries too terrible for words, the Spirit screaming through us what we could not put into language. We had entered into the process of being saved from the wreckage of old emotional traumas and moving into places of peace and healing.

Thriver Soup Ingredient:

If Shamanic Breathwork interests you, check the list of shamanic ministers at the Venus Rising Association for Transformation, co-founded by Linda Star Wolf and Bradford Collins (shamanicbreathwork.org/shamanic-ministers/find-shamanic-minister). Star Wolf has written several books featuring shamanism, including *Shamanic Breathwork: Journeying Beyond the Limits of the Self*.

~~~

Starbucks Virgin

Therefore if anyone is in Christ, he is a new creature; the old things passed away; behold, new things have come.

—II Corinthians 5:17, New American Standard Bible

After the diagnosis, I decided I needed to let old things pass away and become a new creature. It was high time I brought some novel experiences into my life.

When my brother, Walter Bright, found out I had never sipped a coffee from Starbucks, he encouraged me to try one of their small black coffees for a special treat.

So in March of 2010, when I had a guest from Europe, we wandered into a Starbucks. I asked the man at the counter if he could provide me with a sample because I had never tried their coffee before. A woman in the store exclaimed, "A Starbucks virgin!"

Well, he gave me both an espresso and a black coffee. I didn't care for either. I soon found myself at the bar adding a bit of cocoa powder, vanilla powder, raw sugar, and creamer. Then it tasted all right.

This event, however, signaled a change. I was moving toward rebirth. The old was passing away, and the new was growing.

During that week, my guest introduced me to celery root and fennel while I introduced her to jicama root and sweet potatoes.

That fall, I finally dug out my Kansas State University varsity letter jacket. It had lain crushed at the bottom of the cedar chest for decades. I got it dry-cleaned because I realized I needed to start wearing clothes I liked rather than allowing them collect lint for years while I waited for other garments to wear out first.

Among other things I had put off for years was attending local events. I was too busy raising kids and working. When I heard the Vienna Boys' Choir would be singing in Cincinnati, I leapt at the opportunity. Even though I had never heard them before, in the past I would not have gone for any number of reasons—ticket prices, weather, darkness, not wanting to go downtown, not wanting to spend the time. No more! My then-husband, my friend Laura Dailey, and I went. We had a nice time, and the boys' voices were exquisite—especially when the high notes at the ends of songs echoed through St. Peter in Chains Cathedral for several seconds.

I thought about how beautiful voices must sound in heaven.

Nah. On second thought, I would rather wait another fifty years for that concert. In the meantime, I want to be a new creation right here, right now, letting the old things pass away while gathering novel experiences.

Thriver Soup Ingredient:

Drop the virgin status. Get together with your family or friends to do things you've never done before, and have a great time!

∽∽∽

Water: Obey the Thirst

We send down Pure water from the sky,—That with it We may give Life to a dead land, And slake the thirst Of things We have created.
—Qur'an 25:48b-49a

I needed pure water to be revived when the landscape within my body was dying. One of the first things my then-husband and I did after the diagnosis was select a good water filter. He installed it in our kitchen. Oh, how much better the filtered water tasted! I found pint-sized glass bottles to carry the water in when I left the house.

I began to realize the necessity of keeping hydrated during cancer treatment. One morning, after starting chemotherapy, I woke up feeling pressure in my chest and an irregular heartbeat. With trepidation, I called the ankhology nurse. She, however, thought the problems stemmed from dehydration. That made sense, since I had been so focused on eating properly that I hadn't paid much attention to drinking.

I spent the day drinking as much as I could stand, and my chest soon felt better.

Friends enhanced my water experiences. Norma Gracia Munive-Prime came by with holy water from the Dead Sea that had been blessed and had a million prayers instilled within it. I dabbed it on my forehead before meditating, and used it to make the sign of the cross on my body right before my chemosabe infusions.

My friend Judy Merritt, PhD, gave me a bottle of spring water blessed with energy for transformation. My friend Mim Grace Gieser brought me water blessed by Amma, the hugging saint, which I used to refill the spring water bottle. I taped a photo of the healer Bruno Gröning to the outside. I wrote words like "joy," "faith," "love," and "gratitude" on the glass. Each day I added a drop of healing flower essence, from Vince and Connie Lasorso, to what I drank.

Maria Paglialungo suggested I bless my drinking water with love and gratitude, and to have the faith that it was changing the vibration of the fluids in my body so the sarcoma cells would shrivel up. Pure water could revive my dead internal landscape.

Many drops of water were in the bottle I received; the blessing given to the water in the bottle was contained in each drop. It is the Divine who understands these secrets, and by acknowledging this, I can move deeper into oneness with the Spirit.

Thriver Soup Ingredient:

Make sure you have a good source of pure, clean, filtered water. Some water pitchers with filters are inexpensive and portable.

Avoid drinking out of plastic containers that have been hot, or putting hot liquids into plastic containers such as cups, as the chemicals infiltrate the water. If the water in the bottle smells like plastic, don't drink it. I use glass water bottles when I leave home.

Drink often to keep hydrated.

≈≈≈

Your Child and Your Cancer

People were bringing little children to Jesus for him to place his hands on them, but the disciples rebuked them. When Jesus saw this, he was indignant. He said to them, "Let the little children come to me, and do not hinder them, for the kingdom of God belongs to such as these. Truly I tell you, anyone who will not receive the kingdom of God like a little child will never enter it." And he took the children in his arms, placed his hands on them and blessed them.

—Mark 10:13-16, Christian Bible, NIV

Jesus seemed to enjoy holding children and blessing them. When my mother was diagnosed with cancer, I was eleven years old and certainly wasn't invited to sit with her, be held by her, or be blessed with a listening heart. No one talked much about her situation, what was going to happen, or how it might affect me. I remember being told she had breast cancer and had several surgeries, but little else.

Ironically, when I was diagnosed with cancer, my youngest son was eleven years old. Both of my children sat in the surgical waiting area for at least nine hours when the cancer was found and the doctors debulked my insides. I can't imagine their level of dread or sense of powerlessness during that agonizing time, nor was I in any condition afterward to think about them. I was barely holding onto life myself. Sitting with them, holding them, and blessing them with a gracious listening ear would come later.

Based on my childhood experiences, I knew I needed to keep my children informed every step of the way, letting them know what treatments I was undergoing, how I felt, and what my physical symptoms were. I felt they had a right to know, because the more they knew, the less fodder they would have for creating dreadful fantasies.

I encouraged my children to ask questions and talk about their feelings. I focused on listening carefully to them. Then I tried to mirror their experiences back to them, validate their feelings, and empathize with them, based on a process I had learned called Imago Relationship Therapy. Imago therapy was developed by Harville Hendrix, PhD.

As soon as the program was offered at the Cancer Support Community, our whole family attended "Walking the Dinosaur." My sons got to know one of the women working for a local organization called Cancer Family Care, and she counseled them at school a few times.

At one point I sent my youngest son to Camp Courage, a one-day camp in northern Kentucky designed for children touched by cancer. It took him a while to start enjoying himself. His favorite part was writing what he was angry about on a raw egg and throwing it at a wall to watch it burst.

A friend of mine with metastatic breast cancer has done a great job working with her daughter to maintain openness and loving communication. Tami Boehmer has a blog, and her daughter once wrote a helpful guest entry. She encouraged other kids to talk about their thoughts and feelings. "You are not alone," she wrote. "There are countless kids just like you who have parents with cancer and sometimes talking to people who know what it feels like can stop you from wallowing in your misery. There are many ways to find kids just like you, just look online. One that I highly recommend is www.campkesem.org."

She also offered tips for their parents. "One common misconception is that it is better to hide their cancer from their kids than to be open. Due to my mom being open about her cancer with me, I am able to understand what is going on and see how I can help. This allows me to build a trusting relationship with her rather than making false assumptions.

"Set an example. If you stay positive about your situation, your child will most likely do the same. It may be difficult at times, but if you keep an open mind you will not only be helping yourself, but helping your son or daughter."

Tami is acting like Jesus for her daughter: inviting, holding, and blessing her so together they can find the good in their situation.

Thriver Soup Ingredient:

A good parental resource is the book, *When a Parent Has Cancer: A Guide to Caring for Your Children*, by Wendy S. Harpham, a cancer survivor, mother, and physician.

If you have a young child at home, this little activity can be done with him or her. My son did it as part of a Cancer Support Community program for children called "Walking the Dinosaur."

What you'll need:

A variety of colored sands, possibly eight or ten colors

A clear glass jar with a lid

A funnel that fits into the mouth of the jar and is large enough for the sand to pass through

A surface that can easily be cleaned up, such as newspaper or a plastic tablecloth

Place the funnel in the jar and lay out the different colors of sand on your surface.

Talk to your child about your feelings associated with the cancer, such as when you experienced fear, anger, grief, and/or powerlessness. As you talk about each emotion, encourage your child to talk about his or her similar feelings. Then suggest to your child that he or she pick out a color of sand to represent that experience or feeling. Ask your child to pour that color of sand into the jar.

Move slowly, and cover each emotion that comes to mind that your child might be experiencing.

Then talk to your child about a positive emotion you have while with him or her, such as love, joy, peace, and/or comfort. Perhaps you could relate the feeling to an activity you share, such as watching a movie, going to the park, or playing a game.

Then ask your child to pick out sand colors that suggest these happy feelings to him or her, and what brings about those happy experiences.

After you talk about each feeling, ask your child to pour those colors of sand into the jar.

Explain to the child that it's okay to have all these feelings inside, just like the jar has all these colors inside. When your child feels the anger, he or she might be able to remember that sometimes there are more comfortable feelings as well.

F. Soaring with Spirit

Introduction to Soaring with Spirit: Wrestling with the Divine

So Jacob was left alone. Then a man wrestled with him until daybreak. When the man saw that he could not defeat Jacob, he struck the socket of his hip so the socket of Jacob's hip was dislocated while he wrestled with him. Then the man said, "Let me go, for the dawn is breaking." "I will not let you go," Jacob replied, "unless you bless me." The man asked him, "What is your name?" He answered, "Jacob." "No longer will your name be Jacob," the man told him, "but Israel, because you have fought with God and with men and have prevailed." Then Jacob asked, "Please tell me your name." "Why do you ask my name?" the man replied. Then he blessed Jacob there. So Jacob named the place Peniel, explaining, "Certainly I have seen God face to face and have survived."
—Genesis 32:25-31, Christian Bible, NET

One dark night, the Jewish patriarch Jacob found himself wrestling with a man, even though he hadn't invited or initiated combat. Jacob probably had to fight or be killed; he fought so hard his opponent wounded him to end the conflict. Jacob realized he had struggled with the Spirit, had possessed commanding power, and had prevailed. He demanded a blessing, and when the Divine granted it, his entire identity was transformed.

The cancer diagnosis was similar for me. Like Jacob, I hadn't invited the wrestling match. When it assailed me, I felt deeply vulnerable. I had to decide—was I going to fight with commanding power and prevail, or was I going to let go and die? Either way, I faced hell.

I chose to command all the power at my disposal so I could prevail. I didn't come out of cancer treatment unscathed, as the enemy was more powerful than me. Like Jacob, I received bodily injury to my own hips. About nine months after treatment ended, I had both hips totally replaced, as chemotherapy treatment had cleaned the last of the cartilage out of my hip sockets.

I also chose to face my inner wounding, and consciously moved through the emotional pain as a rite of passage into deeper realms. There, I encountered personal demons, profound mysteries, and inner light. I died to my former self. My mental constructs shattered, granting me the opportunity to reorganize my thought processes and rebuild my life on a more grounded basis so I could recognize my inherent wholeness. The Divine interacted with me at my deepest levels, and the dark journey turned numinous—opening a portal into greater realms of transcendent awareness.

In the depths of pain and despair, we can demand the blessings that only deep internal work can manifest within us. If we manage to find meaning in our journeys, or experience glimpses of the ineffable nature of the Spirit, we can use the cancer process as a means of transformation, even if we end up, like Jacob, with a permanent physical reminder of our wrestling match with eternal forces.

Thriver Soup Ingredient:

Try viewing the cancer experience as a divine injury or as a profound invitation to wake up to your true Self. Pray and journal about it until you find some meaning in your experiences. It might take some time to live your way into an answer. For me, the significance shifted as I continued moving along my personal path. The wounding created an entryway for divine light to enter more deeply into my life.

～～～

Acceptance of Death: Jephthah's Daughter

Freedom is not a matter of place, but of condition. I was happy in that prison, for those days were passed in the path of service. To me prison was freedom. Troubles are a rest for me. Death is life. To be despised is honor. Therefore was I full of happiness all through that prison time. When this release takes place, one can never be imprisoned. Unless one accepts dire vicissitudes, not with dull resignation, but with radiant acquiescence, one cannot attain this freedom.

—'Abdu'l-Baha, *Divine Art of Living*

Fear imprisoned me, and the prospect of a painful death created abject terror in my body. There was no acceptance, no freedom in my vocabulary after the diagnosis.

To deal with the potential of an agonizing death, I was reminded of the story in Judges 11 of the Jewish Bible about the daughter of Jephthah. Her father made a foolish vow to the Divine to make a burnt offering of the first thing to meet him after returning home from a war victory. Upon arriving at his house after winning, the first thing to greet him was his joyful daughter, who was singing and dancing. She bowed to her father's vow and to the masculine (not male) principle, or way of being in the world, that insisted on keeping a promise even when it involved murdering an innocent victim.

I felt incensed when I read this story. Not only was the woman never given the dignity of a name, but no angel appeared with a ram at the last moment to save her from an agonizing death (as it did for Isaac in the Jewish book of Genesis).

This daughter understood herself well enough to relish the joy of music and dance. She loved her father. She knew she needed time to prepare for her demise and required support—so she asked for what she needed. With great courage, she spent two months in retreat, contemplating her impending agony. She must have felt rage, terror, grief, and powerlessness during those two months. She did not run away from fulfilling her role. She faced it with grace. She mourned the things she would never experience in life.

Where was the purpose behind such a tragic, senseless death? It seemed totally insane. Yet the Spirit allowed it to happen. The daughter showed a profound acceptance of "things as they are." Not many types of death are worse than being burned alive. She did not cajole, bargain, try to influence or control, give up, or deny the situation.

She must have died in great equanimity with radiant acquiescence. She had much to teach me.

I came to understand that sometimes illness and death are part of the ultimate plan. The Spirit walks and weeps with us, and can offer us strength and courage even as we pass into the next existence. At about this time I read Paramahansa Yogananda's introduction to his commentary on the Hindu holy book, the Bhagavad Gita. He mentioned that his first editor would become ill and pass away, and then his second editor would finish the work. Yogananda certainly had the power to heal his first editor, yet he chose not to. Possibly she had the power to heal herself as well, and did not.

We do not always understand the circumstances of our lives and why things happen as they do. Sometimes simply accepting things as they are is the best solution, along with learning to be, to breathe into the moment, and to allow.

Later, I talked to Vince Lasorso about an upcoming scan. What if it wasn't clear? He said, "Then you'll just go into more chemo." He reminded me that when it is time for me to go, there's nothing I can do to prevent it. He told me a couple of stories about people who most likely should have died in a particular situation but didn't—so they died soon afterward in similar situations. He said two men who should have been at their desks in the Pentagon on September 11, 2001, were on the plane that hit their offices in the Pentagon. What incredible irony! But it points to the fact that there is an Ultimate Planner. And that when it's my time to go, it's my time to go, and there isn't much I can do about it. Everyone has an expiration date. Some are lucky enough to see it coming ahead of time. On the flipside of that coin, if it wasn't time, I would survive. I heard stories of people who did things like smoke and eat Twinkies during cancer treatment and still came out cured. Ultimately, it wasn't up to me. Therefore, my compulsion to control the situation served no purpose. I also knew that I could be cured at any moment—in the twinkling of an eye—if that was what was right and best for everyone concerned.

The point I gained from all of this was to love myself and to experience myself as the Spirit experiences me—whole, and healthy, and healed, and whether that means I am cured or not is not up to me. I was moving closer to release into freedom, into equanimity, and into radiant acquiescence.

Thriver Soup Ingredient:

If fear of death itself raises its ugly head, perhaps you have some unfinished business to take care of before you can feel equanimity.

Dawna Markova, in her book *I Will Not Die an Unlived Life*, proposes four questions that might help bring clarity.

1. What's unfinished for me to give?
2. What's unfinished for me to heal?
3. What's unfinished for me to learn?
4. What's unfinished for me to experience?

Give each question a page in your journal. Sit with the questions, and write responses as they arise throughout your days.

~~~

Active Imagination: Inner Adventures

Now to him who is able to do immeasurably more than all we ask or imagine, according to his power that is at work within us...

—Ephesians 3:20, Christian Bible, NIV

We can dream up a lot, and use our thoughts to bring about healing. A process called active imagination is a tool we can use to explore our unconscious minds and learn more about our situations.

Active imagination involves moving ourselves into a deeply relaxed state, then entering into a make-believe situation. There we interact with other characters and objects, as if they are real, while we seek greater understanding of ourselves and our experiences.

I used active imagination often during the course of my journey. One way I liked to enter this realm was to get completely relaxed. Then I would visualize myself walking with my power animals and spirit guides up wide steps until we reached a giant doorway into an enormous European cathedral. The sanctuary was surrounded by gorgeous, brightly colored stained-glass windows. We walked over to a side wall and entered a door which led down a spiral stairwell. During my first journeys here, the walls were lined with mosaics of golden-winged angels dressed in turquoise robes. Eventually, the images became real angels who walked down the steps with us.

The light in the stairwell gradually would fade, until it had disappeared entirely at the bottom of the stairs. We had to walk ahead into the darkness to encounter whatever I needed to meet to learn something new. Often I was frightened by an enormous animal representing some repressed aspect of my psyche—a huge black viper, a gigantic hungry wolf, a looming bear.... Sometimes I screamed and hit pillows, or wailed with the voice of a young child, or captured and caged the beast. By facing these creatures and either talking or wrestling with them, they lost their fearsome aspects and I gained insight or courage. One time I even was handed a heart of courage to wear. I honored the experience by cutting a large red heart out of paper and attaching images of three of my animal totems.

We also can use active imagination to shrink ourselves down to a size through which we can get into our bloodstreams and visit our tumors. Then we can ask the cancer cells questions, explain their predicaments to them, and get help bringing them back in line. My friend Mica Renes, a naturopath, compared sarcoma cells to rebelling teenagers who needed social workers to show them healthier options. My psychotherapist said to be a firm parent to the nodules.

The Divine can work with and through our imaginations to bring about immeasurable good in our lives. We just need to make time and have the energy for the adventure.

Thriver Soup Ingredient:

Active imagination is best tried with a mental health professional or an experienced witness who can guide you through the process. Set a clear goal about what you want to address or explore, even bringing a list of questions you would like answered. When your session is done, find a way to honor the experience, whether through art, journaling, dance, or other creative expression.

~~~

Allowing: Loving the Questions

The highest excellence is like (that of) water. The excellence of water appears in its benefiting all things, and in its occupying, without striving (to the contrary), the low place which all men dislike. Hence (its way) is near to (that of) the Tao.

—Tao Te Ching, 8

Water does not resist changes to its path, nor does it strive against blockages in its way. It simply flows forward. Water allows things to be as they are, and moves without resistance, which brings it closer to the Tao, or the way of everything.

This seems so peaceful to me; water has a way of being in the world that usually benefits all things.

How different I was; I wanted to control my life as well as others'; I wanted to force a healing through great effort. Yet, I realized, that would not bring me closer to my true desires.

Lynne McTaggart talked about healers who behaved like water in her book, *The Field: The Quest for the Secret Force of the Universe*. Their healing methods were largely irrelevant; instead, their intentions for patients to heal were what mattered most. All the healers seemed to share an ability to make their intentions known, and then get out of the way by surrendering to a healing energy.

The healers placed themselves in a receptive, feminine mode and allowed healing energy to pour into the patients. They simply let natural healing take place, without expectation or goal.

There is a time and a place for setting goals, yet those objectives can create barriers and boundaries to true healing. For example, if I had reached my goal of a clean scan early in my treatment, I would have missed some incredibly valuable healing opportunities and beautiful experiences later during the process. If we let go of determinedly reaching specific objectives, we probably will experience more freedom and entertain more possibilities. This allows for the mystery of life to unfold, moving us into a state of awe and wonder.

Fifteen years before the diagnosis, I saw this quote from poet Rainer Maria Rilke (1875–1926) on someone's wall, and it stayed in my heart. Sometimes, of course, it needed a little dusting off.

I want to beg you, as much as I can, dear sir, to be patient towards all that is unsolved in your heart and to try to love the questions themselves *like locked rooms and like books that are written in a very foreign tongue. Do not now seek the answers, that cannot be given you because you would not be able to live them. And the point is, to live everything. Live the questions now. Perhaps you will then gradually, without noticing it, live along some distant day into the answer.*

There is a vulnerability and a relaxation in this concept that greatly appeals to me. It enables me to be more open to what is happening right now, right in front of me, or right inside my body. It helps me see that control is not necessary; it's really impossible to manage life's circumstances anyway. I can, however, influence my life by living in the moment and making wise choices. Then I can leave the results up to the Divine.

If, like me, you have trouble letting go of even one expectation, then allow that expectation to be what it is, without passing judgment on yourself. When I try to let go of an expectation, I have noticed that I might start rubbing my face, stroking my hair, or getting some chocolate to eat because my body is experiencing feelings of shame and powerlessness. When I am awake enough, I try to feel that shame and powerlessness in my body. The craving for chocolate might not pass, but there is more consciousness in my choice of whether to snap off a square or let it sit. It is my sense of powerlessness that gives rise to my desire to control rather than allowing life and circumstances to be what they are.

And while I'm at it, I can let go of the goal of letting go of an expectation. I can be like water, flowing through my expectations rather than striving, allowing them to be what they are, yet growing in awareness and deepening into the Tao.

Thriver Soup Ingredient:

In your journal, make a list of all the expectations you have of yourself. This is not for judgment; it's simply to raise awareness. Review your list and see if there is one item you can let go of this coming week. See how your body feels when you select an expectation to drop. Give yourself loving attention and allow whatever shame or sense of powerlessness you experience to be what it is. If you still find dropping that expectancy difficult, see if you can select one that feels easier.

During the following week, practice being playfully open to any new possibilities that might emerge around your letting go and allowing in this one area. See if it provides you with a feeling of expansion, joy, and happiness.

≈≈≈

Big Dharma

From the Dharma should one see the Buddhas, From the Dharmabodies comes their guidance. Yet Dharma's true nature cannot be discerned, And no one can be conscious of it as an object.

—*The Diamond Sutra*, 26b

Dharma can mean "the way things are." While undergoing treatment, I read an article by a widely known author and speaker who was diagnosed with cancer. He said he probably had big dharma because he experienced big challenges in life.

My initial reaction to the man's statement was, "Well, I must have big dharma because of my cancer diagnosis and life events."

After a few hours, I went back to that initial reaction and saw it for what it was—for me, it was a self-righteous, ego-based response, not in keeping with a virtuous path toward enlightenment. I look around me and see in the news so many other people who have suffered terrible tragedies, many of them far worse than mine. I am no more special than anyone else. I have my path, others have their paths. My hell is just as much of a hell as the next person's, no matter what makes up that hell. Her hell might not be hell for me, yet it is her experience of it that makes it hell. Cancer doesn't have the corner on wreaking havoc in someone's life. In my opinion, all paths eventually include trauma and lead us back to our Source. Everyone has big dharma at some point.

My friend Mica Renes, a counselor, said life is just plain messy. As people on the spiritual path, we usually are expected to be happy, wealthy, and healthy, and are told we can create our realities if we just have enough faith. Yet I don't think that's why we are here. I believe I chose my body and life experiences for specific lessons. Being healthy all my life might have caused me to circumvent exactly what my soul came into this body to learn. Perhaps cancer was the electric cattle prod I needed to get myself on board the truck of life that was heading toward the Elysian pastures. The goad might be something else for a different type of person. As Paula, an acquaintance who had cancer, said to me, "We're all just on our journeys."

My dharma happened to include suffering, pain, and sorrow; a long road-trip into hell and back. I could allow the suffering to rule over me, or I could learn to move beyond self-defeating pity and into greater light. It all depended on my choices along the way.

I chose to learn how to use the dharma of cancer's hell to find joy in my beautiful, hidden Buddha-nature.

Thriver Soup Ingredient:

I take comfort in what Kahlil Gibran (1883–1931), a Lebanese-American writer, said: "The deeper that sorrow carves into your being the more joy you can contain. Is not the cup that holds your wine the very cup that was burned in the potter's oven?" Take this idea with you to a pottery class. Create something with the clay that represents you—perhaps a cup or bowl carved out to hold the new wine of your beautiful Buddha-nature. Think about Gibran's comment as your piece is burned in the oven.

To find a pottery class in your area, try contacting art centers, art museums, art supply stores, colleges, and potteries.

≈≈≈

Claiming: Mine, All Mine

To Him is due The primal origin Of the heavens and the earth: When He decreeth a matter, He saith to it: "Be," And it is.

—Qur'an 2:117

If we are made in the image of the Divine, and the Spirit speaks things into being, then we can, too, though I think there are a few caveats.

My first month into treatment, my then-husband and I took a quick trip to Colorado. At a restaurant in Breckenridge, we sat at a table with a sign on the wall that said, "Miracles happen every day." I decided to claim that statement as true for me.

One of my affirmations was "I deserve the best." I wanted to return to Cincinnati Sunday night in time for the Bruno Gröning lecture, so we had to catch our flight. When we arrived at the airline gate in Denver, the door to the plane had already been closed...and I felt so grateful they opened it for us. And, because of my then-husband's many business trips, we received a complementary upgrade to first-class seats, a first for me. I was delighted to receive these affirmations of my affirmation.

When it comes to claiming something, I learned to recognize that thoughts can be argued about, while our feelings reflect what is true for us. Our thinking can trap us in the past, yet emotions hold us in the present moment, a place where infinite possibilities exist. It is at the feeling level that we can bring about the most internal changes. What would set off fireworks in your life? What would make you say "ahhh," filling you with wonder?

For me, being cured filled these spaces. How did it feel to imagine myself cured? Joyous! Lively! Freeing! Luscious! Invigorating! Energizing! Those are the emotions that revitalize the body.

Spend time every day feeling those good feelings. Verbalize them. Claim them. Bring them into be-ing within yourself, and see how they manifest in your life. Ask others to do the same for you.

Thriver Soup Ingredient:

Vince Lasorso had suggested I use my writing ability to create a Hallmark-style, happy, fairy-tale ending for my personal story. So I did, and it was fun. If you are so inclined, write your own happy ending in your journal. Fill it with passionate feeling and vivid visual images.

For fun, follow author Elizabeth Gilbert's idea from her book *Eat Pray Love* and turn your story into a petition to the Spirit. Then pretend you are each of your supporters, and sign each of their names on the petition.

~~~

Dark Night: Abduction into the Depths

Kore...suddenly came upon a flower never seen before.... The young woman was amazed and reached for the hundred-headed blossom in delight but as she did, the earth opened wide and up from its chasm leapt the Lord of the Underworld. He snatched the girl and carried her off in his chariot....[a] way to his kingdom under the earth.

—The myth of Persephone

The Greek goddess Persephone was called Kore, or young maiden, in the beginning of her mythological story. One day she was lured away from her mother's sight by a gorgeous flower. The king of the land beneath the earth, Hades, abducted her and took her down to his kingdom. She entered into the first shadowy period of her life.

After experiencing a dark night of the soul during my twenties, I believed, from what others had reported, that if I continued on the spiritual path, I most likely would endure a dark night of the spirit. I had no idea when or what it would involve. I felt frightened by the thought, yet didn't dwell on it.

Like Kore, the innocent maiden, I was shocked when cancer abducted me and dragged me into blackness. Okay, I believed a dark night was part of the spiritual ticket price, but end-stage cancer? Really? I had been so healthy; on the physical level, I had done everything right. The Spirit could not have arranged a more fitting blow. The seeds of death were sown in my uterus, the womb where life itself begins.

After my health collapsed, so did my marriage. I became death's bride.

Unknowingly, I followed Kore's example in the Underworld. She bravely rebelled through her only option—to starve herself, thereby encouraging the gods to eventually permit her passage back into the light of day. Like this determined woman, I resisted Hades every step of the way—I desperately wanted to return to the land of the living.

According to the Christian Bible, in Matthew 12:40, Jesus spent time in the Underworld between his crucifixion and resurrection. The Underworld, perhaps, can be seen as a birth canal. After being kidnapped, Kore died to her maiden self and eventually rose back onto the earth as Persephone, a mature woman. Jesus died to his physical life, visited the Underworld, and was reborn with a resurrected body. My time in the world of shadows provided me with an opportunity to bury old parts of myself that no longer served life. It was necessary for me to emerge a wiser woman.

Do not let Hades have his way with you. Resist his advances. Stand firm in your convictions. Start your journey, one step at a time, back into the world of the living, carrying your treasures from the dark night of the Underworld back into the light of day. Allow the Spirit to bring about your resurrection.

Thriver Soup Ingredient:

If you are experiencing a dark night, try not to waste this opportunity; look for the coal down in the depths of your mine shaft. Bring the lumps up into awareness, one by one. Remember, with enough pressure, they can be turned into diamonds. Work with each as if it were a diamond in the rough. Spend time with it. Feel it. Experience it. Allow it to be what it is. Cry, scream, and rant about it. Journal about it. Talk about it. Then surrender it to the Divine to do with as only the Divine can, to bring about your highest possible good.

∾∾∾

Directed Prayer

Then Jesus said to them, "Suppose you have a friend, and you go to him at midnight and say, 'Friend, lend me three loaves of bread; a friend of mine on a journey has come to me, and I have no food to offer him.' And suppose the one inside answers, 'Don't bother me. The door is already locked, and my children and I are in bed. I can't get up and give you anything.' I tell you, even though he will not get up and give you the bread because of friendship, yet because of your shameless audacity he will surely get up and give you as much as you need."

—Luke 11:5-8, Christian Bible, NIV

Directed prayer is pounding on heaven's door with shameless audacity.

Paramahansa Yogananda, founder of Self-Realization Fellowship, concurred in his 1929 version of *Whispers from Eternity: A Book of Answered Prayers*. When praying, don't ask. Instead, make demands of the Divine. We are not beggars; we are made in the image of the Spirit. Our mistake in prayer is ignorance of our greatness.

So expand your view of yourself and of prayer. Here are some things I learned:

1. Be persistent. I delight in the parable of the widow pestering the judge in the Christian Gospel according to Luke, chapter 18. Jesus tells his disciples to always pray and not give up. We must want life with enthusiastic passion and be more persistent and audacious than those confused rebel cells making trouble in our bodies.

2. Demand a cure. Yogananda wrote, "Every begging prayer, no matter how sincere, limits the soul." As children of the Divine, it is our birthright to partake—to lovingly demand—our share of the Spirit's perfection and abundance.

3. Pray with belief. Both Jesus and Yogananda cautioned against mechanical repetition. Yogananda said to repeat your prayer with deep conviction while focusing your attention at the point between your eyebrows—the spiritual center of willpower, divine self-confidence, and endless possibilities.

4. Have faith in the outcome. "Believe absolutely that your demand has been heard, and you will know that what is God's is yours also," wrote Yogananda. Perhaps this will inspire your faith; it vastly increased my trust that I am receiving a cure. Early in my process, I had a dream in which my lungs were clear and I was cured. I felt such peace and assurance that it was natural to receive this cure, and also felt so tired, that I fell back asleep without writing out the dream in my journal.

My friend Maria Paglialungo wrote, "One of the most important knowings is that healing at the highest level is possible, beyond probable, simply because you demand what is rightly your inheritance."

Insist on getting back your health. If you lack faith, demand faith as well. Follow the instructions given by Jesus: Pound on the doors of heaven with shameless audacity.

Thriver Soup Ingredient:

Scientific Healing Affirmations, by Paramahansa Yogananda, provides this sample directed prayer you might try: "Heavenly Father, Thou art present in every atom, every cell, every corpuscle, every particle of nerve, brain, and tissue. I am well, for Thou art in all my body parts."

≈≈≈

Embody the Divine: Transformers

Look, it cannot be seen—it is beyond form. Listen, it cannot be heard—it is beyond sound. Grasp, it cannot be held—it is intangible.

—Tao Te Ching, 14

Just as the Divine is formless Spirit, so we inhabit bodies that are primarily composed of energy fields below the subatomic level that defy our macro-world understandings of form. Our souls, as well, cannot be seen in the world of objects. I believe they are intangible, timeless, and deathless.

This opens a way for our spirits to embody the Divine. I understood this better after watching a 2008 film, "The Moses Code." Director James Twyman retells how Moses encountered a burning bush and heard the Divine speak from it. When Moses asked what to call this presence, the Divine said, I Am That I Am. Twyman suggests the phrase isn't fully understood without adding a comma after the word "that": I Am That, I Am. Then he explained that the phrase could be spoken about anything Moses saw: I am that child, I am; I am that sheep, I am; I am that tree, I am. Twyman was pointing toward how everything is linked, and everything is connected with the Divine, so everything embodies an aspect of the Divine.

My belief system is similar. I think we are like little holographic images of the Spirit. Each point on a holographic image contains information that comes from every point in the scene it depicts. If a holographic image of a human is cut in half, you will simply see a smaller version of the exact same human on the half piece of the image you look at. If you cut off a little piece, you still have the same full image of the human, only at a lower resolution. Likewise, we are small, yet complete—even if fuzzy—images of the Spirit.

This means I am whole—a holographic image of the Divine—just the way I am. Because I am a reflection of the Spirit, I am worthy of re-experiencing wholeness in my body and of receiving a cure.

I have read in more than one place that it is possible for cancer cells to revert back into healthy cells (I don't know if this is true for sarcoma cells). My Ayurvedic doctor, Hari Sharma, MD, conducted research with the supplement Maharishi Amrit Kalash and said it showed a "reversal of the malignant process" in a laboratory setting. If a supplement can reverse cancer, maybe I could as well by conversing directly with the cancer cells. I tried to bring these concepts into physical form by talking to the straying cells in my body. I told them to either transform back into healthy cells or they would die. After the chemotherapy die-off period and before the next infusion, I visualized sarcoma cells filled with transmuting love so they could revert back into a healthy state. After chemotherapy ended, on the advice of Dr. Sharma, I added Amrit Kalash to my daily nutrient intake.

My psychotherapist and I talked about my issues and came to an affirmation that encompassed these concepts, along with others I needed to learn: "I am worthy." I speak this affirmation a great deal and try to feel that worthiness in my body as I say the words.

As I grow in awareness of my worthiness, I believe I will naturally embody more and more of the attributes of the Divine—that which is beyond form, beyond sound, and beyond senses.

Thriver Soup Ingredient:

As an embodiment of the Divine, you are worthy of a cure and of healing. As energy intuitive Maria Paglialungo wrote, see the healing in your body as you play, shout, sing, and dance. Send love and restorative energy into the cancer. Lay the palms of your hands over the diseased locations and ask for Divine light to send therapeutic energy through your hands.

≈≈≈

Enlightenment: Knockin' on Heaven's Gate

God is the Light Of the heavens and the earth. The parable of His Light Is as if there were a niche And within it a Lamp: The Lamp enclosed in Glass: The glass as it were A brilliant star:
Lit from a blessed Tree, An Olive, neither of the East Nor of the West, Whose Oil is well-nigh Luminous, Though fire scarce touched it Light upon Light! God doth guide Whom He will To His Light: God doth set forth Parables For men: and God Doth know all things.

—Qur'an 24:35

The experience of enlightenment sometimes is described with the metaphor of light. Thomas Merton, OCSO (1915–1968), a Trappist monk, mystic, and writer, said when we go through our dark night of the Spirit, we feel as if we are groping in the night. This perception of darkness, however, is simply caused by a temporary blindness from the intensity of Divine light as we draw near.

My friend Judy Merritt, PhD, performed a chakra energy clearing session for me. When I came out of a trance, I picked up some chalk and drew a medieval fortress on black paper. Weeks later, while working with energy intuitive Maria Paglialungo, I decided to enter the mysterious structure. In my mind's eye, I walked through the blackness with my three animal companions, Mafdet, Cinnamon, and Owl.

We approached the fortress and I opened the door. Intense brightness nearly blinded us, bursting out the door and filling the night. We entered into this light and walked toward the center of the stronghold. My body filled with and radiated the same light. I heard a voice say, "You are the Christ, a child of the Living God."

Please understand I am not saying I am THE Christ, like Jesus who walked the earth 2,000 years ago. I am, however, a human being who also is a holographic image of Christ; made in the image of the Divine; and made to reflect the Spirit in all that I do. Jesus did tell his disciples, "Has it not been written in your Law, 'I SAID, YOU ARE GODS'?" (John 10:34, New American Standard Bible).

I felt I was being reminded to radiate the light of God throughout my body as well as my life. When I reach the point where I do this in every moment, I will be enlightened. By Spirit's timing, which is not bound by our linear ideas about time, I already am enlightened. While in this body, I have a road to travel to reach this destination, because my humanity is bound by my physical experience of linear time.

The process reminded me of the character Dorothy in the movie "The Wizard of Oz" relying on her three friends as she entered into the presence of the wizard. The Great Oz told Dorothy she had to kill the witch before he would help her. Dorothy and her friends faced the demon and used water to melt the witch, just as I needed to learn to use emotions (typically symbolized by water) to help melt away what ailed me.

After our work, Maria pulled out a treasure map she had made at about the time we had met many years before. Right on the center of the map was the word "Enlightenment." The dot over the letter "i" was a bright yellow smiley face. I experienced a moment of deep reverence for the processes of life. I have made a copy of the image for myself. Even though Maria and I are such different personality types, we are both moving toward the same goal: enlightenment. She has been a tremendous help along the way, shining the light where she has tread on her own, with little assistance. I find her to be both an amazing and a remarkable human being.

Just as I experienced a profound moment of light, I also had plenty of moments of darkness. Enlightenment, according to naturopath Mica Renes, comes like a blinking light—it usually turns off and on rather than holding steady. A couple of weeks later I witnessed the perfect metaphor for this phenomenon. I was sitting outside and saw a single two-inch strand of spider webbing strung between a seat and a support bar. A slight breeze moved the strand up and down. When the strand was lifted up, it glistened brightly with shimmering sunlight cascading along its tenuous length. When the breeze dropped its support, the strand descended back into the darkness of shadow and became invisible. And so it is for the typical human being. A little breath of the Spirit's choosing, and we are lifted into the Divine light; a small letting go and we descend back into shadow. It doesn't mean the light's not there anymore. It's simply not within our realm of experience at a particular moment. As we traverse this earth, may we become more and more luminous.

Thriver Soup Ingredient:

When Siddhartha Gautama became the Buddha, he described himself as one who had awakened. He had experienced enlightenment by becoming fully awake to himself, others, and the entire universe. As Mica said, we can experience an awakening into wholeness in bits and pieces, right where we are, right this moment. This can be done as we go through our days by taking occasional pauses in whatever we do. During these pauses we stop everything, get back into being fully present within our bodies, and note any tension, any emotion, any sensation. Awaken to your experience for a few moments before continuing on with your day. Tara Brach, PhD, in her book *Radical Acceptance*, suggests a few ideas such as taking these pauses before getting out of a car, while sipping tea, or when brushing your teeth.

∼∼∼

Faith and Trust

He replied, "Because you have so little faith. Truly I tell you, if you have faith as small as a mustard seed, you can say to this mountain, 'Move from here to there,' and it will move. Nothing will be impossible for you."

—Matthew 17:20, Christian Bible, NIV

Having faith is nearly impossible when I am filled with terror and dread. No, it's completely impossible—for me, anyway. I'm no saint. How can I have faith when I feel like I've failed another chemotherapy regimen and the scan shows even more nodules? When I am facing another surgery or another type of chemo? When I feel like I'm on the slippery-slope into death's deep pit?

My friend Kathy Nace showed up with a wonderful metaphor for faith that helped me through that shadowed valley. She watched a troupe of women aerial performers with thirty-foot lengths of purple silk attached to a pivot ring on an overhang at the Lawrence Arts Center in Kansas. "They would begin to climb these like ropes, then they would begin to twist or wrap the cloth around legs, arms, or torso. Suddenly, they would let go and 'unroll,' striking a pose as the 'knot' they had created so subtly held them. Some routines featured two, each in turn standing on the other, or leaning out to create balance for the other. At times they appeared to be out of control and free falling, but the knots they had woven held them in the end—at times just inches from the impact of the ground. It struck me that this is a wonderful visual metaphor for a life of faith. Woven tightly and with skill of the right materials, sometimes singly and at others in concert with fellow travelers, it will hold us at the essential moment(s). We sometimes begrudge the 'knots' in our lives, but without this preparation, we would not be ready to fly."

Shortly after reading this, I took an unplanned side trip to a different library and looked for SpongeBob DVDs on the shelf. My eyes fell upon a 2006 movie called "Peter Lundy and the Medicine Hat Stallion." When I was a child, I had been moved by a book with this name, written by Marguerite Henry. As I stood in the library holding the DVD, I felt a strong sense of the order of our world—that events are not haphazard but orchestrated. The diagnosis was not some random evil event, but an experience that somehow was useful for Divine purposes. I felt a deep sense of peace, as though I was being woven into a knot that would eventually hold me. How odd that finding a movie on a shelf could trigger such a response. I checked out the movie and, as I watched it, realized it was based on Henry's book.

I wrote about this on my CaringBridge blog. Gary Matthews, a supporter, responded to my post: "You're hinting at a possible truth that real faith is not an action or a doing of the will, but rather a spontaneous arising from the Soul, that Being part of us, our Divine core, and as such, Faith is a Grace."

I suppose that's why it doesn't take a lot of faith or trust to move mountains. It only takes a little because a little bit is everything, and it brings a sense of order to one's world. It is the purple silk cloth weaving a tapestry from my life of knots and keeping me from crashing. It is faith the size of a miniscule mustard seed that contains the power to propel peaks.

Thriver Soup Ingredient:

Judith Broadus, one of my friends, sent me this little poem by Voltaire (François-Marie d'Arouet, 1694–1778, French writer and public activist):

Be like a bird
On limb to light,
Who feels the branch give way beneath?
Yet sings,
Knowing she has wings.

Sit awhile with this poem, turning it over in your mind until it settles in your heart. Know that the air—the Spirit—is supporting you.

Field of Dreams

The thirst for a dream from above, without this you are nothing. This I believe. It is like the prophets in your Bible, like Jesus fasting in the desert, getting his visions. It's like our Sioux vision quest, the hanblecheya.... *Your old prophets went into the desert crying for a dream and the desert gave it to them. But the white men of today have made a desert of their religion and a desert within themselves. The White Man's desert is a place without dreams or life. There nothing grows. But the spirit water is always way down there to make the desert green again.*

—Lame Deer, Minneconjou Sioux medicine man, in 1970

I thirsted for a dream after the diagnosis. I yearned for the spirit water deep down that would provide guidance about treatment and complementary care. I paid careful attention to every nighttime adventure, writing each down, looking for a glimmer of hope for a long-term future. Within five months, two dreams appeared in which I experienced a cure. In the second dream, I walked down two flights of stairs into a heavenly green meadow bursting with violet flowers. I was swathed in brilliant, white, soft blankets...and cured.

Drawing this image on paper, I added cottony stuffing from supplement bottles to supplement the blankets and placed a small photo of my smiling face in it. Several months slipped into the past before I realized I had created an image of myself enclosed in a cocoon.

During a conversation about two years later, a fellow patient referred to uterine sarcomas as demons. Within days, I dreamt I was Harry Potter, the fictional character developed by J.K. Rowling, riding on the train to the Hogwarts School of Witchcraft and Wizardry. The demon-wizard Voldemort found me and we fought—both so worn down by our lives that we were reduced to an ineffectual hand-to-hand struggle. Somehow, I managed to push him off a bridge. I ran down to him and we continued fighting. My heavy arms did little damage and my legs barely held my weight. As I weakened to the point I felt doomed, two dwarves, like the Western cavalry, raced onto the scene. According to Jungian psychoanalyst Marie Louise von Franz, dwarves represent "the creative power of the unconscious." They helped me hold Voldemort's head down in a puddle until he drowned.

The struggle ended. So perhaps, with others' help, I had defeated the uterine demon.

During March 2013, I dreamt I was walking through the middle of a thirsty desert and came upon gorgeous wildflowers—bluebells, daisies, and cottage pinks—about three feet high, blooming on a dry patch of ground. Beauty and color were bursting out of the parched wasteland that had been my life.

My dreams had provided answers I wanted and needed, just as a vision quest opens channels for those who seek Divine guidance. The Spirit water had not only drowned the demon in me, it watered my desert and brought forth vibrant new life.

Thriver Soup Ingredient:

While chemotherapy and other drugs can affect what shows up in dreams, your nightly excursions can still be mined for treasures. Robert Moss (author and the creator of "active dreaming") says people can consciously dream and even enter into their cells' mitochondria to be cured.

Our sleep-time visions are activated about every ninety minutes while we snooze, so if you want to recall your dreams, pave the way with an intention directed toward the Divine or your heart. Help activate your brain by placing your journal and pen beside your bed.

If you wake up and know you had a dream, keep your body still. Mentally retrace the dream, piece by piece—even if all you have is a tiny fragment of information, an image, a word, or a feeling. After you have gathered the parts in your mind and recalled the feelings in your body, turn on a night light, and write everything down that you can remember.

Assistance with dream interpretation can come from dream analysts, dream-sharing groups, books, and perhaps most importantly, from your own intuition.

~~~

Intention Statement

Whoever submits His whole self to God, And is a doer of good, Has grasped indeed The most trustworthy hand-hold And with God rests the End And Decision of (all) affairs.

—Qur'an 31:22

If we submit our intentions to the Divine, and do our part to live well, we are gaining support from the most trustworthy source of all, the Spirit. While this does not guarantee the outcome we might most desire, it sets us up for success better than anything else we can do.

It took me awhile to understand that there is a difference between affirmations and intentions. Affirmations are attempts at changing our core beliefs so we have better experiences of life. Intentions involve decisions that help us move in particular directions.

For example, my intention might be "I want to be healthy and whole," so I arrange my life to reflect that intention: I eat well, exercise, and take good care of my body. By acting on my intention, I am letting the Spirit know I am committed to making it a reality. When we submit our good intentions to the Divine, the Qur'an says we have the most trustworthy form of support. My intention might be further reinforced by an affirmation repeated frequently: "My body is designed to support my health and wholeness."

If you are interested in practicing setting intentions, try a small one first. Here are some ideas. "Today I will eat some steamed broccoli." "Today I will write in my journal." "Today I will pray for the strength to move toward forgiving the person who hurt me."

Then take a step in that direction. Each morning, plant your intention firmly in your mind, and then follow through with supporting behavior. Baby steps will help us arrive at our destinations more quickly, they show our intentions are true, and if they are for the good, we will be supported by the Spirit as we progress.

When you feel confident enough in fulfilling small intentions, create an intention statement that will help you reach an important goal. Then write it down in your journal and intend to remember and work with it each day.

I set my intention to get this book traditionally published because I believed it could provide assistance to others. Nearly every day I worked on it, even if only for five minutes. This let the Spirit know I was serious about making my intention a reality, and the support came to assist me during the process.

Thriver Soup Ingredient:
Create a personal Buddhist prayer flag that states your most desired intention. I learned

how to do this through a Cancer Support Community program. Several of us made flags together, adding an element of community to the experience.

What you'll need:

A piece of cotton fabric on which you can write

Paper and pencil

Fabric pens

A thin dowel rod or twig

Decorative items, such as ribbons, beads, and/or buttons

Fabric glue or needle, scissors, and thread.

What to do:

Write your intention statement with a pencil on regular paper. Draft how you want the words to appear and ways you would like to embellish them.

Fold the top of the fabric down and glue or sew it around a dowel rod or small stick. Tie string around each end so the flag can hang.

Write the intention statement on the fabric following your draft. Decorate with string, beads, buttons, or more drawings.

I wrote my intention statements around in a circular formation, flowing outward from the center. I glued strips of ribbon to the bottom for more flutter. I keep it hung on my bedroom door handle so I see it every morning as a reminder of my firm intentions.

<center>~~~</center>

Intuition: Let Your Heart be Your Guide

O Nanak, this alone need we know, That God, being Truth, is the one Light of all.

—The Japji, 4

If the Spirit is truth and light, and I am made in the image of the Divine, then I am filled with truth and light. I simply have to learn to access it.

Easier said than done. I didn't think I had a lot of intuition. I gradually learned over the years that everyone has intuition. It's more a matter of developing it, listening to it, and learning to trust it.

My friends told me many times that I had all the answers to the cancer within me because I am part of the all-knowing Spirit. That was hard to accept, because I kept asking, praying, meditating, and getting little response.

Maybe it wasn't time. Maybe I wasn't listening well enough. Maybe I wasn't really interested in the truth because I was too terrified of it. Maybe the Spirit didn't even want me to know.

The thirteenth-century Sufi mystic Jalāl ad-Dīn Muḥammad Rūmī came to my aid in a poem that encourages the reader to keep walking without fearfully looking into the distance, and to let our hearts guide us.

My body most certainly was hesitant and full of fear. I needed patience to walk this road and to allow my heart to guide me. My friend Paula Overstreet urged me to pray, "Teach me how to distinguish Your Voice from my own." And the Qur'an supplied more encouragement: "But to those who receive Guidance, He increases The (light of) Guidance" (Sura 47:17).

I began to experiment with asking one of my spirit guides for yes and no indications for little everyday things, like which supplements to take and what to eat. Sometimes I visualized an angel, and if its wings lifted up, I took that as a yes; if the wings drooped, I accepted it as a no.

Gradually, slowly, painfully, I began to develop more of a sense of when I was receiving true information and when my mind got in the way. I continued making many mistakes, yet felt gratified when I seemed to be on the right path. Elizabeth Kübler-Ross, MD, author of *On Death and Dying*, said, "[I]ntuitive decisions make us feel good, even if others think we're crazy. But, as we become authentic, we no longer worry about what others think." Truth is truth, and as we move deeper into the light, not much else will matter.

Thriver Soup Ingredient

If you want to develop your intuition, and feel you have the time, make a game out of it. This idea came from a friend, Paula, who learned it from her teacher.

Get a deck of playing cards and select eight of them. Include two from each suit, and no two with the same face value. Shuffle them and pick one up and, without looking at it, see if you can sense whether it's red or black. If you are correct, place the card in one pile; if incorrect, start another pile. Then pull the next card and try again. Keep practicing. The worse you get at it, I'm told, the better you actually are, yet you might be resisting knowing. Eventually, if you practice long enough, you probably will get good enough to start sensing the suit, then the number.

Relax, have fun, and make a game of it.

Then stretch out and try other games. In the back of the grocery store, sense which checkout lane will be fastest, and try it out. Or see if you can determine who is calling your phone before you check who it is.

∾∾∾

Mindfulness Meditation: Lose Yourself

A tamed mind brings happiness.

—*The Dhammapada*, 3:37

I didn't have a tamed mind, especially while undergoing chemotherapy. Rather, I had what Buddhists call monkey mind because of the constant chatter that would drown out the sublime sensing of my soul.

The day after one chemotherapy session I wanted to spend a lot of time in meditation. First attempt: slept for two hours. Second attempt: slept for one hour. I wasn't even alert enough for monkey mind. Sigh.

A year later I noticed some progress. I had been doing mindfulness meditation daily, thirty minutes in the morning and thirty in the afternoon. I started by asking the Spirit to lift my doubts and fears, grant me faith and trust, and infuse me with divine healing energy. Then I would sit upright, palms facing upward on my lap, and watch my mind chatter. Occasionally a blissful lapse in thinking occurred. I've talked to other chemo patients who had the same experience while meditating. Now I understand why the meditation is called transcendental—one transcends the thinking mind. I also found the gaps rather peaceful, perhaps because I didn't have the energy to get bored or fidgety. I soon realized that at times I had been fighting my thoughts. I needed to back up and simply notice them as an observer would watch clouds passing through the sky. And so I continued learning.

Ainslie Meares, MD (1910–1986), an Australian psychiatrist, studied people who meditated while undergoing conventional cancer treatment. He found that meditation without thought or image had the most healing effect for the cancer patients with whom he worked. Some believe mental stillness during meditation will enable one's natural vital energy to arise, which can cure many types of illnesses. One study demonstrated that significant changes take place in the brains of those who practice mindfulness meditation, even after only eight weeks of daily practice. Their moods lifted and their immune systems were strengthened.

Since I had been meditating for an hour each day during the half year before landing in the hospital, and the tumor was growing rapidly, I doubted meditation would produce a cure for me. I believed, however, that meditation still could be of assistance in my situation, and so I continued. I began attending a few meditation groups. Many told me meditating in groups raises everyone's vibration. While I didn't experience any vibrations, I did find my level of concentration much improved. This increased my capacity to tame and quiet my mind. I can't say it brought me happiness, but it did reduce my experiences of stress and fear. At least it helped me move in the right direction.

Thriver Soup Ingredient:

If you can, find a meditation group to join. It might help you focus more clearly and also might provide some pleasant companionship.

To meditate, sit comfortably in a chair or lie flat so your spine is straight. Take a few slow, deep breaths. Relax, letting go of any unnecessary tension. Bring your attention to your breath. Breathe naturally and experience the air moving in and out of your lungs. As soon as a thought enters your field of awareness, notice it, and let it go, like letting go of a helium-filled balloon. Then return your attention to your breath. Perhaps start by practicing for one minute each day, and gradually increase, as you are able, to twenty minutes twice each day.

~~~

Mothership: Feminine Transformative Substance

Jesus said to the servants, "Fill the jars with water"; so they filled them to the brim. Then he told

them, "Now draw some out and take it to the master of the banquet." They did so, and the master of
the banquet tasted the water that had been turned into wine. He did not realize where it had come
from, though the servants who had drawn the water knew. Then he called the bridegroom aside and
said, "Everyone brings out the choice wine first and then the cheaper wine after the guests have had
too much to drink; but you have saved the best till now."

—John 2:7-10, Christian Bible, NIV

Jesus openly demonstrated his miraculous powers for the first time when he attended
a wedding in Cana of Galilee. The event's purpose, according to Self-Realization Fellowship
founder Paramahansa Yogananda, was to "demonstrate to his disciples that behind every diversity of matter is the one Absolute Substance."

This gospel story dramatically increased in personal potency for me when I had a powerful, numinous dream in January 2011, one and one-half years into treatment. In my dream, a
young girl and her mother handed me a "substance" that, with practice, could be manipulated
into anything I wanted. At first I fumbled with it, yet gradually improved until I could turn a drop
into a tiny clipper ship.

Toying with the dream symbols for months, I eventually came to see that the substance
represented feminine alchemy—creatively forming, out of the imagination, something for beauty's sake, rather than mentally experimenting with actual physical elements to get rich, which
historically was a main goal of alchemy.

After a while it dawned on me, with prodding from energy intuitive Maria Paglialungo,
that in a more broad sense, I could alchemically alter cancer into a new life for myself. The one
substance in my dream was love, the greatest transformative ingredient of all, and granted to me
for working miracles, Maria had said. The first miracle I needed was a cure.

Yogananda further explained the miracle-working power of the Substance: "[U]nderlying
and controlling all atomic matter is the one unifying and balancing power of Divine Intelligence
and Will…. [O]ne form of matter could be changed into another…by the power of Universal
Mind. By his oneness with the Divine Intelligence…Jesus changed the arrangement of electrons
and protons."

With his mind stayed on the Divine, I believe Jesus knew how to rearrange energy at the
subatomic level to create new substances, like transforming water into wine. I can imagine that
for him it was like child's play, just like it was for the girl in my dream. I feel awe at such mastery
over the physical universe.

Some of that mastery was passed on to me, because by the end of my dream, I had created
a tiny clipper ship. Perhaps this ship represented my mothership, a drop of the Divine feminine I
had internalized and could use to transform my life and my surroundings. I filled my internal jar
with water to be miraculously transmuted into the wine of a new life.

Thriver Soup Ingredient:
Sit for a while with the idea that you, as a being made in the image of the Divine, also have

the ability to transform substances at the subatomic level. I believe there have been some individuals through history who have unlocked this ability within themselves. Enjoy daydreaming about what you would do if you developed this ability enough to create miracles for yourself and others.

~~~

Not Suffering

O Son of Kunti (Arjuna), the ideas of heat and cold, pleasure and pain, are produced by the contacts of the senses with their objects. Such ideas are limited by a beginning and an end. They are transitory, O Descendant of Bharata (Arjuna); bear them with patience!
—*God Talks with Arjuna: The Bhagavad Gita*, 2.14

The Bhagavad Gita teaches that physical sensations are only temporary, and not to place a lot of stock in them. Spiritual master Paramahansa Yogananda, who wrote an interpretation of this Hindu classic, said that while adopting reasonable measures to overcome external discomfort, we should gradually develop mental "aboveness" in response to the inevitable pains and disappointments of life. If we succeed, we will experience less suffering.

Well, I'm no yogi. I find such an exercise far easier said than done. Yet I also decided I could at least give it a go.

A year into my treatments, I jammed something under a fingernail and didn't think much of it. Within a few days it started hurting, so I allowed the sensation to be and yet did not suffer from it. I felt pleased that this seemed to work.

The next night the pain dial turned up and my finger throbbed. I hardly slept. So much for allowing the pain to be and not suffering.

The next morning I called my nurse, Vicky, who urged me to have my finger looked at by my doctor. Later that morning, my doctor sliced open my finger right at the nail bed. I was able to stay centered in my body until she did the final slice. When she squeezed out two drops of pus, I screamed. Then my finger felt much better. I got the antibiotics and started them immediately. My finger healed nicely.

The doctor's office called to say I had strep bacteria in my finger. No wonder the infection got out-of-hand.

My response to the pain was normal, yet it demonstrated how little mastery I have over physical sensation. On the other hand, I did find that when the pain was less intense, I could surrender in the moment and not fight the pain. My body relaxed, which helped reduce the raw sensations. By reminding myself of the transitory nature of pain, I continued to learn to bear the discomforts of cancer treatment with patience.

Thriver Soup Ingredient:
As much as we cancer patients are cut, burned, and poisoned, practicing patience and for-

bearance can ease suffering. When you experience physical pain, remember it is only a sensation. See if you can relax your muscles, stay in the moment, and allow the pain to be what it is. Perhaps then your sense of suffering might diminish. Or perhaps you might benefit from Jon Kabat-Zinn's book, *Full Catastrophe Living: Using the Wisdom of Your Body and Mind to Face Stress, Pain, and Illness*, available in a variety of formats.

≈≈≈

Reincarnation: I'll be Back

By diligently following his path, the yogi, perfected by the efforts of many births, is purged of sin (karmic taint) and finally enters the Supreme Beatitude.
— God Talks with Arjuna: The Bhagavad Gita, 6.45

I believe I have experienced many human births, so I think it is possible to access memories of my soul's previous lives to better understand my current circumstances. I presume we carry some sort of pattern forward from lifetime to lifetime. If true, it's possible the sarcoma developed out of a multi-lifetime pattern that blossomed this time so I could fully resolve it.

A year after the diagnosis, I explored some of my past lives to gain insight into any possible causes of the cancer that had roots in previous experiences. To receive information, I placed myself in a deeply relaxed state and asked my psyche several questions, recording the answers in my journal with my non-dominant hand. It provided a good starting place.

One answer reminded me of a vague past-life memory of my soul occupying a different body several centuries ago in what is now Scotland. During that lifetime I had accepted the role of a severely abused female. I am fairly certain I did not heal those negative sexual experiences during that lifetime. I thought it was plausible that the "I" who moved from lifetime to lifetime carried forward a pattern of dysfunction and self-rejection that manifested during my current lifetime through a cancer that occupied a sexual organ. If true, the pain had raised its ugly head to provide me with an opportunity to heal the damage on a cellular level. Using active imagination, I wanted to further explore that life on an emotional level so I could understand, forgive myself and others, and heal the pattern.

After some deep, relaxing breaths, I began approaching, in my imagination, a huge cathedral in the sky. Inside, the Voice of a Presence invited me into a hall of records. There I met an old, wizard-like librarian. We went to my personal section in the stacks, and I asked for the record of the Highlands lifetime. For the first time ever, when I attempted to access a previous life memory, I was told, "No." Not to be deterred, I asked in two or three different ways. Always, the answer came: "No."

Why?

He said I wasn't ready yet. It was horrific and ended with my being burned at the stake.

Oh, hll. More layers to peel. I could only pray I would be granted enough time and courage to heal without accessing this lifetime. I don't think it was a mistake that a previous lifetime involved a burning. Through chemotherapy, I was voluntarily allowing myself to be scorched. Otherwise, I didn't have the karmic explanation for the cancer that I had wanted to find, with the hope that the new information would contribute to a cure. Um, not now, anyway. I guess I had more to learn.

I hoped that during this lifetime I was healing whatever old wound I carried so I could open up room for a cure in my current body.

My friend Charley wrote, "The phoenix reborn arises from the burning mass, but only after it has crashed into the flames. And you surely did crash. That you awoke from the dream of burning means that you are the phoenix reborn. A new day (is) staring you in the face."

As I resolve the issues in my current life, I am reincarnating myself, taking more steps closer to entering the supreme beatitude—infinite bliss consciousness, an ever-new, love-permeated oneness with the Divine in which there is no lack, no disease, and no death.

Thriver Soup Ingredient:

Exploring past lives can be tricky and psychologically dangerous. If you are inwardly led to investigate your past lives, please seek professional assistance rather than attempting to self-regress. I started out with professional past-life regressionists whom I trusted. I relied on them for many years before feeling comfortable about pursuing information on my own.

To select a past-life regressionist, start by looking for a licensed clinical hypnotherapist. The American Psychotherapy and Medical Hypnosis Association provides certificates for professionals in medicine and mental health who complete coursework. Also consider members of the American Society of Clinical Hypnosis (ASCH) and the Society for Clinical and Experimental Hypnosis.

To receive a directory of professionals practicing hypnotherapy near you, contact the American Society of Clinical Hypnosis at www.asch.net, the Society for Clinical and Experimental Hypnosis at www.societiesofhypnosis.com, or the American Association of Professional Hypnotherapists at www.aaph.org.

Look for someone with years of reputable experience, especially in assisting people with integrating what they learned during the process. Ask the hypnotherapist what sorts of questions will be asked during the session. If the practitioner asks open-ended questions, such as "What do you look like?" this is a good sign. If the therapist asks closed-ended questions, such as "Is your hair brown?" you might want to interview another practitioner.

Follow your instincts. They probably will be correct.

~~~

Remission: Sustainable Hope

He took the blind man by the hand and led him outside the village. When he had spit on the man's

eyes and put his hands on him, Jesus asked, "Do you see anything?" He looked up and said, "I see people; they look like trees walking around." Once more Jesus put his hands on the man's eyes. Then his eyes were opened, his sight was restored, and he saw everything clearly.
—Mark 8:23-25, Christian Bible, NIV

In this story, Jesus cures a blind man in stages, not all at once. It seems to me that cures normally come about like this. According to the Bruno Gröning teachings, there often is a crisis involving even more pain and difficulty before the cure manifests. My psychotherapist called this an extinction burst.

Deepak Chopra said in his CD, "Magical Mind, Magical Body," that one's cancer from three months ago is not the current cancer, because the current cancer is made of completely different raw materials. To get better, we need to expunge the memory of the illness at the cellular level. I wondered for months how to do this. I eventually realized that manipulating my emotions would not accomplish this. However, I later learned that one method we can try involves transcending both our emotions and our thoughts. This can be accomplished by becoming silent witnesses of our bodies through the practice of meditation.

The Institute for Noetic Science has a record of 3,500 spontaneous remissions from cancer. I found the book about it on their website and skimmed. A common theme seemed to be the use of "intensive meditation."

Intensive meditation was not explained, so I did an internet search. Basically it is image-less, emotionless, mindfulness meditation like the Buddhists practice. One website suggested practicing at least one hour per day. It noted studies in which visualization and the use of imagery actually interfered with the healing process. Australian psychiatrist Ainslie Meares, MD (1910–1986), reportedly found that meditation inhibited the growth of tumors in ten percent of the cases he studied. When people let go of their thoughts, this allows masculine life-force energy to arise in the body, which has the potential to cure illness.

I'd say a ten percent chance for a cure is better than most cancer prognoses. Did I like mindfulness meditation? I had avoided it for years. I found focusing on an image far easier. After much searching and thinking, I finally settled on the Bruno method (see Bruno Gröning: Access the Divine Healing Stream in the section GPS: Guides Providing and Sustaining, even a Donkey), which really isn't meditation, yet it was the most suitable practice for my history and temperament.

The next question was—how do I change the cellular memory of the disease? I think it might involve, at least in part, stimulating my senses with pleasure, such as pacifying smells, classical music, and delicious food. Painting my model horses gave me a lot of enjoyment, which also might have helped shift things in my body.

I looked up the word "remission" and found it meant an abatement of intensity. In a Christian context, the word re-mission referred to receiving a pardon or forgiveness. This definition fit well with the emotional healing work I was doing. I was learning to forgive myself for a womb issue that had colored my whole life.

Larry Dossey, MD, in his book *Healing Words*, listed the characteristics that five Japanese cancer patients, who experienced spontaneous remissions, had in common. These characteristics included:

1. Having an existential crisis while living with cancer and choosing to resolve their crises themselves.

2. A surprising lack of anxiety and depression after their diagnoses. For four of the patients, this was connected with a strong religious faith.

3. Giving themselves completely to the will of the Divine and renewing their commitment to former activities and new interests. They intuited more meaning and a bigger picture in life's experiences, including the cancer.

4. Improving their relationships with others, which involved both personal growth and introspection.

5. A conspicuous spiritual viewpoint.

I felt I fit all five of these characteristics to some degree.

For me, a spiritual point of view is the source of my hope. To sustain this hope, despite contradictory medical evidence, is life-affirming. Even if we hold onto hope until the bitter end, we can still accomplish more than if we give up, said Bernie Siegel, MD. He called the refusal to hope "a decision to die."

Whatever is occurring with your treatments, you can take hope from the fact that sometimes things just get worse before they get better; and as in the case of the man cured of blindness, sometimes the cure—and the miracle—takes some time to manifest.

Thriver Soup Ingredient:

In your journal, write out Dossey's list of five characteristics the patients had in common and that might have brought about their spontaneous remission experiences. Write out how you do or don't match up with each item. If there are any you don't match up with, create a plan to work on that item. For the first item, if there was no existential crisis leading up to the illness, view the illness itself as an existential crisis to be resolved.

≈≈≈

Screaming at the Spirit

Leaving that place, Jesus withdrew to the region of Tyre and Sidon. A Canaanite woman from that vicinity came to him, crying out, "Lord, Son of David, have mercy on me! My daughter is demon-possessed and suffering terribly." Jesus did not answer a word. So his disciples came to him and urged him, "Send her away, for she keeps crying out after us." He answered, "I was sent only to the lost sheep of Israel." The woman came and knelt before him. "Lord, help me!" she said. He replied, "It is not right to take the children's bread and toss it to the dogs." "Yes it is, Lord," she said. "Even the dogs eat the crumbs that fall from their master's table." Then Jesus said to her, "Woman, you have great faith! Your request is granted." And her daughter was healed at that moment.

—Matthew 15:21-28, Christian Bible, NIV

What was I willing to endure to be cured? Vince Lasorso reminded me that even being called a dog looking for scraps didn't stop the Canaanite woman in the Christian Gospels. She didn't mutely accept things as they were. That uppity woman angrily shouted for help from Jesus. She even successfully challenged his understanding of his mission. And she got what she wanted.

Her faith in God drove her to demean herself before Jesus. Was I willing to do what the Canaanite woman did—scream, be compared to a dog looking for scraps, and challenge the Divine—to be cured?

I did. I had screaming fits. I allowed conventional cancer treatments to dehumanize me. And I challenged the Divine. "Hey, You! What *are* You doing? Why are You allowing this to happen to me? I need to be living my life, not sitting in a chemo chair."

I never quite felt that the Divine caused the cancer within me, just as the Canaanite woman didn't see her daughter's predicament as a punishment from God. She took up her banner and assertively challenged rather than surrendering to the situation like a victim.

I did continue to see the Divine as ever-present to comfort and heal, if not to cure. I wanted what the Canaanite woman received—healing. And I would do whatever it took to get a response from the Spirit.

Thriver Soup Ingredient:

Whenever you are pissed off at the Spirit, feel free to go somewhere private and scream into a pillow. Pour out your rage and pain, hurt and confusion. The Divine already knows and won't be offended. You, in turn, get to be more genuine and authentic.

Sin Big

Being and nonbeing create each other.

—Tao Te Ching, 2

A balance between being and nonbeing, and between being and doing, existed, yet I had not found it.

One step I took along this see-saw evolved from reading about radical feminist and author Mary Daly (1928–2010) when she passed away. She said the word "sin" was derived from the Indo-European root "es-," meaning "to be." She encouraged women to "sin big" because it meant to fully be.

With my background, I experienced an aversion both to sinning and to being. This reluctance needed to be overcome for me to find greater internal balance and harmony.

My psychotherapist loaned me psychoanalyst Marion Woodman's book *Addiction to Perfection*. It reminded me of my addiction to work as one way to avoid truly feeling. In my desperation for a cure, I wanted to heal that propensity immediately. My friend Vince Lasorso cautioned me not to stress over working through all my emotional issues so quickly. Other friends encouraged me to stop grasping for answers and forcing information.

I learned that relaxing, being open and quiet, and having fun would have greater positive influence toward a cure than my driving to resolve everything. Daly would have encouraged me to sin big—to enjoy being as much as doing, to trust life, and to trust myself. Information would spontaneously appear when the time became right for me.

A month later, I dreamt that I moved out of an office building where I had been living and into a nice home with a man I admired. My psyche was moving in the right direction.

The following winter, in preparation for surgery, I finally gave myself permission to sin big. I went on a nine-day silent retreat at Grailville conference center in Loveland, Ohio. I only got out of bed when my body moved of its own accord. When I ate, I focused only on my food. Each day filled with rich gifts that only silence could bring. It took a few days to let go of the compulsion to "get up and do something useful" and spend more time in quiet receptivity.

While crunching through snow on the retreat center's labyrinth, I realized that when I was doing, my ego usually had a firm grasp on my mind. I became its slave. When I would simply be, my thinking and judging mind slipped its grip, allowing the gates of both the unconscious and superconscious aspects of myself to crack so tidbits could gently enter into my awareness.

Such realizations can be frightening when they have been pushed out of our conscious awareness for a long time. Truth can hurt, inciting fear and further shut-downs. On the other hand, we sometimes run from the beautiful truths because we are afraid of our greatness, our light, our tremendous inner power and strength. I believe we are tiny, individual, holographic images of the Divine. How terrifying and, at the same time, how glorious.

Balancing this glory with our deeper humanity that occasionally arises from the unconscious takes practice. Sinning big—nonjudgmentally allowing ourselves to fully be the wondrous creatures we are—helps us enter the process. By being, we create non-being, which then gives rise to being. They balance each other out and help create harmony and wholeness, which draws our bodies into healthier states of being.

Thriver Soup Ingredient:

Sometimes it's hard to break an ingrained pattern of doing by deliberately being. Spending time on retreat provides a great opportunity to break up old ways and experiment with simply being. So go sin big—take a retreat and give yourself permission to do nothing.

∽∽∽

Surrendering: Offering no Resistance to the Divine

If they surrender, then truly they are rightly guided.

—Qur'an 3:20b, Rodwell edition

I have a difficult time with the idea of surrendering to the Spirit, even if it brings guidance. This stems from a deep fear of losing control over my life—as if I ever had any real control. This makes grasping the concept of surrender hard for me. My friend Clark Echols, MDiv, helped me understand what surrender is not: giving up or turning the course of your life over to someone or something else. My friend Lois Clement said what surrender is: opening up your heart to the Spirit, allowing, trusting, believing, and having faith.

According to ParamahansaYogananda, founder of Self-Realization Fellowship, when one surrenders, one offers no intellectual or emotional resistance to the Divine yet trusts that the Spirit will answer and bless every sincere prayer and endeavor.

As I prayed one night, I realized surrender involved telling the Spirit about every concern and asking the Divine to lead, guide, and direct it all toward a resolution for everyone's highest good. Then my place was to do my best and let go of any attachment to outcome. Surrender also involved living in conscious awareness of the Spirit's presence at every moment, allowing the light of Divine love to flow through me and spill over into the world.

My psychotherapist added that surrender is not permanent—invitations to yield arrive as we move through our days. My role is to influence—not control—what I can, accept life's circumstances, and be aware of what's happening inside my body. What messages are my cells giving me? How am I responding to them? If I follow these suggestions, my mind will still. My awareness will yield to the present moment, in all its messiness and mystery. Then I will be open to the guidance already present.

Thriver Soup Ingredient:

Mary Beth Hall, author of *Lessons from a Bald Chick*, provided me with a good image for surrendering to the Spirit. She said she placed her book on Jesus' lap and told him to do whatever he wanted with it, even if that meant it fell off his lap when he stood up and it got kicked under a table and forgotten. Modify this image to suit your needs. Allow the mystery of life to be what it is, even with all your pain, confusion, and questions.

≈≈≈

The Present Moment: It's Now or Never

When you conquer the mind, You conquer the world.
—Meditation 28, *Japji: The Path of Devotional Meditation*

My mind has remained an unconquered beast, running around me in circles, taking me wherever it pleases. I watch it, day in and day out, wandering repeatedly over the same thoughts, reinforcing them without adding freshness or originality. I would expect to get bored with the same repeated nonsense, but no, my brain mindlessly chatters away. I wanted to be more conscious of my thoughts so I could choose to stay with them, change them, or discard them.

It takes a lot of concentration to tame this brainimal. Learning to live in the present moment helps a great deal with this training.

All anyone ever has is this moment, right here, right now. Not a moment in the past, and not a moment yet to come. Simply here. Now.

This became even more significant for me while I learned to patiently wait, wait, wait after the diagnosis. Wait for test results, wait during treatments, wait through recovery periods.

Not one of us is promised a tomorrow, my friend Diane Faul reminded me. "All any of us need to do for a fulfilling and rewarding life is simply use the time, the day we have at the present moment, to give and receive love ~ for we truly came here for learning and sharing the gifts of love."

Gradually, I learned that when I'm in my thinking/judging mind, I'm not being present to others around me or even to myself, much less giving or receiving love. One way of letting go of the ego and being present is to focus on one's breath.

I took to sitting outside all during the spring and summer, watching tree leaves unfurl, hickory buds sprout, and light speckle the trunks and ground. How pleasant it all was...something I had missed most of my adult life.

It brought to mind this little vignette by poet Elizabeth Barrett Browning:

Earth's crammed with heaven,
And every common bush afire with God;
But only he who sees, takes off his shoes,
The rest sit round it and pluck blackberries.

I wanted to conquer my mind. I wanted to see the bush afire with the Divine. I wanted to take off my shoes and forego plucking blackberries.

Thriver Soup Ingredient:

We can transform the mundane into the sacred by setting our intention and attention. As you move through your day, practice stepping back mentally and seeing what you are doing or noticing what you are thinking. This will assist you with stepping outside of the ego and moving into the present moment. Perhaps set the intention of doing this once each day for a week, then gradually step up your practice so you can live more and more in your body and in the present moment.

~ ~ ~

Undirected Prayer: Help, Thanks

... yet not my will, but yours be done.

—Luke 22:42b, Christian Bible, NIV

Undirected prayer involves letting go of control and getting into harmony with Divine purpose. Jesus eloquently expressed it when he knelt among the olive trees in the Garden of Gethsemane, not asking for anything specific, all the while awaiting what he knew was an un-mitigated disaster for himself as a human being. He had been betrayed by Judas and knew the authorities were coming after him and probably would crucify him. Who wouldn't want to get out of such a horrific situation? Yet Jesus had the strength to surrender to Divine will.

Jesus had the confidence that comes from deeply knowing who he was. According to Larry Dossey, MD, remembering our true nature, who we truly are, is the purpose of prayer. This Self-knowledge enabled Jesus to let go of any preconceived or desired outcome so he could carry through with the impending agony.

In my own agony during treatment, months would go by without my uttering a single prayer. No way could I pray as Jesus did in the garden. Part of my silence stemmed from a deep sense of betrayal and abandonment by the Spirit; part from a sagging faith; and part from simple, perpetual exhaustion.

My friend Mim Grace Gieser reminded me I could offer a general prayer and then express gratitude for Divine provision. I like how writer Anne Lamott puts it: there are three basic prayers, which are "Help me," "Thank you," and "Wow." Simple, heartfelt, undirected. No specific outcome is requested.

I could do this. In fact, it came naturally to me, without much conscious awareness, as it would to anyone drowning.

If we pray with deep emotion, no matter what words might come out of our mouths, then our bodies' cells can pick up on the prayers and intentions. Candace Pert, PhD, neuroscientist and pharmacologist, explains in her book, *The Molecules of Emotion*, that our feelings turn into chemicals that communicate information to our cells. It reminds me of a favorite passage from the English Standard Version Christian Bible: "Likewise the Spirit helps us in our weakness. For we do not know what to pray for as we ought, but the Spirit himself intercedes for us with groanings too deep for words" (Romans 8:26).

The Divine knows our hearts and desires and how best to assist us. By letting go of the need to control any outcomes, we can better come into harmony with our inner selves and with Divine purpose. This makes it easier for us to pray like Jesus, "...yet not my will, but yours be done."

Thriver Soup Ingredient:

If you find yourself unable to pray, or too weak to pray like you might ordinarily do, simply accept that it's too hard to pray, and let it go. Thomas Merton, a Catholic monk, once wrote, "True love and prayer are learned in the hour where prayer has become impossible and the heart has turned to stone."

If you have a little energy, then perhaps you can mutter, like Lamott, "help me, help me, help me," and maybe follow it with "thank you." Or simply sit with the emotions in your body. Such a prayer is more than enough.

❧❧❧

Upside-down Trees

The Blessed Lord said: They (the wise) speak of an eternal ashvattha tree, with roots above and boughs beneath, whose leaves are Vedic hymns. He who understands this tree of life is a Veda-knower."
—God Talks with Arjuna: The Bhagavad Gita, 15.1

The ashvattha tree, or holy fig tree, is pictured upside-down in this passage from one of Hinduism's sacred writings. Its roots reach into the heavens, or the divine world of light and love, so the sap flows downward to penetrate our everyday physical world. The branches descend into the dark soil, connecting heaven with earth. It's under the fig tree, also called the Bodhi tree, that Buddha received his enlightenment. In the Jewish mystical tradition, there are two different tree of life symbols: one is right-side-up while the other, like the sacred fig tree, is upside-down. It is our work to awaken and begin climbing the tree to its roots to reconnect with Divine source.

Trees quickly took on significance during my cancer journey. My friend Maria Paglialungo visited me after the hysterectomy and drew a tree on the board in my hospital room. For my next birthday she gave me a poem, "Miracle Grow," comparing the Divine to a master gardener who has planted a seed within me. With peace, love, and patience, Spirit waters, shines sunlight, weeds, and prunes so that seed can grow into a tree. She warned me not to try to get out of this dark night of the soul prematurely—I was being pruned and needed faith and willingness to surrender to the Divine. When the deep roots of faith take hold, only then will I grow into whatever it is I am to do and will drop the fear. "What we think is harmful is often 'Miracle Grow' and for our greatest good," she concluded.

About eight months after the diagnosis, I sat outside to absorb spring. Daffodils cheered our home with their sunny yellow faces. I found it interesting how the trees didn't have their buds yet. The giant sentinels woke up slowly, allowing the vigorous flowers, small plants and grasses to soak up as much sun as possible early in the spring. Each had its place, each took its turn. I had my place, and I would take my turn.

The following winter, as I walked a labyrinth in a field, I stopped and laid hands on a sleeping tree and asked that my juices rise from my own dark depths during the coming spring, full of strength and life. Yet that spring still was not my time.

During the summer, I pulled out an older photo taken of me standing inside a giant, empty tree at Glacier National Park. The womblike trunk had felt warm and soft, muffling every sound like the protective shelter of a uterus. The photo graced my altar as a reminder to allow myself to rest in the healing womb of mother earth, waiting for the sap of spring to flow upward through my body.

Soon afterward, while visiting the Great Serpent Mound effigy in Peebles, Ohio, a woman suggested I stand with my back against a particular tree. I did, and images quickly and powerfully flooded my awareness—pictures of my own roots deep in the earth, drawing energy up into my body while my spine was supported by a tree of life embracing me.

Trees have energy centers, or chakras, according to Alberto Villoldo in *Shaman, Healer, Sage*. He suggested scanning the surface of a tree with your hands until "you feel the tingling sensation that indicates the presence of a chakra." I haven't experienced that sensation, yet he says you can gently nudge the tree's chakra to align with one of yours so you can energetically connect with it.

Trees link the earth, through their roots, with the heavens, through their branches. And like the Jewish idea, there also is the Tree of Life that joins the heavens, through roots in Divine eternal existence, with the earth, through branches. As we connect to both, we obtain more spiritual wisdom.

Thriver Soup Ingredient:

Find a tree you really like. Stand with your spine against its trunk and imagine your feet are like vibrant roots traveling underground. Draw up Divine healing light and energy from mother earth, like sap surging through roots. Experience the tree's life-force energy supporting you in your process, connecting your humanity with your inherent divine nature.

∽∽∽

Visualizations: Just Imagine

May the God of hope fill you with all joy and peace as you trust in him, so that you may overflow with hope by the power of the Holy Spirit.
—Romans 15:13, Christian Bible, NIV

One needs to feel hope to be motivated to visualize. I found it took a lot of energy that I often didn't have, yet I continued anyway as I believed it would be helpful. There are probably as many visualizations one can use as there are people. I came across many ideas for putting my imagination to work while dealing with cancer.

One's imagination triggers the most primitive part of the brain, getting it into direct contact with the body, according to Ken Wilber, author of *Grace and Grit*.

Bernie Siegel, MD, added, "Our emotions and words let the body know what we expect of it, and by visualizing certain changes we can help the body bring them about."

During the 1970s, Carl Simonton, MD, an ankhologist, decided to study the impact of visualization on cancer patients. He taught patients to imagine the cancer cells or tumors as accurately as possible. He told them cancer cells are chaotic and weak, helping impart confidence that their bodies could innately defend against cancer. He also urged patients to imagine their treatment as potent and successful, able to generate the desired results. Even more important, he encouraged patients to imagine that their white blood cells formed a powerful army that was destroying the disease. He found these patients lived longer and experienced improved quality of life.

I've heard of white blood cells being imagined as snow flurries, popcorn, and even white killer rabbits. According to Bernie Siegel, MD, some of the most successful visualizations involved images of white blood cells eating tumors as if they were food. The image, however, must be chosen by the patient, must be seen clearly in her or his mind, and must be one with which the patient feels totally comfortable.

One hospitalized cancer patient was hypnotized and asked "to find the room in his brain that had the valves controlling the blood flow to his tumor. He did, and the tumor shrank to one-fourth its original size." He was discharged from the hospital.

Studies have demonstrated that those with the liveliest immune cells had the best chances for survival. It appears that visualizing those cells as active and powerful enhances our abilities to fulfill our desires for longer survival.

During my cancer journey I tried out a variety of visualizations. One visualization I particularly liked was seeing every cell in my body as a bright yellow smiley-face radiating Divine light. Doing periodic visualizations boosted my sense of hope, and gave me strength to keep on moving toward my desired goal of regaining my health. Eventually, joy and peace emerged from the process.

Thriver Soup Ingredient:

Spend some time selecting a visualization that feels right for you. Find a way to represent that image in physical form, such as a drawing or cutting out pictures from magazines. Set aside five minutes each day to relax in a comfortable chair or in bed and, with strong emotion, play out the scene in your imagination.

~~~

Walking the Labyrinth: 'Round 'n' 'Round We Go

Great is the fruit, great the advantage of earnest contemplation when set round with upright conduct. Great is the fruit, great the advantage of intellect when set round with earnest contemplation.
—"The Book of the Great Decease," 2:4

The Buddha taught that upright conduct forms a backdrop for earnest contemplation. When one behaves in a seemly manner, there's little or no remorse to plague one while attempting to meditate. Intense reflection, in a similar way, feeds the desire to behave uprightly. Both produce great fruit and great advantage, both for ourselves and for others.

One centuries-old method for practicing sincere contemplation is walking a labyrinth. A labyrinth consists of a winding path that leads into a central area and back out again to the starting point.

While awaiting my second major surgery, I wanted to take a silent retreat to prepare. The nearby Grailville conference center in Loveland, Ohio, provided the perfect location for me. Daily I walked the large labyrinth laid out in their meadow. As I wound around, the trail meandered close to the center, then farther away, then nearer again, then outward a few times before finally depositing me in the center. This experience provided a great little metaphor for the spiritual life. When I embarked on my inner journey, I had many exciting experiences at the beginning. These gave me a taste for what lay ahead. Yet as I neared my goal, I was pulled back away with dry periods when prayer and meditation became tasteless and rote, meaningless as the jabber of an excited monkey. By continuing on the path set before me, however, eventually I would travel close to the center again. Then be drawn outward. Finally I got so close I could almost touch the center; in this labyrinth, I easily could have stepped into the round center from my path. To do so, however, would have short-circuited the process and kept me from the full strength that could be garnered from the journey. Without the foundation of deep inner work, the experience of reaching the core of our souls could prove overwhelming.

There are no real shortcuts in the spiritual life. For most people, it can be a long and arduous task, dancing around the focal point like a moth orbiting a lit candle. Get too close too soon, and the person gets singed.

It's similar to peeling an onion. We pull back each individual layer as it presents itself. Pushing through the layers and jumping to the middle can leave us blind with tears. The process brings to my mind St. Teresa of Avila's book, *The Interior Castle*, which describes the circling one experiences while moving more and more deeply into the center of our spiritual homes.

Finally, when fully prepared, we can enter into the stillness of the One, the central room, the eternal silence of true being. Like Buddha, we can stay a little while and bask in the brilliance.

When we enter into the light, we receive the great fruit of the intellect—an experience of our cells soaking in pure intelligence, wrote Hari Sharma, MD, my Ayurvedic physician. "This can help correct the flaws in the DNA.... When you have the most intelligence awake within your cells, you are best positioned to derive the most profound level of nutrition from the plants."

Then, like Buddha, we dust ourselves off and begin the journey back out—out of the center, out of the labyrinth, out into the world. Yet now there is a difference. The candle flame is within us; it cannot be snuffed out. Pure intelligence has washed our cells. Our light bulbs have turned on, and we are inspired to glow outward by offering our gifts to others through upright conduct and loving service.

Thriver Soup Ingredient:

Do an internet search to find a labyrinth, possibly using labyrinthlocator.com/locate-a-labyrinth to find one in your area. When you go to a labyrinth, walk the path with a quiet, attentive, prayerful heart. Pause in the center to listen with your heart, express yourself, present a small gift, or make a request. Then wind your way back out and into the world.

If you cannot find a labyrinth close enough to where you are, obtain a picture of one. Place yourself into a meditative state. Then slowly trace the path with your fingertip.

G. GPS: Guides Providing and Sustaining

Introduction to GPS: Guides Providing and Sustaining, Even a Donkey

In those days Hezekiah was stricken with a terminal illness. The prophet Isaiah son of Amoz visited him and told him, "This is what the Lord says, 'Give instructions to your household, for you are about to die; you will not get well.'" Hezekiah turned his face to the wall and prayed to the Lord, "Please, Lord. Remember how I have served you faithfully and with wholehearted devotion, and how I have carried out your will." Then Hezekiah wept bitterly. The Lord told Isaiah, "Go and tell Hezekiah: 'This is what the Lord God of your ancestor David says: "I have heard your prayer; I have seen your tears. Look, I will add fifteen years to your life."'"

—Isaiah 38:1-5, Christian Bible, NET

Only the Divine heals, as Hezekiah knew. If I'd been this Hebrew king living long ago, however, I probably would have pleaded with the prophet Isaiah, bearer of bad news. "Please!" I'd say. "Tell the Divine there's been a mistake. I'm supposed to live."

The king, however, remained mute toward the human prophet. He turned his back to Isaiah, and to all other humans, and instead faced a wall—perhaps to better focus on contact with the Divine. He took his sorrow straight to the Spirit.

The Divine alone cures and heals. Yet just as we receive information into our lives through a variety of means, the Divine chooses a plethora of pathways and guides to deliver information and revitalizing experiences to those who demand it.

For example, Bruno Gröning (1906–1959), a spiritual teacher in Germany, stated over and over that he was only a channel for healing energy—never the One who healed. He passed away decades ago, yet promised to always assist those who ask him for help. Many spiritual guides are included in this section because they either devoted their human lives to the Divine and now work in spiritual realms to help humans, or because they represented a particular type of energy I wanted to enliven within myself. I wanted to place myself in the best possible position to receive a cure. As my friend Melinda said, "Pray as if everything depends on God; act as if everything depends on you."

Having enough faith in a guide does not guarantee a cure, or even healing; ultimately it's not up to us or the level of faith we possess. It is up to the Spirit, and the Spirit uses medical and complementary interventions as well as our spiritual guides and our faith. Heck, even the Jewish Bible contains a story of the Divine using a donkey to get a verbal message across to a stubborn man (in Numbers 22:28).

The guides in this section are only those with whom I have a personal connection. They provide examples for how to work with whatever guides feel right for you. Perhaps you prefer Moses or Muhammad, Inanna or Isis, Buddha or Baha'u'llah. Maybe you only want to feel the arms of Divine Mother wrapped around you while Divine Father stands guard beside you. Or you don't want any guides—you turn your face directly to the wall and go straight to the Source. Whatever way you choose, move forward with faith, trust, and persistence.

Thriver Soup Ingredient:

Create a home altar. What you will need:

A location in your home where you can place a small altar.

A table, small cabinet top, or space on the floor.

A cloth covering that speaks to you.

Objects that serve as symbols or reminders of your devotion and desires. These can include images of your guides.

My altar includes photos of my guides placed in wire leaves of a tree sculpture; a crystal bowl with rose petals and butterfly wings I found; and several candles, among many other objects.

Place the cloth on your table, cabinet top, or floor space, and add your images. Sit by the altar during your prayer and/or meditation time and use it as a reminder to keep focused on your positive outcome.

~~~

Asclepius: Lucky Strikes

Moshe made a bronze snake and put it on the pole; if a snake had bitten someone, then, when he looked toward the bronze snake, he stayed alive.

—Numbers 21:9, Complete Jewish Bible

Snakes show up in many cultures as symbols for healing. The Hebrew prophet Moses was instructed to hold up a fiery serpent on a pole so those who looked upon it could live. Meso-American societies depicted their highest god, Quetzalcoatl, as a flying serpent with feathers. Quetzalcoatl was a dying god who would someday return, a symbol of resurrection. The ancient Greeks went to temples devoted to Asclepius to seek cures for what ailed them. Asclepius, now believed to have been an historical person with exceptional ability to cure diseases, was elevated to divine status as a god of healing. His symbol is a single snake wrapped around a staff.

I never liked snakes. My first memory of them is from about age five when two rattlesnakes slithered onto our driveway. My parents transmitted their terror into my body when they warned me to stay away.

I worked with my fear of snakes through the years, yet it still held sway over me. Less than a month after the hysterectomy, energy intuitive Maria Paglialungo suggested I do active imagination with snakes to see what would show up.

During the visualization process, I was joined by a fat, stubby, brown-and-vanilla-striped snake—yet I did not fear it, even when its fangs bit into me. Immediately I thought of Asclepius.

In ancient healing shrines, those who were ill would come to sleep overnight and ask for dreams from Asclepius. Priests would interpret the dreams and recommend remedies or give advice.

Then a word popped into my head—cinnamon. Cinnamon? With a snake? Well, he did have cinnamon-colored stripes. I decided to look up the health benefits of cinnamon, and found this surprise: "Its mild anti-inflammatory, anti-spasmodic, and anti-clotting properties are believed to be due to its content of cinnamaldehyde.... Cinnamon extracts have also inhibited the growth of cultured tumor cells. This effect may be due to the presence of procyanidins and eugenol in the bark extract."

My friend Judy Merritt, PhD, who occasionally has had pit vipers appear in her outer life, wrote that the snake bite initiates a shaman into death to transmute all poisons, be they mental, physical, spiritual, or emotional. The bite also indicates the power of creation, sexuality, psychic energy, alchemy, reproduction, and ascension.

At about the time of my visualization, an injured rattlesnake lay in the road leading to Judy's house. She picked it up, put it into her car, and drove it home. She spent the next two days sitting with the rattler, waiting for it to die. She wrote, "You could say her colorations were cinnamon. I am getting the sense that there is a connection between the Snake who came to me and the Snake who came to you.... [T]here is some powerful healing magic there."

Maria quoted to me from Ted Andrews' book *Animal Speak*: "Anytime a snake shows up as a totem, you can expect death and rebirth to occur in some area of your life." Hmm.... Cinnamon was my second powerful representation of resurrection from the dead.

The snake symbolizes this radical transformation because it outgrows its old skin. When the snake prepares to shed, the covering over its eyes starts to turn opaque or adopt a bluish appearance. To many ancient people, this indicated an ability to enter into a trance-like state and move between the realms of life and death. Once the dead skin is off, the eyes once again are clear, indicating a new view of the world.

The snake totem also can symbolize the awakening of one's kundalini, or life force. This energy lies coiled at the base of the spine until awakened. Then it moves up one's back, activating the body's chakra centers to release new levels of health, creativity, and intuition.

There is one aspect of snake medicine I especially like. Those who survive snake bites receive the ability to transmute poison into healing energy. This was what I wanted—a strong symbol that could heal rather than destroy the sarcoma cells.

While not on chemotherapy, I asked Cinnamon to surround my chest with coils of healing golden light, helping the fast-growing cells to transmute into healthy cells.

To honor Cinnamon and seek more healing energy from the symbol, my friend Rebecca Woods and I visited the Great Serpent Mound effigy in southwest Ohio. It is the world's largest-known prehistoric serpentine-shaped mound, almost a quarter-mile long when measured by the centerline of its curves. Taking someone's suggestion, I meditated by lying on the ground successively within each of the five coils, which park management allowed at the time. Powerful images came quickly at each location. I felt like the serpent's energy entered my body to attack the sarcoma cells, biting at them with sharp fangs and injecting them with deadly poison.

Later, I ordered a rattlesnake cake (similar to a crab cake) while dining in Denver, living my intention to absorb more snake medicine.

I added a new visualization when I started taking the chemotherapy agent paclitaxel. This drug keeps microtubules (tiny tubes within each cell) from unforming. By gumming up the different processes in the cell, the cell dies. With this treatment, I visualized Cinnamon transforming into millions of Cinnamons, each entering their own sarcoma cells to surround the microtubules so they could not unform. This gazing upon my cinnamon-and-vanilla-colored snake infused from an IV pole helped me live.

Thriver Soup Ingredient:

Purchase some Crayola Model Magic modeling compound in whatever color you prefer. Use it to sculpt a creature with whom you can identify healing properties. Snakes are easy to sculpt. I got a piece of wire, shaped it into a striking position, and then rolled out segments of model magic to wrap around the wire. I used broken-off tips of black-headed sewing pins for eyes and broken-off and bent bits of paper clips for fangs. Be creative and have fun.

$$\approx\approx\approx$$

Amma: Are You My Mother?

Like someone comforted by his mother, I will comfort you; in Yerushalayim you will be comforted.
                                        —Isaiah 66:13, Complete Jewish Bible

The feminine aspect of the Divine can provide us with comfort if we are open to receiving it. One human manifestation of the Divine comforting mother is the Hindu hugging saint known as Amma (Mātā Amṛtānandamayī Devī). Amma travels the world as an embodiment of the Divine Mother. "My sole mission is to love and serve one and all," she says on her website, www. Amma.org.

My friend Mim Grace Gieser made arrangements for me to see Amma in Detroit around Thanksgiving 2010. Mim's friend Nancy Lawlor proved an invaluable advocate, encouraging me to get into the sitting area set aside in the hotel meeting area for those with special needs. Within an hour of the hugging time, I felt Amma's loving embrace and asked her for a cure. "My daughter, my daughter, my daughter," she whispered into my ear.

Nancy lined up with dozens of volunteers who took turns handing out a chocolate kiss and rose petal to each hug recipient. Amazingly, of the hours and hours of hugging time offered to thousands of people, and the dozens of volunteers helping out, Nancy happened to be the one handing Amma the kiss and petal when I received my hug. Nancy made sure I received a bag of blessed ashes as well.

On Sunday I learned Amma was answering questions for twelve people. Nancy encouraged me to participate. Amma responded to my quest for a cure by telling me to do what the doctors suggested for my cancer treatments. Even better, she said she would pray specifically for me. Mim said when Amma promised her the same, she received exactly what she had asked for. I felt deeply fortunate and grateful.

Whatever the outcome of my visit, I felt blessed for having been in her presence. I relished her arms comforting and surrounding me, symbolizing the feminine side of the Spirit enfolding me in love.

Six months later, I happened to see Mim's copy of the book, *Messages from Amma*, by Janine Canan. One message struck me: "When you go on a trip, you carry your bags to the station; once on the train, you set them down and relax. If you have faith in the Supreme, place all your baggage at God's feet and let God take care of it." Even though I still was in the thick of treatment, her message was clear: I had asked for Divine intervention, and placed my burden at Amma's feet. She had prayed for my cure. I could relax and feel the comfort of the Divine Mother.

Thriver Soup Ingredient:

If you are interested in receiving a hug from Amma, visit her website, www.Amma.org, to look for tour dates. If you are unable to go, look for her address and write her a letter explaining your situation and requesting prayer.

~~~

Angels Watching over Me

For each (such person) There are (angels) in succession, Before and behind him: They guard him by command Of God.

—Qur'an 13:11a

Imagine that—each of us has a succession of angels going in front of us to clear our paths, and behind us to watch our backs, all with Divine orders to protect us. I find this most encouraging.

Archangel Michael, mentioned in the Hebrew and Christian Bibles and the Qur'an, developed a reputation for defeating evil and bringing healing. I wanted his curative powers to protect my cells from the inside out, not just from the front and back. I visualized myself ensconced in a bubble of Divine light with this heavenly being, sword drawn, protecting me on every side.

Practically every time a heavenly messenger appears to a human being in the Bible, the first thing said is, "Fear not." Fear not! I had lived life carrying around a boatload of dread, and I certainly hadn't had any visions of angels floating before my eyes. At the time I most needed to punt my fears, angels began appearing in my life. The gift shop in the MD Anderson Cancer Center in Houston had a sale on large prayer candles depicting angelic beings. A local church had an Angel Tea, during which we ate cookies imprinted with angels, listened to harp music, and shared our experiences with angels. Seven large, stunning, Tiffany stained-glass windows, depicting heavenly messengers from the Christian Bible's book of Revelation, appeared on display at a local museum. Later, at a thrift store, I found an old-fashioned framed print of a golden-winged angel. She has joined two other framed angels hanging over my bed.

Since the diagnosis, my life has been filled with a succession of angels. I call upon them to protect my body, slay cancer cells, and bring healing.

Thriver Soup Ingredient:

Find an angel prayer candle you really like. These candles can be found for sale in many grocery stores (especially Mexican), Mexican restaurants, and Catholic bookshops. Light it while inviting heavenly beings into your prayer time and ask them to protect, defend, and cure you.

Black Panther and Feminine Energy: Bringing Light into Darkness

Oh Midnight Jaguar...[w]ash me with your courage and steel me with your grace, so I may know the value of The Void of time and space. Teach me all your lessons, how to face the dark unknown, then let me bravely leap into the shadows all alone.

—Jamie Sams, medicine teacher

Seemingly disparate stories, involving a black panther, all come together in the end. I am holding the black panther with great love and affection. Our love, even through many stories disconnected by time and distance, remains deep and strong.

This dream came to me in 2008—when the cancer probably had started growing in my uterus. I didn't know the symbolism of black panthers at the time, so I read the panther section in Ted Andrews' book, *Animal Speak*. This big cat brings a period of darkness, suffering, and death on some level. Panther can assist the heroine through these experiences and can help her eliminate her fears. Following the death will come a rebirth and the reclaiming of one's true power.

I didn't know what to make of this symbol. My life seemed rocky but okay. Certainly nothing life-threatening was going on.

Ah, but the black panther had arrived because she knew what lay on the horizon.

Later, I named her Mafdet after the Egyptian panther goddess of the First Dynasty (beginning 3100 BCE). Egyptians prayed to Mafdet for protection against snakebites and scorpion stings. Her claws were used against enemies in the underworld.

Her role became clear after the cancer diagnosis. As a symbol for the feminine, including the dark mother, the black panther possesses the life and power of the night. She would become part of the resurrection of my true feminine nature.

Further describing the panther totem, Andrews wrote that early woundings that caused suffering and a loss of creativity and internal power are "about to be reawakened, confronted and transmuted," giving rise to a reclamation of one's authentic power.

Soon after chemotherapy started, I began seeing a psychotherapist. Mafdet's role clarified more as I began confronting my old issues. I learned to roar like a mother panther protecting her cubs. This enabled me to let go of old resentments trapped in my body.

For some fun, I went to a party store and purchased a plain mask and a black panther snout. I colored the mask black. One day, I put on the mask and nose and sat in black panther energy. After several deep breaths, in my visualization Mafdet entered my mouth and went down into a lung, standing in front of a nodule. She empowered me to face the dark unknown, and bravely leapt into my psychic shadow by asking the nodule for the original cause of the cancer. After several minutes, I heard the painful screaming of the sarcoma cells. They told their story of how they had spent nearly five decades as normal cells, being squeezed, constricted, and deprived of oxygen until they finally flipped into an anaerobic state to survive. They told me the psychological basis for the constriction and when it began.

Through Mafdet, I asked how to help the cells transform back into healthy, oxygen-burning cells. It was my understanding that they wanted to return to a normal, balanced state, and to do this, they needed me to send them light and love.

Mafdet, one who brings light into darkness, accepted this role between chemotherapy treatments. She gave me courage and grace to value the contents of my inner void and helped me face, and leap into, the dark unknown.

Thriver Soup Ingredient:

Before chemotherapy, my sister-in-law and I found a black panther pendant with diamond-like eyes that glittered beautifully. I began wearing it daily. Perhaps you can find a pendant to represent an animal totem with feminine healing energy to wear between conventional treatments to assist with bringing love and light into your cells.

≈≈≈

Black Panther and Masculine Energy: Night Stalker

Mafdet leaps at the neck of the in-di-f-snake, *she does it again at the neck of the serpent with raised head. Who is he who will survive? It is I who will survive.*
                                        —Utterance 295, *The Ancient Egyptian Pyramid Texts*

When ancient Egyptians were bit or stung, they called on Mafdet to invoke healing so they could survive. Mafdet was the panther goddess of the First Dynasty (beginning around 3100 BCE). Mafdet entered my life less than a year before my diagnosis. I had experienced a numinous dream involving a beloved black panther, and felt Mafdet was the only name for her.

I invoked her power to eliminate sarcoma cells, calling in her healing abilities. Before starting chemotherapy, I sent her hunting for loose sarcoma cells within my bloodstream and putting them into a sarcophagus that Jesus and Glinda (the good witch in the movie "The Wizard of Oz") would lift into Divine light.

My niece, Grace Bright, drew a black panther for me and, with the help of her mother, Trish Bright, placed the image on the cover of a tote to remind me of my new panther roar and my visualization of her hunting. I used the carrying case for my equipment every time I went to chemotherapy.

During chemo and for several days afterward, I invited Mafdet to sniff out and enter into the center of each nodule to eat, digest, and mulch the toxic energies, assisting the chemotherapy agents in their work. Jaguar's mulching allows the dead sarcoma cells and their attendant energies to compost and become a source for healthy, new life.

I also learned how my particular chemo agents worked. Certain drugs, called alkylating antineoplastic agents, attach an alkyl group (C_nH_{2n+1}) to the guanine base of DNA. (DNA is a nucleic acid molecule, shaped like a twisted double helix, which carries genetic information within cells. One of the four main nucleobases found in DNA strands is called guanine.) When an alkyl group is attached to a strand of DNA, the strand no longer can uncoil and separate. This prevents DNA replication, and the cell soon dies.

Among the alkylating agents are ifosfamide. When I took ifosfamide, I asked Mafdet to divide into millions of black panthers. My beautiful hunters journeyed into individual sarcoma cells and clutched guanine nucleotides with their paws so the DNA strands could not separate.

The archetypal masculine energy of Mafdet, the midnight jaguar, granted me courage to face the dark unknown shadows of my cancer journey and walked with me through the great Void. She assisted me with my lessons brought about by the cancer, and offered the hope of survival on the other side.

Thriver Soup Ingredient:
Select an animal that represents inner masculine and/or resurrection power for you. Go to a party store and purchase an inexpensive mask, or create your own with papier-mâché. When alone, shape shift into the energy of that animal and act it out in safe ways to engage the power it brings. Experience the strength; use it to move the energy of old wounds; and ask the animal to bring that gift into your daily life.

Perhaps you might enjoy making a papier-mâché mask.

Ingredients:

Plain plastic mask from a party store, or round balloon, or aluminum foil

Flour

Water

Masking tape

Lots of newspaper

Scissors or knife

Acrylic paint

Paintbrush

Ribbon or elastic

Decorative items such as yarn for hair or fake fur

Optional: salt, bowls, plastic wrap, a container with lid for storing the glue, and cinnamon.

To start:

Create a work area where you can get messy. Use old newspaper or an old plastic table cloth to cover your work surface.

Make your papier-mâché paste by thoroughly mixing one part flour with two parts water. It should be the consistency of thick glue—not runny and not thick like paste. If you live in an area with high humidity, add a few tablespoons of salt to help prevent mold. You can add a few sprinkles of cinnamon to sweeten the smell. The glue can be stored in a covered container in the refrigerator for a few days.

If you are using a balloon as a mold for your mask, blow it up and tie it closed. Find a bowl or cup for your balloon to sit on while you work on it. Completely cover the cup or bowl with plastic wrap to help prevent the papier-mâché from sticking to it.

If you are using your face as a mold, tear off a piece of aluminum foil at least twice as long as your face and fold it in half. Gently press the double layer of foil over your face. Remove it, and then place wads of newspaper inside the curved section of the foil mold. Lay it on your work surface.

Now you are ready to begin. Tear newspaper into strips about one or two inches wide and four to eight inches long. Run each strip through the paste and attach it to your base mask.

If you are working with a balloon, you will only want to cover half of the balloon with papier-mâché unless you want to make an entire head.

If you are working with a foil mold, avoid pressing too hard or it might lose its shape. Cover the foil mold with at least four or five layers of papier-mâché, letting it dry completely between layers.

Once your first layers of papier-mâché are dry, cut out eye and nose or mouth holes. Punch a hole on each side of the mask to add ribbon or elastic to fit the mask around your head.

Use various supplies, such as cardboard, newspaper, and foil, to make dimensional features on the mask, such as a snout, fangs, or ears. Masking tape can be used to hold these items in place while you add strips of newspaper. Add three to four more layers of papier-mâché.

Once the papier-mâché is dry, the mask can be painted and decorated however you like. If you used a balloon base, pop the balloon and remove any loose pieces. Use a variety of craft supplies to add personal touches to your mask, such as yarn for hair, fake fur, fabric scraps, beads, glitter, and paper. Let your imagination flower.

<p style="text-align:center">~~~</p>

Bruno Gröning: Access the Divine Healing Stream

By David: Bless ADONAI, my soul! Everything in me, bless his holy name! Bless ADONAI, my soul, and forget none of his benefits! He forgives all your offenses, he heals all your diseases, he redeems your life from the pit, he surrounds you with grace and compassion, he contents you with good as long as you live, so that your youth is renewed like an eagle's.

—Psalm 103:2-5, Complete Jewish Bible

It is the Divine who heals all illnesses, who redeems our lives from the pit of despair, and who renews our youth. We can trust the Divine for healing and help. Nothing is incurable, according to Bruno Gröning (1906–1959). "God is our greatest physician," he said. "Trust and believe that Divine power helps and heals!"

Bruno quickly became a phenomenon in Germany during 1949. He had been visiting the Hulsmann family when nine-year-old Dieter was cured of muscular dystrophy. Dieter's family members had naturally expressed their gratitude for their son's health to others. Word quickly spread. Soon, thousands of people arrived at the Hulsmann's home, where Bruno still was staying, bringing with them the hope of receiving healings for themselves. Bruno spoke to the crowd, and many people received healings.

A media blitz turned Bruno's gift controversial. Officials banned him from the healing work, and he ended up dying in France while on trial.

His healing work lives on, however, through the Bruno Gröning Circle of Friends that has spread throughout the world.

Bruno said, "Every illness comes from evil, is evil, and can only be removed by goodness." He compared a person with a battery. Both burn up energy. Batteries need to be recharged to continue providing power. However, with people, the charge often is insufficiently absorbed. Eventually, the body battery becomes depleted, resulting in exhaustion, anxieties, and illness.

Bruno taught his circles of friends how to access the healing stream from the Divine: Sit upright in a chair, with feet flat on the floor, hands upturned on your lap, and your spine straight. This allows the free flow of the energy throughout your body. Invite the healing stream into your body. Clear the mind of all negativity, letting go of fears and doubts. Focus on something pleasant. Then leave your thoughts behind and move your attention into your heart. Focus on how your body feels as you open to the sensations you experience. Allow divine energy to saturate and recharge every cell.

Do this for at least ten minutes twice each day. The more time you spend recharging your body, the healthier you probably will become. The Divine healing energy will seek out any sick areas of the body and begin purifying them. Sometimes this causes temporary pain.

I began doing the practice, though not consistently at first. Early during chemotherapy treatment, I lifted a heavy book. Pop! went the infusion vein in my forearm. I followed the suggestion of our circle's co-leader, Judi Winall, by inserting a picture of Bruno into a piece of gauze and placing it on top of the bruise. I also applied arnica homeopathic ointment.

Yes, it's a bizarre thing to do. Yes, it sounds like magical thinking.

Yet, the vein healed well.

A few weeks later, I put Bruno's picture in a piece of gauze and taped it to my right hand at the infusion point, leaving it on for several days. Amazingly, for the first time, my infusion point and accompanying veins were free of the typical docetaxel-induced rash, even though I never iced it. I also had used arnica homeopathic ointment two or three times.

While some of the things I did might seem strange and ridiculous, with a little magical thinking thrown in, I knew I had nothing to lose and everything to gain. While this activity didn't always produce the desired result, I felt if nothing else, the placebo effect—when one's mind, rather than the treatment, controls the outcome—wouldn't hurt. I had read many anecdotes about cancer patients who either lived or died, depending on how they believed something would or would not work. I knew that simply holding the intention that a particular activity could help would transmit a positive idea to my cells, and my body would respond in a positive way.

Some people who follow Bruno's teachings regain their health over a span of time, while others receive spontaneous cures. I have found that the focus on feeling my body helps me live more consciously within my own skin. My body, in response, loves the attention it receives. This can only result in good energy for my body to absorb and use to improve my health.

Among those who practice what Bruno taught, thousands of cures have been medically verified. The Spirit is capable of healing all our illnesses and redeeming our lives from the pit of cancer. The Divine wants to grant us kindness, mercy, and goodness. As we imbibe in Divine healing energy, our youth might be renewed so we can become like eagles and fly once more.

Thriver Soup Ingredient:

Joining a local Bruno Gröning Circle of Friends can provide support and encouragement. Doing the technique taught by Bruno in a group setting adds more energy to the experience. For more information, visit www.bruno-Gröning.org/English/.

Butterflies are Free to Fly

Once upon a time, Chuang Tzu dreamed that he was a butterfly, flying about enjoying itself. It did not know that it was Chuang Chou. Suddenly he awoke, and veritably was Chuang Chou again. He did not know whether it was Chuang Chou dreaming that he was a butterfly, or whether it was the butterfly dreaming that it was Chuang Chou. Between Chuang Chou and the butterfly there must be some distinction. This is a case of what is called the transformation of things.

                                          —"The Butterfly Dream," *Chuang Tzu*

Because of their ability to completely transform themselves after dying in their chrysalides, butterflies symbolize rebirth for many people.

Drawing butterflies turned out to be my first art project after the diagnosis. I wrote "I am Alive!" on a large sheet of paper. As I started painting big butterflies around the words, I realized the top wings on their bodies could be painted in the shape of hearts. It took months for me to realize how cramped the wings looked. This indicated to me that I needed to learn to stretch my inner wings a lot more before I could learn to fly.

A week later I felt like creating something using my fingers. I got out some modeling clay and made a beautiful butterfly. The wings still looked small and cramped.

Several months later I dreamt I was lying in a field of purple flowers and cocooned in a soft, white material, like a cloud. It took some months for me to realize I was like the pupa in a cocoon. No wonder my wings looked cramped.

Someone explained to me that a caterpillar in its chrysalis will digest itself, dying from the inside out, dissolving into soup.

Oh, I could really identify with that metaphor.

Remnants of the caterpillar's former tissues inside the cocoon are combined with digestive juices and consumed by what remains of the pupa to build a butterfly body. Once the butterfly is formed, it still must work to remove itself from its chrysalis. Without this struggle, the butterfly would not become strong enough to survive outside its protective shell.

The same is true for a chick. To live, it must develop strength by pecking at the shell from the inside. If the shell is opened from the outside, the chick probably will die.

Less than a year into my process, Vince Lasorso asked me, when I am resurrected, who will I be? I knew I needed to be someone different from the person who went into the chrysalis the year before. I wrote down a list of characteristics into which I wanted to more fully move.

For another year I swam in a chemotherapy soup. My cells constantly broke down and endured various assaults. Healthy cells, like a butterfly's imaginal cells, knew instinctively how to recreate my body in their image. I even had a dream in which I was handed an egg containing a transformative substance with which I could creatively form whatever I chose. It took a few years for it to dawn on me that the substance was like the imaginal cells in a cocoon, waiting to form a butterfly.

Eventually, my body solidified and I grew little imaginary wings. I began the work of emerging.

One year after I started having clean scans, I took a short hike and encountered a butterfly sitting next to the trail. As I drew close, it fluttered farther along the trail. This happened three times. Then it flew off into the sky. Joy filled my chest while my arms spontaneously and gracefully began floating up and down as if they were my own butterfly wings—my manner of grateful prayer and praise to the Divine for my new body.

Thriver Soup Ingredient:

There is a pose in yoga called the butterfly. My friend Diane Faul explained how to do it:

Sit on the soft earth, soles of the feet together, knees falling out to the sides, and eyes gently closed. Begin feeling the freedom and transformation that is within you as it is with the butterfly. Allow your knees to gently move skyward and earthward as if you are beginning to take flight. After some time, allow stillness to enter your being and begin feeling the spaciousness within. Let the expansion between your hips and rib cage be a symbol of your willingness to receive healing on a deeper level. Coming out of the pose, bring your knees to your chest, wrap your arms around your knees, and bow your head forward in gratitude.

∾∾∾

Glinda: You have Always had the Power

"Very truly I tell you, whoever believes in me will do the works I have been doing, and they will do even greater things than these, because I am going to the Father."
—John 14:12, Christian Bible, NIV

Jesus tells us we are capable of doing even more than he did. That's a pretty potent statement. Add to that the wisdom offered by Marianne Williamson in her book, *A Return to Love:* "We are powerful beyond measure." Glinda, good witch of the North in the movie "The Wizard of Oz," would concur.

As part of an effort to heal my uterus during the summer, right before landing in the hospital, I had decided the best image for my inner feminine was Glinda. She wears a lovely, feminine, peach-colored dress with a silver butterfly choker necklace and a huge, silver butterfly pin on her shoulder.

The main movie character, Dorothy, spends most of her time trying to get to the Emerald City so she can hitch a ride back home to Kansas on the Wizard of Oz's hot-air balloon. During her travels she fought her demon, the wicked witch of the West, before receiving her gift. At the end of the movie, the wizard takes off without Dorothy. Devastated, she turns to Glinda for advice on how to return home. Glinda tells her, "You have always had the power within you."

A life-sized cardboard cutout of Glinda greeted me as I walked for the first time into Whatever Works Wellness Center, in Cincinnati, Ohio. I was searching for advice for my journey, which had started a few weeks earlier with the cancer diagnosis.

"Glinda is the ultimate archetype for a positive attitude," co-owner Vince Lasorso told me.

So I adopted her energy as a guide for my journey.

My friend Laura Dailey gave me a Glinda figurine which held space for me on my altar, reminding me that the power of the Spirit that already lives within me can bring about my cure.

During my first type of chemotherapy, I felt inspired to draw a picture of Glinda filling up an empty hole in my lung (left by a nodule that had died) with Divine light. I also visualized healthy new cells filling in the space. The process felt complete. Two months later, a CAT scan showed two of three lung nodules had died.

Months of chemo dragged into years. I fought my own demons, both physical and psychological, to receive the gift of recognizing the power within me to be cured of the disease and healed of mental and emotional baggage. This great power comes from the Divine, and enables us to do more than Christ was able to do during his lifetime.

Thriver Soup Ingredient:

Consider purchasing a Glinda wand for your altar. You can find them at party stores. My sister-in-law Janet Bright and her daughter Mindy Bright made a lovely wand for me. If you want to make one, here's what you will need:

1 wooden star shape (available at craft stores)

1 dowel rod for a handle

White and silver acrylic paint

Gloss varnish

Brush

Wood glue

Super glue

Three-dimensional round rhinestone jewels (available at craft stores)

¼-inch-wide ribbons, including possibly white, gold, silver, and/or peach

Newspaper or old plastic table cloth

Lay down newspaper or an old plastic table cloth for a work surface.

Use the wood glue to attach the dowel rod to the star, about halfway up one side of the star. After the glue dries, paint it all white.

After the wand dries (about 20 minutes), paint it all silver. Wait another 20 minutes before applying the varnish. Allow to dry for at least three hours.

Glue the jewels to the star, starting with larger gems at the center and working out to small rhinestones around the edge of the star. Glue ribbons to the bottom of the star and tie them in a bow with long streamers.

When completed, wave your magic wand over your body and say, like Glinda, "I have the power within me to heal." Imagine divine healing light flowing from the wand into every cell in your body.

Goldfinches: Harbingers of Miracles

"Do they not look at The birds, held poised In the midst of (the air And) the sky? Nothing Holds them up but (the power Of) God. Verily in this Are Signs for those who believe."

—Qur'an 16:79

On August 14, 2009, Maria Paglialungo, an energy intuitive, shared about her "audience" with a goldfinch. She had been walking with her friend Debbie, talking about me, when she saw the beautiful golden bird.

"It was, to me, the most, most beautiful sight to behold. I squealed like a child." She told Debbie, "This is a most auspicious moment...to behold such a vibrant, radiant bird, and she came back twice."

She excitedly referred to Ted Andrews' *Animal Speak* for goldfinch's symbolism. It represents an amplification of opportunities, new experiences and encounters with people from all walks of life, and beautiful singing, which could include vibrational healing.

Two weeks later, Karen Wagner wrote on my CaringBridge blog about her son Matthew, who was in sixth grade. Each Easter, Karen added flower or vegetable seeds to her boys' baskets. This year Matthew received red sunflowers. They grew into a few plants. "Two days ago we noticed goldfinches sitting on the sunflower blossoms, enjoying the feast. Matthew said, 'I hope the Heidi in our prayers has red sunflowers, too.' I asked why, and Matthew said, 'Well, first, they are beautiful. Second, they make fences look lots better. And third, they are home to goldfinches.' I kept listening because I didn't understand the part about the goldfinches. Finally, I asked. Matthew looked at me as if I'm the most clueless person in the world. 'Mom, look at the goldfinches. Don't you see God in our garden? When you see them, don't you think that angels and miracles are really, really, really close?' He paused and then added, 'I think those goldfinches can carry anything to Cincinnati.'

"We're sending you an abundance of mental images filled with red sunflowers, goldfinches, angels, miracles, prayers, and blessings."

Maria read the entry and responded to Matthew. "I work energetically with Heidi with a free form of healing energy that comes from a place beyond this world, like your garden where you saw God. Two weeks ago, I had a visit from a goldfinch, and Matthew, my heart leaped right out of my chest with such joy. I said to my friend, 'This is a message from God, and it has to do with Heidi.'"

She asked Matthew to see a photo of me on CaringBridge that had recently been posted. In the photo, a light spot showed on my third eye, the point on the center of the forehead right above the eyes. "Ask your mom to show you...where the third eye or spiritual eye is, see if you can see the image, and if you can, you will know that truly God and the angels have come into Heidi's life. One day we will see with eyes that only belong to the childlike wonder of magic and miracles.... [A]nd yes, Matthew, miracles do happen because of our love. Let's together keep praying for a miracle for our beloved one Heidi."

Soon afterward, I was in Manhattan, New York, with family for an appointment with a leiomyosarcoma specialist at Memorial Sloan-Kettering. We toured three cathedrals. First we went to Holy Trinity, which had a box of folded fans in the back of the sanctuary. I unfolded one and saw a picture of a bird. I unfolded a second and it showed a different kind of bird. Having received the CaringBridge entries about Matthew's and Maria's goldfinch sightings, I wanted to see if there might be a goldfinch among them. Sure enough, the third fan I opened had a picture of a goldfinch! So I told Matthew his prayer for a miracle in Cincinnati and in Houston came true; and now the goldfinch had brought a blessing to me in New York City.

My two main miracles up to that point were: 1. My surgeon expected my CAT scan to show spots all over my lungs. There was only a small spot that could be seen. 2. The two ankhologists in Houston expected to see spots all over my lungs and in my abdomen. The PET scan showed only one small spot on my lung, and only moderate cell activity. And there were many other miracles along the way, such as housing provided for my medical travels.

Two weeks later, while I was sitting for chemotherapy in Columbus, Karen wrote, "Yesterday morning around 6:15 a.m. I saw three goldfinches on the red sunflowers. I woke Matthew and then his older brother. We watched for at least ten minutes and none of us said a word. When the birds flew off, Matthew said, 'How far do the prayers need to go today?' I responded, 'Just to Columbus, only two hours away.' In the midst of the turmoil, blessings and hope abound!"

Several months later, as I took a walk in a nature sanctuary, four goldfinches—a number of completion—flew in front of me, as if leading the way for me to believe in more miracles.

Thriver Soup Ingredient:

If you like the symbolism of goldfinches, purchase a bag of yellow feathers from a craft store. Use them as bookmarks, put them in vases, or lay them around your home to remind you that goldfinches can carry miracles and blessings.

$$\sim\!\sim\!\sim$$

Horses: Reclaiming Your Power

Hast thou given the horse strength? hast thou clothed his neck with thunder? Canst thou make him afraid as a grasshopper? the glory of his nostrils is terrible. He paweth in the valley, and rejoiceth in his strength: he goeth on to meet the armed men. He mocketh at fear, and is not affrighted; neither turneth he his back from the sword. The quiver rattleth against him, the glittering spear and the shield. He swalloweth the ground with fierceness and rage: neither believeth he that it is the sound of the trumpet. He saith among the trumpets, Ha, ha; and he smelleth the battle afar off, the thunder of the captains, and the shouting.
—Job 39:19-25, Christian Bible, King James Version

This biblical passage has always captivated my attention. How strong this horse is—fierce, courageous, laughing in the face of death. Horses represent power, and I needed to reclaim mine.

For decades I had dreams about wanting horse figurines, yet they always eluded me. Finally, after more than two years of cancer treatment and three major surgeries, I had a dream in which five rare ceramic Arabian horses were given to me. I woke up feeling delighted. Perhaps I was finally coming into my personal power.

This dream might also have been triggered by my final choice of art therapy. About a year before this dream, a new idea formed through discussions with my psychotherapist. I had looked for a spirit horse figurine at a recent model horse festival—I wanted it to be turquoise, like the painting of a spirit horse gracing the July 1959 issue of *Arizona Highways* magazine I'd treasured since childhood. I could not find one among the tens of thousands of horse figurines I saw.

Then an idea surfaced. I realized I could combine my love of horses with spirituality and create something entirely new. I dug into some old cardboard boxes and pulled out a few scratched horse figurines that had patiently waited in paper wrappers for decades. Yup, I could do this. I bought some primer, acrylic paints, brushes, glue, and rhinestones. I found and ordered sculpting clay for building up the horses' manes and tails.

Sitting out on the deck, I brought the horses back to life. The feel of paint flowing off the brush brought deep satisfaction. I added sacred geometrical designs—mandalas, mandorlas, pentagonal stars, third-eye stars, and labyrinths. I drew the eye of Horus, a healing symbol from ancient Egypt, around each eye. Attaching rhinestones added just the right touch.

Following my psychotherapist's suggestion, I obtained a copyright on the designs, and began buying more horses to transform into Bright Spirit Horses. I also figured out a way to add feathered and butterfly wings.

The metaphor was perfect for me—I was taking worthless "bodies" in need of transformation, like my body, and transmuting them into beautiful, bright, spiritual bodies. The process of going deep within during my cancer journey provided access to my inner well of creativity, bringing forth more of Spirit's light and a deep sense of fulfillment and joy. The horses were helping me regain access to my power and exercise the courage to face and do battle with my inner enemy.

Thriver Soup Ingredient:

If you are physically able, see if you can find a horseback riding stable where you can go on a trail ride. As you ride, feel the power of the horse beneath you, and imagine transposing that power into yourself.

If you are unable to ride, perhaps visit a barn where you can pet horses and see if you can feel a connection with their strength and power.

My psychotherapist suggested watching the movie "The Horse Whisperer" because of its theme of humans and horses bringing healing to each other. Or perhaps enjoy Walter Farley's "The Black Stallion," and imagine how you would feel in your own body if you experienced the fierceness of the horse's indomitable will, his powerful strength, and his scorn of fear.

Jesus: Wounded Healer

Jesus went throughout Galilee, teaching in their synagogues, preaching the good news of the kingdom, and healing every disease and sickness among the people. News about him spread all over Syria, and people brought to him all who were ill with various diseases, those suffering severe pain, the demon-possessed, those having seizures, and the paralyzed; and he healed them.

—Matthew 4:23-24, Christian Bible, NIV

Jesus cured every person who came to him, no matter what the illness. According to the

Christian scriptures, he later was crucified, placed in a tomb, and raised from the dead. At that point, he became an archetypal wounded healer—one who understood deep pain and thereby could compassionately relate to others' suffering.

For me, there was no greater guide for the cancer pilgrimage than someone who had overcome excruciating pain and death. I knew Christ could relate on a personal level to my journey.

First, Jesus expressed his emotional agony one night by sweating drops of blood. While I've never sweated drops of blood, after the diagnosis I sank into a cesspool of dark emotions—shock, terror, rage, powerlessness, insecurity, and sorrow.

Jesus' physical pain before the crucifixion began when deep slashes were gouged into his flesh by a Roman flagrum, a whip which had at least two short leather strands with metal tips. A long gash creased my abdomen following the hysterectomy. At least I had morphine to take the edge off the pain.

After the scourging, soldiers crushed a crown of thorns onto the Christ's head. When paclitaxel took my hair, my scalp hurt, as if someone was yanking out my hair at the roots, and I knew Jesus would empathize.

Nails were driven into Jesus' wrists in preparation for the crucifixion. The scarred veins in my purple-and-red forearms and hands reminded Vince Lasorso of this damage done to Jesus.

Finally, the injurious stab of the sword thrust into Jesus' side while he hung helpless on a cross was not unlike my bleeding surgical wounds from two separate lung resections.

Through Christ's vulnerability and acceptance of his own pain, I knew he could identify with my afflictions and offer compassionate salve.

Even while Jesus endured his trials, without hope for a normal life and without anything external to assuage the pain, he steadfastly focused his attention on his ultimate healing. He paved the way for me to endure the death of my own self-injuring thought and behavior patterns in my pursuit of resurrection into a more empowered and whole self.

Before dying, Christ cried out to the Divine, "Why have You forsaken me?" After resurrection, he moved ever deeper into the Divine, telling his followers he had entered into his glory. Christ serves as my beacon, shedding light on the purposes behind my need to die to my old self—even while feeling abandoned by the Spirit during the dark night of cancer treatment—to be reborn into the glory of a resurrected life. This new, healed life includes a generous outpouring of love and connection, both internally with the Spirit and externally through my relationships with others. The wounded healer gave me back the life I was created to live.

Thriver Soup Ingredient:

When Jesus' disciple Peter attempted to walk on water, he locked his attention on Jesus. When he looked away, he began to sink (Matthew 14:29-30, Christian Bible). Lock your attention on the Divine, in whatever form you feel comfortable addressing, with unswerving devotion. Allow yourself to feel the Spirit's healing balm within your soul. Perhaps you also might receive the miracle of a physical resurrection.

≈≈≈

Martha: Subduer of Dragons

Jesus, once more deeply moved, came to the tomb. It was a cave with a stone laid across the entrance. "Take away the stone," he said. "But, Lord," said Martha, the sister of the dead man, "by this time there is a bad odor, for he has been there four days." Then Jesus said, "Did I not tell you that if you believe, you will see the glory of God?" So they took away the stone. Then Jesus looked up and said, "Father, I thank you that you have heard me. I knew that you always hear me, but I said this for the benefit of the people standing here, that they may believe that you sent me." When he had said this, Jesus called in a loud voice, "Lazarus, come out!" The dead man came out, his hands and feet wrapped with strips of linen, and a cloth around his face. Jesus said to them, "Take off the grave clothes and let him go."

—John 11:38-44, Christian Bible, NIV

"But Lord," said Martha, questioning and challenging Jesus, pushing the boundaries of convention by courageously speaking her truth. Martha was not the typically submissive woman of her culture—she boldly claimed her rights and her dignity. In this story, she witnessed the resurrecting power of the Divine moving through Jesus.

After Christ completed his earthly sojourn, legend reports that Martha and her sister were forced into a rudderless boat on the Mediterranean Sea. They were left to die, yet washed ashore in what is now France. Martha began preaching and healing. One man, who traveled to hear her, drowned while attempting to cross a river. Mirroring the resurrection experience Martha had witnessed for herself, she accessed Divine power and raised the man from the dead.

Martha eventually arrived in a village terrorized by a dragon. Unlike St. George, who wore spurs and killed his dragon with a lance, this saint remained barefoot and used her sash—something feminine—to wrap up the dragon's legs, subduing it so it couldn't move.

I find the story of her approach an interesting mix of doing and being—going after evil, represented by the dragon, yet using a softer, more feminine, and equally effective method that I suspect required a deep access to the experience of being.

I needed this new set-point. About nine months after the diagnosis, as I drew hot water in my bathtub, I lit a Catholic patron-saint candle depicting Martha subduing a dragon. When I sank into the hot water, I fell into an anxious mood. The urge to get out of the bathroom and start doing something worthwhile tugged at me. Fortunately, I stayed conscious enough to check in with my body. Sure enough, my thighs had tightened—an unconscious fight or flight reflex. Why was I stressing so much when being in warm water, at that moment, called for relaxation? When my express purpose in doing this was to simply be? I sank my awareness more deeply into my body and went into the emotion that registered as tension. Ah, it was my old acquaintance, fear—fear of not getting enough done. It was time for me to face this lurker. I shifted into fully experiencing fear's expression in my taut muscles. I avoided thinking. A few minutes later I found myself thinking—and realized my body had relaxed. A peaceful sensation arose. Ironically, by simply being with my emotions, I actually had done something worthwhile—I had allowed the tension to move effortlessly and naturally out of my body. Around the candle flame, Martha continued glowing above her dragon, her approval of my transformation lighting up her figure.

According to my psychotherapist, when we are transformed, four things are experienced:

1. Time seems to stop.
2. One's view of reality shifts.
3. One's view of one's self shifts.
4. Synchronicities—seemingly unrelated events that are connected—appear.

All of these occurred, and I had moved one step closer to becoming a human being, shedding my grave clothes and embracing my internal resurrection.

Thriver Soup Ingredient:

Consider reading the children's book, *Brave Martha and the Dragon*, by Susan L. Roth. Ponder how you might be able to use your feminine power of being to subdue the cancer dragon.

~~~

Mary: From Annihilation to Glorification

And the pains of childbirth Drove her to the trunk Of a palm-tree: She cried (in her anguish): "Ah! would that I had Died before this! would that I had been a thing Forgotten and out of sight!" But (a voice) cried to her From beneath the (palm-tree): "Grieve not! for thy Lord Hath provided a rivulet Beneath thee; And shake towards thyself The trunk of the palm-tree: It will let fall Fresh ripe dates upon thee[.] So eat and drink And cool (thine) eye."

—Qur'an 19:23-26a

In this scene from the Islamic holy book, Mary the mother of Jesus is about to give birth. Her pain is so terrible she wishes she had already died. She has spent her pregnancy in seclusion, and now this.... Her ego was receiving its final annihilation before she could give birth to the great inspiration, Jesus. In her agony, Mary clung to a palm tree and voiced her terrible grief. Another Voice encouraged Mary to look down and see a stream beneath her. Now she could receive divinely provided nourishment and drink for her upcoming ordeal.

The Christian Church also greatly esteems Mary. My friends Rebecca Woods, Laura Dailey, and I did a short stained-glass window tour of Cincinnati. We found it fascinating how many Catholic churches venerated Mary in their art and windows. I think this arises from our human need for a balancing feminine aspect of the Divine—a mother who is full of loving compassion. As my book, *Hidden Voices: Biblical Women and Our Christian Heritage*, shows, there are many images of Divine Mother (pregnant, in labor, giving birth, nursing...) in the Bible. Even though these parts of the Bible have largely been ignored, the Divine Feminine still finds a way to gain human attention and expression.

Especially on the dark cancer journey, fraught with its own agonies. I had moments either wishing I were dead or wishing to escape the pain and sickness of treatment. How did this happen, after I had been so careful with my health and after years of spiritual practice? Having Mary as a guide felt encouraging, knowing she also suffered terribly despite her total devotion to the Divine.

Vince Lasorso had a deck of fifty-four beautiful cards depicting Mary in various situations. He invited me to select three face-down cards from the stack. He explained that the first card I select would show where I'd been in my life; the second, where I was at that time; and the third, where I was heading.

The first card I picked out showed Mary in colors representing the mind and depicting separateness from others. The second was an image of Mary's face filling the front interior of a cathedral in Yugoslavia—"Our Lady of Medugorje," bringer of miracle healings. In the third card, Mary sat, clothed in purple, writing, and Archangel Michael stood overhead, protecting her.

According to Vince's interpretation, I was on the path toward a miracle healing so I could fulfill my spiritual purpose of writing to share what I learn.

I felt jubilant. I had hugged the palm tree trunk, was traveling along the deep stream, and would soon be eating the fruit of my labors.

Thriver Soup Ingredient:

If you can find it, consider reading the children's book, *The Lady of Guadalupe*, by Tomie de Paola. It tells the story of Mary appearing to an indigenous man to teach true peace and bring miraculous healing. Contemplate Mary's healing powers and demand a cure from her.

Other Guides: The Seen and the Unseen

But ask the animals—they will teach you—and the birds in the air—they will tell you; or speak to the earth—it will teach you—and the fish in the sea will inform you.

—Job 12:7-8, Complete Jewish Bible

All of nature can speak to us. It's up to us to pay attention so we can learn. I found guidance for my journey from many sources. Here are a few I found interesting, and who might be beneficial to others.

Bucks represent the rise of masculine life-force energy and can lead one into altered states of consciousness. While I have often seen does, I encountered two young bucks in one week. I found this significant and a springboard for doing active imagination.

Buddha experienced extreme privation, nearly dying of self-induced starvation. He found a way out of suffering through mindfulness and awareness.

Fr. Damien was a priest who worked on the Hawaiian leper colony for many years until passing from the illness. My friend Judy Merritt told me a woman who had a sarcoma that had metastasized to her lungs had prayed at Fr. Damien's grave. She was cured.

Guru Nanak taught compassion and kindness, bringing together Hindus and Muslims to live in harmony. He might provide guidance for bringing together disparate parts of yourself to help you journey toward greater personal wholeness.

Krishna taught Arjuna to fight even when he didn't want to; he might provide strength for you during conventional treatment.

Moses freed the Israelites from slavery, and can offer assistance freeing people from slavery to cancer cells and from unhelpful habits.

Muhammad repeatedly encouraged his followers to let go of bad habits and attitudes and to turn instead to the Divine for assistance.

Peacocks represent resurrection and wholeness, and are a symbol for meditation and reflection.

Sharks do not get cancer. Ask sharks to journey with you and provide guidance for eliminating cancer from your body.

St. Agatha is the patron saint of breast cancer and will have great compassion and perhaps guidance for those dealing with this disfiguring form of the disease.

This is only a sampling of ideas for you to explore as ways of listening more closely to the Spirit's whisperings in your heart and teachings for your mind. As the text above indicates, the world of the seen and the unseen can provide guidance and support in a myriad of ways as you move through the cancer journey.

Thriver Soup Ingredient:

If you are comfortable with the idea, explore who or what might provide a good role model or guidance for you on your journey. Find one that feels comfortable and beneficial to you. Spend time developing your relationship and getting to know that energetic aspect of your life.

∾∾∾

Owl: It's all Inside Me

The owl is the leading medicine-man among the birds.

—Pawnee saying

Halfway through my first chemotherapy regimen, owl made contact with me, sharing some of his medicine.

I was walking up a path in Isis Cove, North Carolina, near Smoky Mountain National Park, on a trail taken daily by the local residents. I was making plenty of noise when I saw a great grey owl in front of me, perched on a tree limb. I stopped to look at him and ask for his medicine—

wisdom. He stared at me. After a few minutes I continued forward and he flew—not away from the path, as I had expected, but farther up it. So, like in a dream or a fairytale, I followed him up the hillside, and soon saw him again, watching me from a branch. I stopped and again requested a gift. As I moved forward, he flew up the path a third time. I saw him a bit off to the right side, still watching me as I arrived at my destination, a beautiful vista.

It seemed to me that the owl taking three flights ahead, as if to lead me up the trail, was not exhibiting ordinary fowl behavior. So perhaps the owl wanted to bestow its medicine on me, including wisdom, intuition, and even clairvoyance.

Later, I did an active imagination on the great grey owl. With my mind's eye, I hurried after him up the same wooded trail until I stopped to lean, panting, on my knees. I looked up into the nearby tree and asked owl for a message. In my mind, I heard this message: "Your body is a chamber of healing. Live in it." It was time for me to incorporate owl energy into my life by spending time experiencing my body and listening to my own inner wisdom rather than relying on others.

This message harkened to my psychotherapy work. My budding ability to stay in my body while experiencing strong emotions gradually grew. I began to notice how much tension I hold in my body all day. Owl medicine was working.

Thriver Soup Ingredient:

If the owl totem works for you, you can get into its energy with a mask or costume. I purchased an inexpensive plastic owl mask at a costume supply store. Using safety pins, I shaped an old brown sheet, purchased from a thrift store, into a pair of wings.

Wear black, grey or brown clothes, put on the mask and wings, and allow owl energy to come into your body. Perhaps sit on a pretend tree, flap your wings, or swoop around, calling "whoo, whoo." See if any thoughts, images, memories, or intuitive awarenesses arise. Record them in your journal for reflection.

Place an owl image on your home altar if you find significance in the symbolism.

~~~

Paramahansa Yogananda: God's Boatman

Again listen to My supreme word, the most secret of all. Because thou art dearly loved by Me, I will relate what is beneficial to thee.

—*God Talks with Arjuna: The Bhagavad Gita*, 18.64

The supreme word of the Divine, which is beneficial for everyone, can be found in many religious traditions. Paramahansa Yogananda (1893-1952), an Indian yogi, brought me clarity of understanding regarding the word of the Divine in both the Christian gospels of Jesus and Hinduism's Bhagavad Gita.

This guru was introduced to me through my friend Rusty Wells, who suggested I read *Autobiography of a Yogi*. Yogananda brought the practice of yoga to the United States in 1920 and founded Self-Realization Fellowship, now an international organization with meditation groups around the world. Yogananda left behind voluminous teachings through a large number of books.

For me, Yogananda's two-volume *The Second Coming of Christ: The Resurrection of the Christ Within You* clarified many aspects of the gospels, even though I had spent five years in seminary and decades reading about the many facets of Christianity.

Less than a year before the diagnosis, I was reading *The Second Coming of Christ* and had the following dream:

I'm walking along a shoreline at night when an archaic seagoing vessel passes nearby. I jump onto its deck. We skim along the water, heading eastward into the open sea. I am worried that we might bump into something because there is no light from the moon or stars. I guide the vessel the best I can. Finally, at dawn I see land ahead. We reach it and disembark. The sun is rising and I have a whole new, undiscovered continent to explore, and I am eager to start!

I contacted my SRF friend Sam Quick about the dream. He responded by showing me the poem, "God's Boatman," written by Yogananda and set onto a photo of the yogi standing on an archaic boat:

I want to ply my boat, many times,
Across the gulf-after-death,
And return to earth's shores
From my home in heaven.
I want to load my boat
With those waiting, thirsty ones
Who are left behind:
And carry them by the opal pool
Of iridescent joy—
Where my Father distributes
His all-desire-quenching liquid peace.
Oh! I will come again and again!
Crossing a million crags of suffering,
With bleeding feet, I will come—
If need be, a trillion times—
As long as I know
One stray brother is left behind.
I want Thee, O God,
That I may give Thee to all!

I want salvation,
That I may give it to all!
Free me, then, O God
From the bondage of the body—
That I may show others
How they can free themselves!
I want Thine everlasting happiness,
Only that I may share it with others—
That I may show all my brothers
The way to happiness,
Forever and forever, in Thee.

Shortly, during one of the meditation circle meetings, I heard for the first time Yogananda's chant, "Polestar of My Life":

I have made Thee Polestar of my life.
I have made Thee Polestar of my life.
Though my sea is dark and my stars are gone,
Though my sea is dark and my stars are gone,
Still I see the path through Thy mercy.
Still I see the path through Thy mercy.

My eyes watered and my mouth opened with surprise and joy. The Divine was weaving beautiful synchronicities that would serve to sustain me during my cancer journey. As I drifted through my dark night on a sea of terror, rage, sorrow, pain, and despair, I clung to the grace of these Divine messages, especially my dream about coming to the far country where the sun would rise upon a new world and life for me. I called upon Yogananda for assistance with everything, and his photo was among those I always hung on my chemotherapy bags, asking for his blessing. I wanted him, as a representative of the Divine, and because of his dear love for me, to relate all that was beneficial to me.

Thriver Soup Ingredient:
Yogananda wrote a book of prayer-demands called *Whispers from Eternity*. Instructions in the book tell the reader to repeat a selected prayer over and over, with deep feeling, while one's eyes are closed and pointing upward toward the center of the forehead. Here is a favorite healing prayer from his book: "O Divine Spirit, Thou didst create my body. It is well, for Thou art present in it. Thy Being is perfect. I am made in Thine image: I am perfect."

Glossary

Active imagination: This therapeutic process was developed by Carl Jung, founder of analytical psychology. While active imagination can be done in many ways, my preference is to enter into a meditative state and then allow dream or visualization images to appear on the screen of my mind. Then I interact with them as if they are real, without controlling anything about what the characters do or say. I pretend the drama being enacted before my inner eyes is real, and glean insights that arise. I normally attempt to ask questions of the characters as this often provides me with valuable information.

Acupuncture: This ancient form of Traditional Chinese Medicine involves a practitioner inserting tiny needles into various points following energy channels (meridians) in the body. It purportedly assists the body with self-healing, reduces pain, and treats both the causes and symptoms of illness. Acupuncture is used to help the body return to a balanced state so vital energies are restored within the body.
www.ehow.com/how-does_4564041_acupuncture-work.html#ixzz1jdYGlMC1

Alchemy: A precursor to modern chemistry. This ancient art, in the physical plane, involved finding a way to turn base metals, such as lead, into noble metals, such as silver or gold. On the psychological plane, alchemy refers to using symbols from the unconscious to induce psychic and spiritual integration.

Ankhologist: A phrase coined by my nephew James Bright to refer to the oncologists in service of life because the Egyptian word "ankh" means life.

Antihistamine: A drug used to calm a body's allergic reaction to a foreign substance.

Anti-oxidants: These substances are said to protect our cells from free radicals, which can damage our cells and cause aging. Anti-oxidants include vitamins A, C, and E, along with beta-carotene, lutein, lycopene, and selenium.
http://www.nlm.nih.gov/medlineplus/antioxidants.html

Apoptosis: Apoptosis is a natural daily process by which the human body's cells are programmed to die so they can be replaced with young, healthy cells.

Arjuna: Heroic prince of the ancient Hindu epic *Mahabharata*.

Arnica: A homeopathic remedy for bruises, pain, or swelling. It can be purchased as a gel or cream for application on unbroken skin, or as pellets to be taken sublingually. Before surgery, five pellets can be dissolved in a small dropper bottle using filtered water, then shaken ten times and applied behind the earlobes every two hours on the day of surgery.

Bhagavad Gita: This ancient Hindu scripture involves a 700-verse theological and philosophical conversation on yoga between Prince Arjuna and the Hindu god Krishna.

Bhikkhu: An ordained male Buddhist monastic.

CAT/CT scan: Computerized (axial) tomography is a procedure that integrates numerous x-ray images to create cross-sectional views of the body to locate any abnormal structures.

Chakra: In Eastern traditions, the body contains several energy vortexes or centers called chakras. They occur in many places on the body, yet the primary chakras run up the spine, starting at its base and finishing at the crown of the head.

Chemosabe: A word I learned from Connie Lasorso referring to chemotherapy. It's a play on the Potawatomi (a Native American language) word *kemosabe*, which means "faithful friend."

Chi, qi, ki, prana, shakti (energy): Chi is life-force energy that animates every living thing, sort of like the vibration that occurs at the subatomic level. Some people are trained in the ability to move and manipulate this energy in others' bodies to enhance health.

Christian Bible: The Christian holy scriptures, which consists of dozens of books considered divinely inspired.

Clinical trials: Clinical trials involve volunteers participating in a research plan or protocol being investigated for its effectiveness for a particular condition. It might involve the use of drugs, devices, procedures, or behavioral modifications (such as diet). Clinical trials come in phases with different risks at each level of participation. To find out more, visit clinicaltrials.gov/

Corticosteroid: Chemicals, including steroids, produced naturally in the adrenal cortex or synthetically in a laboratory.

Cytoplasm: All of the contents between a cell's membrane and its nucleus.

Decadron: An anti-inflammatory steroid drug taken along with chemotherapy.

Dhammapada: A collection of Buddha's sayings in verse form.

Elysian fields: According to Greek mythology, this is where virtuous and heroic souls exist.

Flavonoids: Compounds found in colorful produce that act as antioxidants, protecting the body from aging.

Glutamine powder: An amino acid.

Guru Nanak (1469–1539): Founder of the Sikh religion and the first of the Sikh gurus.

Hara: Considered by some to be one's physical center of gravity and the seat of one's internal energy. It is located about three finger widths below and two finger widths behind the navel. en.wikipedia.org/wiki/Dantian

Hasidic Judaism: An orthodox branch of Judaism that views mysticism as the fundamental aspect of the Jewish faith.

Helios: In Greek mythology, this god personifies the sun.

Henry Crow Dog: Lakota spiritual man.

Homeopathy: A medical system developed in Germany at the end of the eighteenth century using two theories: "like cures like"—the idea that a condition can be cured by a substance that creates similar symptoms in healthy people; and "law of minimum dose"—the notion that the lower the dose, the greater its effectiveness. nccam.nih.gov/health/homeopathy.

Hydrocodone: A narcotic pain reliever.

Inanna: Queen of heaven and earth and the goddess of love for the ancient Sumerians.

Intention: A goal that a person wants to manifest in her or his life.

Ip6 (inositol hexaphosphate): A component of fiber found in whole grains and legumes. While it is not significantly bioavailable from food, it has been extracted and used as a supplement.

Jainism: An Asian Indian religion that emphasizes non-violence toward all living beings.

Jewish or Hebrew Bible: The canonical collection of Jewish texts considered divinely inspired.

Juicer: A machine that extracts juice from fruits and vegetables.

Khuddaka-Patha: A Buddhist scripture.

Lacriminal tear ducts: Short tubes in the inner corners of the eyelids.

Lame Deer: Sioux medicine man.

Lipoic acid: An organic compound that contains sulfur.

Lymphatic system: A network of conduits that carries a clear yellowish fluid called lymph. The lymphatic system, part of the circulatory system, delivers fats and fat-soluble vitamins to the cells of the body and removes waste. www.lymphnotes.com/article.php/id/151/

Medical Qigong: An ancient form of Traditional Chinese Medicine that views the individual as a whole unit and seeks to treat the root cause of disease. Practitioners are trained in sensing and manipulating a person's vital energies.

Meditation: Concentration of one's mind, either on emptiness or on a particular object, such as one's in-breath and out-breath.

Megace: A man-made chemical similar to the female hormone progesterone.

Meridians: According to Traditional Chinese Medicine, meridians are energy pathways through the body. When these pathways get blocked, disease can result. Various techniques, such as acupuncture, can be used to open the pathways back up and help restore health.

Mesopotamia: The region of the Tigris–Euphrates river system in the Middle East.

Mudra: A yoga posture done with the hands.

Mystic: A spiritual person who seeks oneness with the Divine.

Native American Ghost Dance: In 1889, the Ghost Dance was given in a vision to Wovoka, a Paiute prophet and dreamer from Pyramid Lake, Nevada. The dance was performed by many tribes.

Nodule: A cancerous growth larger than 0.5 centimeters.

Ophthalmologist: A physician who specializes in eye problems.

Osteoporosis: A disease that weakens one's bones.

Oxycodone: A narcotic pain reliever.

Pain body: A term used by Eckhart Tolle to describe an energy system in the body created from an accumulation of painful and unresolved emotional experiences. www.huffingtonpost.com/eckhart-tolle/living-in-presence-with-y_b_753114.html

Pali Canon: A collection of texts written in the Pali language that forms the basis of Theravada Buddhism.

Persona: The social role or character mask one uses when relating to others.

PET (positron emission tomography) scan: Radioactive particles are used to detect minute alterations in the body's chemical activities and metabolism.

Polyerga: A highly purified extract of peptides from the spleens of pigs that helps the immune system. Unfortunately, patients with metastases do not seem to respond as well as other patients.

Progestin: A man-made version for the female hormone progesterone. womenshealth.about.com/od/womenshealthglossary/g/progestin.htm

Qur'an: The Islamic holy book, as dictated by the Prophet Muhammad.

Sacred geometry: Particular geometric proportions and shapes that are given spiritual meaning or relevance.

Sanskrit: The classical language of ancient India.

Sarcoma: Malignant tumor of the connective tissues.

Self-Realization Fellowship: A worldwide spiritual organization founded in 1920 by Paramahansa Yogananda, widely recognized as the father of yoga in the West. www.yogananda-srf.org

Serpent Mound: The largest serpentine effigy mound yet discovered. It is located near Peebles, Ohio.

Shadow: Aspects of one's personality with which the conscious mind does not identify. en.wikipedia.org/wiki/Shadow (psychology)

Shaman: An indigenous medicine woman or man who connects to the spiritual aspects of people and the world to bring healing.

Spathes: The leafy sheaths on plants that enclose flowers.

Spirit guides: Angels, saints, animals, or other beings who are believed by some people to help heal, protect, and teach us.

Subtle body: A layer of energy that surrounds one's physical body.

Sufi: Someone who adheres to the inner, mystical dimension of Islam.

Sumerians: People living between 3000–2350 BC in southern Mesopotamia.

Sutra: A portion of Eastern religious text.

Tao Te Ching: The Taoist sacred writings, presumably written by Lao Tzu (c.604–531 BC).

Taxanes: Chemotherapy agents, such as paclitaxel and docetaxel, that are derived from yew plants and are used to disrupt the process of cell division.

Taxotere: A chemotherapy medication that interferes with cell division.

Tramadol: An opioid pain reliever.

Visualization: Using the imagination to experience something with one's various senses.

Vitamix: A professional-grade, high-speed blender.

Yang and yin: Yang represents the masculine, active aspect of nature, while yin represents the feminine, passive facet. They are opposing yet complementary forces.

Yoga: A system of exercises, postures, and breathing techniques developed in ancient India to yoke together the body, mind, and spirit.

Sources

Introduction:
Wilber, Ken. *Grace and Grit: Spirituality and Healing in the Life and Death of Treya Killam Wilber.* Boston: Shambhala, 1991.

I. Conventional Methods Introduction

"Sri Raag, Mahala 1." Sri Guru Granth Sahib. Pg. 15, Shabad 55. www.sikhiwiki.org/index.php/Three_Days_in_the_River. Retrieved March 20, 2014.

A. Cushioning Chemotherapy

Antihistamines: Flying the Friendly Chemotherapy Skies
Yogananda, Paramahansa. *God Talks with Arjuna: The Bhagavad Gita, Royal Science of God-Realization.* Los Angeles: Self-Realization Fellowship, 2001:562.
www.drugs.com/benadryl.html. Retrieved March 20, 2014.
Chemo Die-off Phase: O Burn That Burns to Heal
Unlocking the Gate of the Heart, 157-158. www.sacred-texts.com/bhi/bahaullah/pm.txt
Symons, Arthur, trans., Thomas Walsh, ed. *Hispanic Anthology: Poems Translated from the Spanish by English and North American Poets.* New York: G.P. Putna m's Sons, 1920:249.
Chemo Stool: Think Outside Your Buns
www.livestrong.com/article/112838-benefits-fennel-seeds/#ixzz2GdxAR2IZ. Retrieved March 20, 2014.
Aggarwal, Bharat B., with Debora Yost. *Healing Spices: How to use 50 Everyday and Exotic Spices to Boost Health.* New York: Sterling Publishing, 2011:114-115.
Hair Today
Quillin, Patrick. *Beating Cancer with Nutrition.* Encinitas, CA: Nutrition Times Press, 4th Edition, 2005:302.
Baldilocks
"Star Trek: The Motion Picture." Paramount Pictures, 1979.
Hair Regrowth: Fuzzy Wuzzy
www.livestrong.com/article/387715-how-to-turn-grey-hair-back-with-nutrition/. Retrieved March 20, 2014.
Chemo Side Effects: How Can You Spell "Relief"?
www.sacred-texts.com/chr/apo/marym.htm. Retrieved March 20, 2014.
Barnstone, Willis, and Marvin Meyer, eds. *The Gnostic Bible.* Boston & London: New Seeds, 2006:479.
www.clinicaltrials.gov/ct2/show/NCT00477607. Retrieved March 20, 2014.
Yance, Donald R. Jr., with Arlene Valentine. *Herbal Medicine Healing and Cancer: A Comprehensive Program for Prevention and Treatment.* Lincolnwood, IL: Keats Pub., 1999:57-58.
Bee Products: Sweet Healing Gifts
Journal of Food Science. 2008 Nov;73(9):R117-24.
Journal of Clinical Investigation, 2009. Washington University School of Medicine in St. Louis.
nano.cancer.gov/action/news/2009/aug/nanotech_news_2009-08-27a.asp. Retrieved March 20, 2014.
Lansing State Journal, July 30, 1997.
www.ncbi.nlm.nih.gov/pubmed/19021816. Retrieved March 20, 2014.
Mouth Sores: Melt in Your Mouthwash
Cleary, Thomas, trans. "Entry into the Realm of Reality." Volume 3, *The Flower Ornament Scripture: A Translation of the Avatamsaka Sutra.* Boston: Shambhala, 1987:161.
Shaw, Miranda. *Buddhist Goddesses of India.* Princeton, NJ: Princeton University Press, 2006:159.
Simon, David. *Return to Wholeness: Embracing Body, Mind, and Spirit in the Face of Cancer.* New York: John Wiley & Sons, Inc., 1998:82-83.
Booster Shots: Bringing Good Things to Life
Kramer, Samuel Noah. "Inanna's Descent to the Nether World," *Sumerian Mythology: A Study of Spiritual and*

Literary Achievement in the Third Millennium BC. Philadelphia: University of Pennsylvania Press, 1944, rev. 1961:95. www.sacred-texts.com/ane/sum/sum08.htm. Retrieved March 25, 2014.

Heterogenius Cells

Saporito, Bill. "The New Cancer Dream Teams." *Time* Vol. 181, No. 12 (April 1, 2013):30.

Taxanes: Hecate's Slips of Yew

Evelyn-White, Hugh G., trans. *The Theogony of Hesiod*. 1914:404-452. www.sacred-texts.com/cla/hesiod/theogony.htm. Retrieved March 20, 2014.

Bolen, Jean Shinoda. *Goddesses in Older Women: Archetypes in Women over Fifty*. New York: HarperCollins Publishers, 2001:49.

en.wikipedia.org/wiki/Hecate. Retrieved March 20, 2014.

www.spiritus-temporis.com/hecate/symbols.html. Retrieved March 20, 2014.

Yew tree exhibit, Lloyd Library and Museum, Cincinnati, Ohio, 2012.

Murray, Michael. *How to Prevent and Treat Cancer with Natural Medicine*. New York: Riverhead Books, 2002:250, 264, 267.

Ifosfamide: Spa Chemosabe

The Book of Psalms, A New Translation According to the Traditional Hebrew Text. Philadelphia: The Jewish Publication Society of America, 1972, Psalm 16:7.

Neuropathy: Tingle Town

Braverman, Eric. *The Healing Nutrients Within*. North Bergen, NJ: Basic Health Publications, 2003:112-113, 115, 152-3.

Maestri, A., A. Ceratti De Pasquale, S. Cundari, C. Zanna, E. Cortesi, L. Crinò. "A Pilot Study on the Effect of Acetyl-L-carnitine in Paclitaxel- and Cisplatin-induced Peripheral Neuropathy." *Tumori* 2005; 91:135–8.

Moss, Ralph. *Cancer Therapy: The Independent Consumer's Guide to Non-Toxic Treatment & Prevention*. Brooklyn, NY: Equinox Press, 1996:285.

http://www.livestrong.com/article/534545-r-lipoic-acid-neuropathy/ Retrieved March 12, 2015.

Visualizations: Imagination at Work

Kramer, Samuel Noah. *Sumerian Mythology: A Study of Spiritual and Literary Achievement in the Third Millennium BC*, rev. ed. Philadelphia: University of Pennsylvania Press, 1961. www.sacred-texts.com/ane/sum/sum08.htm. Retrieved March 20, 2014.

White Cell Counts: Great White Hope

Palmer, EH, trans. The Qur'ân, part II (Sacred Books of the East volume 9). Oxford: The Clarendon Press, 1880. www.sacred-texts.com/isl/sbe09/023.htm. Retrieved April 25, 2014.

http://www.mcrh.org/Blood-Cells/13589.htm. Retrieved March 12, 2015.

Fatigue: You Snooze, You Cruise

Simon, David. *Return to Wholeness: Embracing Body, Mind, and Spirit in the Face of Cancer*. New York: John Wiley & Sons, Inc., 1998:83.

Corticosteroids: I'm Melting, Melting...

Chen, Ellen M. *The Tao Te Ching: A New Translation with Commentary*. New York: Paragon House, 1989:202.

dailymed.nlm.nih.gov/dailymed/archives/fdaDrugInfo.cfm?archiveid=3162. Retrieved March 20, 2014.

"The Wizard of Oz." Metro-Goldwyn-Mayer, 1939.

Finishing Chemo: Good to the Last Drip

Champion, Bob, and Jonathan Powell. *Champion's Story: A Great Human Triumph*. Leicester, England: Ulverscroft, 1983:168, 173.

Ending Chemo: Take a Licking and Keep on Ticking

Blackman, A.M. *Rock Tombs of Meir, II*. London: Egypt Exploration Fund, 1915:24.

Lesko, Barbara S. *The Great Goddesses of Egypt*. Norman, OK: University of Oklahoma Press, 1999.

B. Softening Surgery: Scarred—>Scared—>Sacred

Introduction to Softening Surgery: Scarred—>Scared—>Sacred

Thomas à Kempis, c. 1380–1471, was a Catholic monk and probable author of *The Imitation of Christ*.

Woodman, Marion K. *Bone: Dying into Life*. New York: Penguin Group USA, 2001:17, 18, 19.

Stomach Tube: Elephant Woman
www.astrojyoti.com/GaneshaGita.htm. Retrieved March 20, 2014.
Psalm 23:1-4, English Revised Version, 1885.
Paying Someone to Knife You
Mitchell, Stephen, trans. *Tao Te Ching: A New English Version.* New York: HarperCollins Publishers, 2000:76.
Pre-operative Testing: Fit for a Queen
Block, Keith. *Life over Cancer: The Block Center Program for Integrative Cancer Treatment.* New York: Bantam Dell, 2009:460, 462.
www.lef.org/protocols/prtcl-026.shtml?source=search&key=tramadol. Retrieved March 20, 2014.
In a study on rats, tramadol was able to block the enhancement of lung metastasis induced by surgery, whereas morphine did not produce this beneficial effect (Gaspani et al. 2002).
Preparing for My First Lung Surgery: Eve's Rib
Thoracic Cardiovascular Surgery. 49:89, 2001.

C. Conventional Companions

Trance Fusions
Herbert, George. "The Agonie." *The Temple,* 1633, as found at www.ccel.org/h/herbert/temple/Agonie.html. Retrieved March 20, 2014.
Levels of Albumin: Blood Will Tell
Yance, Donald R. Jr., with Arlene Valentine. *Herbal Medicine Healing and Cancer: A Comprehensive Program for Prevention and Treatment.* Lincolnwood, IL: Keats Pub., 1999:11.
Guptal, Digant, and Christopher G. Lis. "Pretreatment serum albumin as a predictor of cancer survival: A systematic review of the epidemiological literature." *Nutrition Journal.* 2010; 9:69. www.ncbi.nlm.nih.gov/pmc/articles/PMC3019132/. Retrieved March 20, 2014.
Lien, YC, CC Hsieh, YC Wu, HS Hsu, WH Hsu, LS Wang, MH Huang, BS Huang, "Preoperative serum albumin level is a prognostic indicator for adenocarcinoma of the gastric cardia." *Journal of Gastrointestinal Surgery.* 2004 Dec;8(8):1041-8. www.ncbi.nlm.nih.gov/pubmed/15585392. Retrieved March 20, 2014.
Pain Management: A Time to Kill the Pain
"Raag Sorat'h." Part 065, Shri Guru Granth Sahib. www.sacred-texts.com/skh/granth/gr13.htm. Retrieved March 20, 2014.
Lung Mets or Fungus Among Us?
Veith Ilza, trans. *The Yellow Emperor's Classic of Internal Medicine.* Oakland, CA: University of California Press, 1966. Quoted by McNamara, Sheila. *Traditional Chinese Medicine.* New York: Basic Books, a Division of HarperCollins Publishers, Inc., 1996:132.

II. Congruent Care

DeNial: Playing the Fool
Van Loon, Gabriel, ed. "Su11#56-63." *Charaka Samhita: Handbook on Ayurveda Volume I.* © 2002:2003:295, as found at www.scribd.com/doc/56568096/Charaka-Samhita-2003-rev2-Vol-I. Retrieved March 20, 2014.
Curing and Healing
Villoldo, Alberto. *Shaman, Healer, Sage: How to Heal Yourself and Others with the Energy Medicine of the Americas.* New York: Harmony Books, 2000:20.
Brand, Paul, and Philip Yancey. *Fearfully and Wonderfully Made.* Grand Rapids, MI: Zondervan Publishing House, 1980:44-45.
Eldering: Regenerpause
Conze, Edward. *The Perfection of Wisdom in Eight Thousand Lines and Its Verse Summary.* Bolinas, CA: Four Seasons Foundation, 1975:31.
Shaw, Miranda. *Buddhist Goddesses of India.* Princeton, NJ: Princeton University Press, 2006:168.
www.barbaramarxhubbard.com/site/node/14. Retrieved March 20, 2014.

Why I Needed to Leave the Marriage: Be All You Can Be
Ornish, Dean. *Love and Survival: The Scientific Basis for the Healing Power of Intimacy*. New York: HarperCollins, 1998:112.
Siegel, Bernie S. *Love, Medicine, & Miracles: Lessons Learned About Self-healing from a Surgeon's Experience with Exceptional Patients*. New York: Harper & Row, 1986:76.

Ending of a Marriage: Braveheart
"Born Free." Columbia Pictures, 1966.
www.ted.com/talks/amy_cuddy_your_body_language_shapes_who_you_are.html. Retrieved March 20, 2014.

Legal Documentation: It's the Law
The Cancer Legal Resource Center (CLRC) is a national, joint program of the Disability Rights Legal Center and Loyola Law School Los Angeles.
www.disabilityrightslegalcenter.org/cancer-legal-resource-center. Retrieved March 20, 2014.
www.ehow.com/facts_5366625_power-vs-durable-power-attorney.html. Retrieved March 20, 2014.
www.mayoclinic.com/health/living-wills/HA00014. Retrieved March 20, 2014.

Aging: You're Not Getting Older, You're Getting Wiser
Aggarwal, Bharat B., with Debora Yost. *Healing Spices: How to Use 50 Everyday and Exotic Spices to Boost Health*. New York: Sterling Publishing, 2011:245.

Dying: The Terminator
Chief Aupumut, Mohican, 1725, www.ilhawaii.net/~stony/quotes.html. Retrieved in March 2011.
Ornish, Dean. *Love and Survival: The Scientific Basis for the Healing Power of Intimacy*. New York: HarperCollins, 1998:401-402.
Siegel, Bernie S. *Love, Medicine, & Miracles: Lessons Learned About Self-healing from a Surgeon's Experience with Exceptional Patients*. New York: Harper & Row, 1986:209.
Servan-Schreiber, David. *Anticancer: A New Way of Life*. New York: Viking Penguin, 2008:171.

Death: An Exchange of Raiment
Rinpoche, Lama Sogyal. *The Tibetan Book of Living and Dying*. New York: HarperCollins Publishers, 1992: chapters 11-19.

III. Complementary Therapies

Introduction to Complementary Therapies: Sow Your Seeds
Erdos, Richard. *Crying for a Dream: The World through Native American Eyes*. Rochester, VT: Bear & Company, 2001:35.
Simon, David. *Return to Wholeness: Embracing Body, Mind, and Spirit in the Face of Cancer*. New York: John Wiley & Sons, Inc., 1998:199-203.
Servan-Schreiber, David. *Anticancer: A New Way of Life*. New York: Viking Penguin, 2008:93.

A. Let Food be Your Medicine

Alkalize or Die?
www.chem1.com/CQ/ionbunk.html. Retrieved March 20, 2014.
missourifamilies.org/features/healtharticles/health70.htm. Retrieved March 20, 2014.

Amino Acids: They Will be Assimilated
Braverman, Eric. *The Healing Nutrients Within*. North Bergen, NJ: Basic Health Publications, 2003:112-113, 115, 152-3.
Maestri, A., A. Ceratti De Pasquale, S. Cundari, C. Zanna, E. Cortesi, L. Crinò. "A Pilot Study on the Effect of Acetyl-L-carnitine in Paclitaxel- and Cisplatin-induced Peripheral Neuropathy." *Tumori* 2005; 91:135–8.
Moss, Ralph. *Cancer Therapy: The Independent Consumer's Guide to Non-Toxic Treatment & Prevention*. Brooklyn, NY: Equinox Press, 1996:285.

An Apple a Day
Colum, Padraic. "Iduna and Her Apples: How Loki Put the Gods in Danger." *The Children of Odin*. New York: Macmillan Publishing Co., 1920:15. www.sacred-texts.com/neu/ice/coo/coo04.htm. Retrieved March 20, 2014.

Eder, Carley. "The Awesome Apple." *Life Extension Retail*, July/August 2011:91.

Sharma, Hari, James G. Meade, Rama K. Mishra. *The Answer to Cancer: Is Never Giving It a Chance to Start*. New York: SelectBooks, Inc., 2002:18-23.

Kirschmann, Gayla J., and John D. Kirschmann. *Nutrition Almanac*, Fourth Edition. New York: McGraw Hill, 1996:95.

Buckley, Anne. "Quercetin: Systemic Immune Defense." *Life Extension*, September/October 2012:85.

Ayurveda: Balancing Act

Horner, Christine. *Waking the Warrior Goddess*. Laguna Beach, CA: Basic Health Publications, Inc., 2005:117-119.

Becoming Juicy

"Raag Aasaa," Shri Guru Granth Sahib. www.sacred-texts.com/skh/granth/gr08.htm. Retrieved March 20, 2014.

www.lef.org/magazine/mag2012/aug2012_In-The-News.htm. Retrieved March 20, 2014.

Gamonski, William. "Time to Celebrate Celery." *Life Extension*, November/December 2012:90.

medicalxpress.com/news/2013-05-compound-mediterranean-diet-cancer-cells.html?utm_source=buffer&utm_medium=twitter&utm_campaign=Buffer&utm_content=buffera2850. Retrieved March 20, 2014.

Berries: Be the Berry Best

Van Loon, Gabriel, ed. "Ka1#9." *Charaka Samhita: Handbook on Ayurveda Volume I*, © 2002, 2003:557. www.scribd.com/doc/56568096/Charaka-Samhita-2003-rev2-Vol-I. Retrieved March 20, 2014.

Beliveau, Richard, and Denis Gingras. *Foods to Fight Cancer: Essential foods to help prevent cancer*. New York: DK Publishing, 2007:121.

www.livestrong.com/article/372546-berries-cancer-fighting-super-foods/#ixzz2GCALt8eo. Retrieved March 20, 2014.

Servan-Schreiber, David. *Anticancer: A New Way of Life*. New York: Viking Penguin, 2008:107, 108.

Evans, Susan. "Blueberries Boost Longevity." *Life Extension*, November/December 2012:57.

Aggarwal, Bharat B., with Debora Yost. *Healing Spices: How to use 50 Everyday and Exotic Spices to Boost Health*. New York: Sterling Publishing, 2011:146-7.

Cruciferous Vegetables: Cabbage Patch Dollops

Brown, Joseph Epes. *The Sacred Pipe: Black Elk's Account of the Seven Rites of the Oglala Sioux*. Norman, OK: University of Oklahoma Press, 1953:xx.

Gamonksi, William. "Cauliflower: The Head of the Cruciferous Vegetable Family." *LifeExtension Retail*, January/February 2013:89.

Curcumin: Go for the Gold

Borger, J. Everett. "How Curcumin Protects Against Cancer." *LifeExtension*, March/April 2011. www.lef.org/magazine/mag2011/mar2011_How-Curcumin-Protects-Against-Cancer_01.htm. Retrieved March 20, 2014.

Aggarwal, Bharat B., with Debora Yost. *Healing Spices: How to use 50 Everyday and Exotic Spices to Boost Health*. New York: Sterling Publishing, 2011:243, 248.

Horner, Christine. *Waking the Warrior Goddess*. Laguna Beach, CA: Basic Health Publications, Inc., 2005:94, 96.

Servan-Schreiber, David. *Anticancer: A New Way of Life*. New York: Viking Penguin, 2008:105.

Enlarge Your Circle of Foods

www.vitaminb17.org/. Retrieved March 20, 2014.

Food Preparation: No More Nukes

American Institute for Cancer Research, www.aicr.org/.

Aggarwal, Bharat B., with Debora Yost. *Healing Spices: How to use 50 Everyday and Exotic Spices to Boost Health*. New York: Sterling Publishing, 2011:201.

Lubec, G., Chr. Wolf, B. Bartosch. "Aminoacid Isomerisation and Microwave Exposure." *Lancet*. December 9, 1989:1392-1393.

"Organic Foods: What are They?" Integrative Medicine Clinic notebook. The University of Texas MD Anderson Cancer Center Patient Education Office, 2007:2.

Servan-Schreiber, David. *Anticancer: A New Way of Life*. New York: Viking Penguin, 2008:80.

Fruit: It's Magically Delicious

Bulfinch, Thomas. "Medea and Aeson." *The Golden Age of Myths and Legends*. Boston: David D. Nickerson & Company, Publishers, circa. 1855.

Murray, Michael, Tim Birdsall, Joseph Pizzorno, and Paul Reilly. *How to Prevent and Treat Cancer with Natural Medicine*. New York: Riverhead Books, 2002:183.

Sharma, Hari, James G. Meade, Rama K. Mishra. *The Answer to Cancer: Is Never Giving It a Chance to Start*. New York: SelectBooks, Inc., 2002:39.

Aggarwal, Bharat B., with Debora Yost. *Healing Spices: How to use 50 Everyday and Exotic Spices to Boost Health*. New York: Sterling Publishing, 2011:193.

Servan-Schreiber, David. *Anticancer: A New Way of Life*. New York: Viking Penguin, 2008:108, 127.

www.livestrong.com/article/549783-tart-cherries-and-pancreas/#ixzz2GCMK8YWA. Retrieved March 20, 2014.

www.bing.com/videos/search?q=how+to+eat+a+pomegranate+video&mid=32FA16F3334C6A34976E32FA16F-3334C6A34976E&view=detail&FORM=VIRE3. Retrieved March 20, 2014.

Getting Seedy

Black cumin seeds are also known as Roman coriander, nigella sativa, or kolonji; they are not the common grocery-store-variety cumin.

www.seedsavers.org/onlinestore/Herbs/Herb-Black-Cumin.html. Retrieved March 20, 2014.

www.naturalmedicinalherbs.net/herbs/n/nigella-sativa=black-cumin.php. Retrieved March 20, 2014.

www.livestrong.com/article/71562-chia-seed/#ixzz2GfCQEzZx. Retrieved March 20, 2014.

www.livestrong.com/article/500273-sugar-vs-sugar-alcohol/#ixzz2GdslAQ8A. Retrieved March 20, 2014.

www.livestrong.com/article/418462-the-health-benefits-of-coriander-seeds/. Retrieved March 20, 2014.

Aggarwal, Bharat B., with Debora Yost. *Healing Spices: How to use 50 Everyday and Exotic Spices to Boost Health*. New York: Sterling Publishing, 2011:59 (caraway seeds), 92 and 96 (cocoa), 104 (coriander), 119-121 (fenugreek seeds), 167 (mustard seeds), 197 (Pumpkin seeds), 218 (sesame seeds).

Horner, Christine. *Waking the Warrior Goddess*. Laguna Beach, CA: Basic Health Publications, Inc., 2005:78-80 (flax).

Grab Life by the Herbs

Barrett, Clive. "Frigga, Queen of the Gods." *The Viking Gods: Pagan Myths of Nordic Peoples*. Northamptonshire, England: The Aquarian Press, 1989:42.

Servan-Schreiber, David. *Anticancer: A New Way of Life*. New York: Viking Penguin, 2008:109 (studies on rosemary).

www.livestrong.com/article/514275-nine-spices-that-are-good-for-you/#ixzz2Bv6UE79A (studies done on nine spices). Retrieved March 20, 2014.

Moss, Ralph. *Herbs Against Cancer*. Brooklyn, NY: Equinox Press, 1998:217, 228-229.

Aggarwal, Bharat B., with Debora Yost. *Healing Spices: How to use 50 Everyday and Exotic Spices to Boost Health*. New York: Sterling Publishing, 2011:43, 154 (lemongrass), 187-188 (parsley), 212, 237 (sage).

ebm.rsmjournals.com/content/234/8/825.full. Retrieved March 20, 2014.

Green Smoothies: Liquid Sunshine

"Raag Goojaree." Fifth Mehl, Section 03, So Purakh, Part 001. Shri Guru Granth Sahib.

www.sacred-texts.com/skh/granth/gr03.htm. Retrieved March 20, 2014.

"Crazy Sexy Cancer" DVD. Red House Pictures, 2001.

Here's the Beef

www.cayce.com/beefjce.htm. Retrieved March 20, 2014.

Fallon, Sally. *Nourishing Traditions: The Cookbook that Challenges Politically Correct Nutrition and the Diet Dictocrats*. Washington, DC: NewTrends Publishing, Inc. 2001:124.

Little Sprouts

Fallon, Sally. *Nourishing Traditions: The Cookbook that Challenges Politically Correct Nutrition and the Diet Dictocrats*. Washington, DC: NewTrends Publishing, Inc. 2001:113, 615.

www.livestrong.com/article/460391-list-of-vitamins-in-rejuvelac/#ixzz1i2yqvexV. Retrieved March 20, 2014.

Magic of Mushrooms

Van Loon, Gabriel, ed. "Ka1#10." *Charaka Samhita: Handbook on Ayurveda Volume I*, © 2002, 2003:557. www.scribd.com/doc/56568096/Charaka-Samhita-2003-rev2-Vol-I. Retrieved March 20, 2014.

Lee, William H., and Joan A. Friedrich. *Medicinal Benefits of Mushrooms: Healing for More Than 20 Centuries—Their Effects on Cancer, Diabetes, Heart Disease and More*. New Canaan, CT: Keats Publishing, 1997:28, 37.

Chang, Raymond Y. *Role of Ganoderma Supplementation in Cancer Management*. Ithaca, NY: Meridian Medical Group, 1996. www.alternative2cancer.com/docs/role.pdf (reishi mushrooms). Retrieved March 20, 2014.

Murray, Michael. *How to Prevent and Treat Cancer with Natural Medicine*. New York: Riverhead Books, 2002:177-180.

Horner, Christine. *Waking the Warrior Goddess*. Laguna Beach, CA: Basic Health Publications, Inc., 2005:89-91 (maitake and reishi mushrooms).

www.mskcc.org/cancer-care/integrative-medicine/about-herbs-botanicals-other-products. Retrieved March 20, 2014.

Freuhauf, Bonnard, Herberman. "The Effects of Lentinan on Production of Interleukin-1 by Human Monocytes." *Immunopharmacology*. 1982; 6:65-74.

Varona, Verne. *Nature's Cancer-Fighting Foods: Prevent and Reverse the Most Common Forms of Cancer Using the Proven Power of Great Food and Easy Recipes*. Paramus, NJ: Reward Books, 2001:171.

Shirota, Mike. "What You Should Know about Medicinal Mushrooms." *Explore!* 1996; 7(2).

Microgreens: Behold the Power of These

"Raag Basant." Section 29, Part 004. Shri Guru Granth Sahib. www.sacred-texts.com/skh/granth/gr29.htm. Retrieved March 20, 2014.

Nutrient Density: Thriver Soup

Watson, Burton, trans. "The Parable of the Medicinal Herbs." *The Lotus Sutra*. New York: Columbia University Press, 1993:98.

Horner, Christine. *Waking the Warrior Goddess*. Laguna Beach, CA: Basic Health Publications, Inc., 2005:100 (seaweed), 107-108 (vitamin B12).

Murray, Michael. *How to Prevent and Treat Cancer with Natural Medicine*. New York: Riverhead Books, 2002:242-244 (melatonin), 255-256 (co-enzyme Q10).

Moss, Ralph. *Cancer Therapy: The Independent Consumer's Guide to Non-Toxic Treatment & Prevention*. Brooklyn, New York: Equinox Press, 1996:216, 257, 258.

Yance, Donald R. Jr., with Arlene Valentine. *Herbal Medicine Healing and Cancer: A Comprehensive Program for Prevention and Treatment*. Lincolnwood, IL: Keats Pub., 1999:67.

Drum, Ryan W. "Appendix 1: Sea Vegetables." Gladstar, Rosemary, and Pamela Hirsch, ed. *Planting the Future: Saving Our Medicinal Herbs*. Rochester, VT: Healing Arts Press, 2000:277-284.

Servan-Schreiber, David. *Anticancer: A New Way of Life*. New York: Viking Penguin, 2008:124.

Boik, John. *Cancer and Natural Medicine: A Textbook of Basic Sciences and Clinical Research*. Princeton, MN: Oregon Medical Press, 1996:177.

Gamonski, William. "Bell Peppers: The Ring of Sweetness and Nutritional Value." *Life Extension*. September/October 2012:93-94.

Kelley, Claudia. "Seven Ways Melatonin Attacks Aging Factors." *Life Extension*. September/October 2012:57.

Oil Protein Diet: This Budwig's for You

Singh, Nikki-Guninder Kaur, trans. "Sukhmani." *The Name of My Beloved: Verses of the Sikh Gurus*. New York: Penguin Books 2003:180.

Budwig, Johanna. *Flax Oil As a True Aid Against Arthritis Heart Infarction Cancer and Other Diseases*. Vancouver, BC: Apple Publishing Co. Ltd., 1994:7-22.

Budwig, Johanna. *The Oil Protein Diet Cookbook*. Vancouver, BC: Apple Publishing Co. Ltd., 1994:vii.

Omega-3: Precious Oils

Servan-Schreiber, David. *Anticancer: A New Way of Life*. New York: Viking Penguin, 2008:124.

Boik, John. *Cancer and Natural Medicine: A Textbook of Basic Sciences and Clinical Research*. Princeton, MN: Oregon Medical Press, 1996:179.

Probiotics: Rejoice and be Glad

www.livestrong.com/article/497860-acidophilus-depression/. Retrieved March 20, 2014.

Servan-Schreiber, David. *Anticancer: A New Way of Life*. New York: Viking Penguin, 2008:126.

www.mayoclinic.com/health/lactobacillus/NS_patient-acidophilus. Retrieved March 20, 2014.

Budgar, Laurie. "Supportive Supplements." *Delicious Living*. July 2011:23.

Proteolytic Enzymes: The Bigger Picker Upper

Wilber, Ken. *Grace and Grit: Spirituality and Healing in the Life and Death of Treya Killam Wilber*. Boston: Shambhala, 1991:336-396.

www.dr-gonzalez.com/index.htm. Retrieved March 20, 2014.

Root Vegetables: Buried Treasures

Exodus 16:31, Jewish Bible.

Yance, Donald R. Jr., with Arlene Valentine. *Herbal Medicine Healing and Cancer: A Comprehensive Program for Prevention and Treatment*. Lincolnwood, IL: Keats Pub., 1999:56.

www.jonbarron.org/article/how-do-liver-detox-blood-cleanse. Retrieved March 20, 2014.

Dougherty, Patrick. "Buried Treasures." *Energy Times*. Oct. 2009:34.

Aggarwal, Bharat B., with Debora Yost. *Healing Spices: How to use 50 Everyday and Exotic Spices to Boost Health*. New York: Sterling Publishing, 2011:127-178.

Horner, Christine. *Waking the Warrior Goddess*. Laguna Beach, CA: Basic Health Publications, Inc., 2005:98.

Sometimes You Feel Like Nuts

www.ehow.com/about_6632257_symbolism-almond-trees.html. Retrieved March 20, 2014.

www.edgarcayce.org/are/holistic_health/data/thalmo1.html. Retrieved March 20, 2014.

www.ncbi.nlm.nih.gov/pubmed/17125534. Retrieved March 20, 2014.

www.ncbi.nlm.nih.gov/pubmed/22254047. Retrieved March 20, 2014.

Moss, Ralph. *Cancer Therapy: The Independent Consumer's Guide to Non-Toxic Treatment & Prevention*. Brooklyn, New York: Equinox Press, 1996:122.

keckmedicine.adam.com/content.aspx?productId=35&pid=35&gid=66410. Retrieved March 20, 2014.

Fallon, Sally. *Nourishing Traditions: The Cookbook that Challenges Politically Correct Nutrition and the Diet Dictocrats*. Washington, DC: NewTrends Publishing, Inc. 2001:512, 514, 516.

Spice up Your Life

www2.mdanderson.org/cancerwise/2011/06/cinnamon-common-spice-takes-a-stand-against-cancer.html. Retrieved March 20, 2014.

www.ehow.com/list_6006101_10-antioxidant-spices.html. Retrieved March 20, 2014.

ebm.rsmjournals.com/content/234/8/825.full. Retrieved March 20, 2014.

www.livestrong.com/article/527190-medicinal-nutritional-values-of-nutmeg/#ixzz2Bv3OtHhd. Retrieved March 20, 2014.

www.ncbi.nlm.nih.gov/pubmed/12617584. Retrieved March 20, 2014.

www.ncbi.nlm.nih.gov/pmc/articles/PMC2783227/?tool=pubmed. Retrieved March 20, 2014.

Sunshine Vitamin D

Ozaki, Yei Theodora, ed. "The Story of Prince Yamato Take." *Japanese Fairy Tales*. New York: A.L. Burt Company, 1908. etc.usf.edu/lit2go/72/japanese-fairy-tales/4852/the-story-of-prince-yamato-take/. Retrieved March 21, 2014.

Budwig, Johanna. *Flax Oil As a True Aid Against Arthritis Heart Infarction Cancer and Other Diseases*. Vancouver, BC: Apple Publishing Co. Ltd., 1994:50.

www.health.harvard.edu/newsweek/time-for-more-vitamin-d.htm. Retrieved March 20, 2014.

www.johnshopkinshealthalerts.com/reports/prostate_disorders/3115-1.html. Retrieved March 20, 2014.

Servan-Schreiber, David. *Anticancer: A New Way of Life*. New York: Viking Penguin, 2008:126.

Faloon, William. "Vitamin D Blood Levels in Life Extension Readers 3 Years Later." *LifeExtension Special Winter Retail Edition*. 2012/2013:22-23.

Tea: Fill it to the Brim

www.hopkinsmedicine.org/neurology_neurosurgery/specialty_areas/pediatric_neurosurgery/patient/prepare_procedure.html. Retrieved March 20, 2014.

Moss, Ralph. *Herbs Against Cancer*. Brooklyn, NY: Equinox Press, 1998:108-135, 157-158.

www.mskcc.org/cancer-care/herb/essiac. Retrieved March 20, 2014.

www.livestrong.com/article/111323-concerns-essiac-tea/. Retrieved March 20, 2014.

Moss, Ralph. *Cancer Therapy: The Independent Consumer's Guide to Non-Toxic Treatment & Prevention*. Brooklyn, NY: Equinox Press, 1996:147, 163.

Yance, Donald R. Jr., with Arlene Valentine. *Herbal Medicine Healing and Cancer: A Comprehensive Program for Prevention and Treatment*. Lincolnwood, IL: Keats Pub., 1999:119.

Aggarwal, Bharat B., with Debora Yost. *Healing Spices: How to use 50 Everyday and Exotic Spices to Boost Health*. New York: Sterling Publishing, 2011:201, 202.

Horner, Christine. *Waking the Warrior Goddess*. Laguna Beach, CA: Basic Health Publications, Inc., 2005:91-93.

Servan-Schreiber, David. *Anticancer: A New Way of Life*. New York: Viking Penguin, 2008:120.

cincinnati.com/blogs/cookingwithrita/2013/01/14/try-herbal-teas/. Retrieved March 20, 2014.

Treat Yourself Right
Servan-Schreiber, David. *Anticancer: A New Way of Life*. New York: Viking Penguin, 2008:63, 128.
Aggarwal, Bharat B., with Debora Yost. *Healing Spices: How to use 50 Everyday and Exotic Spices to Boost Health.* New York: Sterling Publishing, 2011:253.
Weighing In
"Raag Basant." Section 29, Part 7. Shri Guru Granth Sahib. www.sacred-texts.com/skh/granth/gr29.htm. Retrieved on March 21, 2014.
en.wikipedia.org/wiki/Gurmukh. Retrieved on March 21, 2014.
Whole Foods: Taste the Whole Rainbow
Cleary, Thomas, trans. The Qur'an: A New Translation. Chicago: Starlatch Press, 2004.

B. Minding the Body

Acupressure: Get to the Point
Mitchell, Stephen, trans. *Tao Te Ching: A New English Version*. New York: HarperCollins Publishers, 2000:42.
www.holisticonline.com/Acupuncture/acp_yin_yang.htm. Retrieved March 21, 2014.
www.acupressure.com/articles/immune_system_boosting.htm. Retrieved March 21, 2014.
www.eclecticenergies.com/acupressure/howto.php. Retrieved March 21, 2014.
www.chinese-holistic-health-exercises.com/exercise-for-lower-back.html. Retrieved March 21, 2014.
Art: Draw it Out
"Raag Raamkalee." Section 22, Part 004. Shri Guru Granth Sahib. www.sacred-texts.com/skh/granth/gr22.htm. Retrieved March 21, 2014.
Body Fullness Meditation
Nhất Hạnh, Thích. *Transformation & Healing: Sutra on the Four Establishments of Mindfulness.* Berkeley, CA: Parallax Press, 1990. www.buddhism.org/Sutras/2/FourGroundsSutra.htm. Retrieved March 21, 2014.
Breasts: Cleaving of Cleavage
Lesko, Barbara S. "Utterance 703, Egyptian text." *The Great Goddesses of Egypt*. Norman, OK: University of Oklahoma Press, 1999:65.
Siegel, Bernie S. *Love, Medicine, & Miracles: Lessons Learned About Self-healing from a Surgeon's Experience with Exceptional Patients*. New York: Harper & Row, 1986:76.
Breath: In-spiring
Woodman, Marion K. *Bone: Dying into Life*. New York: Penguin Books, 2001:121.
Chakras: Raising Life-force Energy
Yogananda, Paramahansa. *God Talks with Arjuna: The Bhagavad Gita, Royal Science of God-Realization*. Los Angeles: Self-Realization Fellowship, 2001:740.
Chiropractic: Make Straight the Way of the Lord
Yogananda, Paramahansa. *The Second Coming of Christ: The Resurrection of the Christ Within You*. Los Angeles: Self-Realization Fellowship, 2008:117.
Detox Baths: You're Soaking in it
www.pureinsideout.com/ginger-bath.html. Retrieved March 21, 2014.
Energy Work
Bahá'u'lláh, *Epistle to the Son of the Wolf.* Wilmette, IL: Bahá'í Publishing Trust, 1953:21-22.
Ornish, Dean. *Love and Survival: The Scientific Basis for the Healing Power of Intimacy*. New York: HarperCollins, 1998:303.
Moritz, Andreas. *Cancer is Not a Disease: It's a Survival Mechanism*. Brevard, NC: Ener-chi.com, 2008:63.
Exercise: Have a Ball
Servan-Schreiber, David. *Anticancer: A New Way of Life*. New York: Viking Penguin, 2008:182-3, 185, 186.
Hand Yoga: Your Health is in Your Hands
Cleary, Thomas, trans. The Qur'an: A New Translation. Chicago: Starlatch Press, 2004.
Mesko, Sabrina. *Healing Mudras*. New York: Ballantine Publishing Group, 2000.
Hirschi, Gertrud. *Mudras*. York Beach, ME: Samuel Weiser Inc., 2000.

Inflammation: Smother the Fire
Harding, Elizabeth U. *Kali: The Black Goddess of Dakshineswar*. York Beach, ME: Nicolas-Hays, 1993:xix-xxii.
Hoffnung, David. "The Inflammatory Factor Underlying Most Cancers." *LifeExtension*. November/December 2011:39-47.
Servan-Schreiber, David. *Anticancer: A New Way of Life*. New York: Viking Penguin, 2008:35, 39.

Qi Gong: Ancient Chinese Secret, eh?
Goddard, Dwight. *Tao Teh King*. New York: Brentano's Publishers, 1919. www.sacred-texts.com/tao/ltw/tao64. htm. Retrieved March 21, 2014.
Sykes, Claire. "Go with the Flow: Tai Chi and Qi Gong are Two Gentle Practices Designed to Keep Your Energy Moving." *Energy Times*. January 2012:14-15.

Sound Healing: Good Vibrations
Harding, Elizabeth U. *Kali: The Black Goddess of Dakshineswar*. York Beach, ME: Nicolas-Hays, 1993:xix-xxii.
Chopra, Deepak. "Magical Mind, Magical Body." Audio CD. New York: Simon & Schuster Audio/Nightingale-Conant, 2003.
McTaggart, Lynne. *The Field: The Quest for the Secret Force of the Universe*. New York: Harper, 2008:50-51.
Yogananda, Paramahansa. *Where There Is Light: Insight and Inspiration for Meeting Life's Challenges*. Los Angeles: Self-Realization Fellowship, 1989:193.

Stress Trek
Tzu, Lao. *Tao Te Ching*. Lexington, KY: Pacific Publishing Studio, 2010:44.
Boik, John. *Cancer and Natural Medicine: A Textbook of Basic Sciences and Clinical Research*. Princeton, MN: Oregon Medical Press, 1996:171.
Servan-Schreiber, David. *Anticancer: A New Way of Life*. New York: Viking Penguin, 2008:41, 61.

Synesthesia: Raiders of the Lost Art
voices.yahoo.com/is-kabbalah-form-spiritual-synesthesia-4121741.html. Retrieved March 21, 2014.
Villoldo, Alberto. *Shaman, Healer, Sage: How to Heal Yourself and Others with the Energy Medicine of the Americas*. New York: Harmony Books, 2000:116-117.

Uterus: Seat of Compassion
Trible, Phyllis, trans. Jeremiah 31:20. *God and the Rhetoric of Sexuality*. Philadelphia: Fortress Press, 1978:50.
Parales, Heidi Bright. *Hidden Voices: Biblical Women and Our Christian Heritage*. Macon, GA: Smyth & Helwys, 1998:140-141.

Yoga: May the Force be with You
J Am Acad Nurse Pract. 2011 Mar;23(3):135-42. doi: 10.1111/j.1745-7599.2010.00573.x. Epub 2010 Nov 5. Banasik J, Williams H, Haberman M, Blank SE, Bendel R.
www.cancer.org/treatment/treatmentsandsideeffects/complementaryandalternativemedicine/mindbodyandspirit/yoga Retrieved March 21, 2014.
Guthrie, Catherine. *Health* (Time Inc. Health). Apr 01, 2005; Vol. 19, No. 3:120-126.
Holtby, Lisa. *Healing Yoga for People Living with Cancer*. Lanham, MD: Taylor Trade Publishing, 2004:8-9.

Your Physical Environment: Freeing Yourself from Chemicals
Servan-Schreiber, David. "AntiCancer Action." *Anticancer: A New Way of Life*. New York: Viking Penguin, 2008:2, 6, 7.
www.panna.org. Retrieved March 21, 2014.

C. Mapping the Emotions

Introduction to Mapping the Emotions: Linking Heart and Body
Berenson, David, and Sheryl Cohen. *A Guide to the Map of Emotions©*, 2011:2-12.

Anger: Eggs of Wrath
Masters, Robert. *The Goddess Sekhmet*. St. Paul, MN: Llewellyn, 1991:45-46.
William Congreve (1670–1729) wrote this in his play, "The Mourning Bride."
Boik, John. *Cancer and Natural Medicine: A Textbook of Basic Sciences and Clinical Research*. Princeton, MN: Oregon Medical Press, 1996:171.
Tolle, Eckhart. *The Power of Now: A Guide to Spiritual Enlightenment*. Namaste Publishing, 2004:158.

Authenticity: Be the Real Thing

Singh, Nikki-Guninder Kaur, trans. Rag Dhanasri Mahalla 1, "Hymn of Praise." *The Name of My Beloved: Verses of the Sikh Gurus.* San Francisco: Harper San Francisco, 1996:140.

Lee, Blaine. *The Power Principle: Influence with Honor.* New York: Simon & Schuster, 1997:166.

Rumi, Maulana Jalalu-'d-din Muhammad. The Masnavi, abridged and translated by E.H. Whinfield, 1898. www.sacred-texts.com/isl/masnavi/msn01.htm. Retrieved March 15, 2015.

Breaking Childhood Contracts: Silence of Lambs

Lazaris channels through Jach Pursel. "Ending Shame II: The Psychic Contracts of Pain." lazaris.com/. Retrieved March 25, 2014.

Childhood Issues: Get a Little Closure

Müller, Max, and Max Fausböll. *Sacred Books of the East, Vol. 10: The Dhammapada and Sutta Nipata.* Oxford, England: Clarendon Press, 1881:1.5. www.sacred-texts.com/bud/sbe10/sbe1003.htm. Retrieved March 25, 2014.

Courage: Saddling up Your Horse Anyway

Siegel, Bernie, with Andrea Hurst. *A Book of Miracles: Inspiring True Stories of Healing, Gratitude, and Love.* Novato, CA: New World Library, 2011:60.

Crying for a Mother

Big Thunder (Bedagi) Wabanaki Algonquin, from www.ilhawaii.net/~stony/quotes.html. Retrieved March 25, 2014.

Daily Excitement: You Deserve a Break Each Day

Emmerick, R.E., trans. *The Sutra of Golden Light: Being a Translation of the Suvarnabhasottamasutra.* London: Pali Text Society, 1970. In Shaw, Miranda. *Buddhist Goddesses of India.* Princeton, NJ: Princeton University Press, 2006:34.

Depression: The Pause that Depresses

Brown, Joseph Epes, ed. *The Sacred Pipe: Black Elk's Account of the Seven Rites of the Oglala Sioux.* Norman, OK: University of Oklahoma Press, 1953:115.

Embracing the Feminine

Sinha, Jadunath, trans. *Rama Prasada's Devotional Songs: The Cult of Shakti.* Calcutta: Sinha Publishing House, 1966:no.6:3.

EMDR: Eye Movement Desensitization and Reprocessing

Goddard, Dwight. *Tao Teh King.* New York: Brentano's Publishers, 1919. www.sacred-texts.com/tao/ltw/tao33.htm. Retrieved March 25, 2014.

www.emdr.com/. Retrieved March 25, 2014.

Emotional Freedom Technique: Free at Last, Free at Last...

Shree Chitrabhanu, Gurudev. *Twelve Facets of Reality: The Jain Path to Freedom.* New York: Dodd, Mead & Company, 1980:xi.

Fear of Dying

Wilber, Ken. *Grace and Grit: Spirituality and Healing in the Life and Death of Treya Killam Wilber.* Boston: Shambhala, 1991:77.

Norwich, Julian of. *Revelations of Divine Love.* Guildford, England: White Crow Books, 2011:68.

"Little Big Man." Los Angeles: 20th Century Fox, 1970.

Gratitude Attitude

Voskamp, Ann. *One Thousand Gifts: A Dare to Live Fully Right Where You Are.* Grand Rapids, MI: Zondervan, 2011:32-36.

Healing the Shame that Blinds You

Ornish, Dean. *Love and Survival: The Scientific Basis for the Healing Power of Intimacy.* New York: HarperCollins, 1998:181.

Berenson, David, and Sheryl Cohen. *A Guide to the Map of Emotions©*, 2011:6.

I Want to Live

Joachim, H. *Papyros Ebers, das älteste Buch über Heilkunde.* Berlin: Walter de Gruyter, reprint, 1973:2. In Lesko, Barbara S. *The Great Goddesses of Egypt.* Norman, OK: University of Oklahoma Press, 1999. Ebers papyrus was written about 1500 BC, but probably copied from texts dating as far back as 3400 BC.

www.womenontheedgeofevolution.com. Retrieved March 25, 2014.

Journaling: Writing Down to Your Bones

J Clin Oncol 20:4160-4168. ©2002 by American Society of Clinical Oncology.

Results: "Compared with CTL participants at 3 months, the EMO group reported significantly decreased physical symptoms, and EMO and POS participants had significantly fewer medical appointments for cancer-related morbidities.

"Conclusion: Experimentally induced emotional expression and benefit finding regarding early-stage breast cancer reduced medical visits for cancer-related morbidities. Effects on psychological outcomes varied as a function of cancer-related avoidance."

Joy: Predictor of Survival

Rinpoche, Bokar, trans. by Christiane Buchet. Stanza 10, "Praise of the Twenty-one-fold Homage in The Seven Hundred Thoughts, The King of the Tara Tantra." *Tara: The Feminine Divine.* San Francisco: Clear Point Press, 1999:89.

Templeton, Sir John. *Wisdom from the World Religions: Pathways Toward Heaven on Earth.* Philadelphia: Templeton Foundation Press, 2002:123.

Goleman, Daniel. Article in *The New York Times.* September 17, 1987. In Wilber, Ken. *Grace and Grit: Spirituality and Healing in the Life and Death of Treya Killam Wilber.* Boston: Shambhala, 1991:291.

Siegel, Bernie S. *Love, Medicine, & Miracles: Lessons Learned About Self-healing from a Surgeon's Experience with Exceptional Patients.* New York: Harper & Row, 1986:96, 97.

Looking Fear in the Face

Cleary, Thomas, trans. The Qur'an: A New Translation. Chicago: Starlatch Press, 2004.

Wolkstein, Diane, ed. Ed Young, ill. *The Red Lion: A Tale of Ancient Persia.* New York: Crowell, 1977.

Love YourSelf

Yogananda, Paramahansa. *God Talks with Arjuna: The Bhagavad Gita, Royal Science of God-Realization.* Los Angeles: Self-Realization Fellowship, 2001:234.

Peggy O'Neill, guest on the online teleseminar series called "Women on the Edge of Evolution." www.womenontheedgeofevolution.com/people/peggy-oneill.php. Retrieved March 25, 2014.

Map of Emotions©: Let it Be

Berenson, David, and Sheryl Cohen. *A Guide to the Map of Emotions©,* 2011.

Feng, Gia-Fu, and Jane English, trans. Lao Tsu, *Tao Te Ching.* New York: Vintage Books, 1972: 76.

Memory or Imagination: Childhood Sexual Abuse

Loftus, Elizabeth. "The Memory Wars." *science&spirit,* March/April 2004:29-34.

Old Griefs

Section 11, Part 011, "Raag Bihaagra." Shri Guru Granth Sahib. www.sacred-texts.com/skh/granth/gr11.htm. Retrieved March 25, 2014.

Schimmel, Annemarie, trans. *Look! This is Love: Poems of Rūmī.* Boston: Shambhala, 1996:102.

Williams, Margery. *The Velveteen Rabbit (or How Toys Become Real).* New York: George H. Doran Company, 1922.

Berenson, David, and Sheryl Cohen. *A Guide to the Map of Emotions©,* 2011.

Opening My Heart

Rodwell, JM. The Koran. London: B. Quaritch, 1876. www.sacred-texts.com/isl/qr/094.htm. Retrieved April 25, 2014.

Saleem, Shehzad. Qur'an 94:1. www.teachislam.com/dmdocuments/8/Surah%20Alam%20Nashrah.pdf. Retrieved March 25, 2014.

www.inplainsite.org/html/quran_miracles_and_prophecy.html. Retrieved March 25, 2014.

Woodman, Marion K. "The Crown of Age" CD. Louisville, CO: Sounds True, Inc., 2005.

Rūmī, Jelal-'d-din, and Shemsu-'d-Din Ahmed, trans. by James W. Redhouse. "The Reed Flute." *The Mesnevi and The Acts of the Adepts.* London: Trübner & Co., Ludgate Hill, 1881:1. www.sacred-texts.com/isl/mes/mes15.htm. Retrieved March 25, 2014.

Paradigm Shift Happens

Spontaneous Remission Bibliography Project of the Institute of Noetic Sciences. www.noetic.org/research/project/online-spontaneous-remission-bibliography-project/. Retrieved March 25, 2014.

www.noetic.org/research/project/spontaneous-remission/faqs/#question7. Retrieved March 25, 2014. There is a free downloadable pdf file of Appendix 2.

Power of Powerlessness

Berenson, David, and Sheryl Cohen. *A Guide to the Map of Emotions*©, 2011:10.

Rock the Block: Warming the Heart of Stone

Barrett, Clive. "Freya and Odur." *The Viking Gods: Pagan Myths of Nordic Peoples*. Northamptonshire, England: The Aquarian Press, 1989:68.

Markova, Dawna. *I Will Not Die an Unlived Life: Reclaiming Purpose and Passion*. San Francisco: Conari Press, 2000:38.

Shadow Work: Dark Night Rises

Wolkstein, Diane, and Samuel Noah Kramer. *Inanna, Queen of Heaven and Earth: Her Stories and Hymns from Sumer*. New York: Harper & Row, Publishers, 1983:59-60, 158, 160-161.

Ornish, Dean. *Love and Survival: The Scientific Basis for the Healing Power of Intimacy*. New York: HarperCollins, 1998:439.

Spiral Staircase

Sangharakshita, trans. *The Dhammapada: The Way of Truth*. Birmingham, England: Windhorse Publications, 2008:9,123.

Tapas Acupressure Technique: The Deed Hunter

www.tatlife.com/. Retrieved March 25, 2014.

Visiting the World of Shadows

Carlson, Kathie. "Hymn to Demeter." *Life's Daughter/Death's Bride: Inner Transformations Through the Goddess Demeter/Persephone*. Boston: Shambhala, 1997:33.

D. Introduction to Mending the Mind: Entering Peace Like an Arrow

Byrom, Thomas, trans. *Dhammapada* 3:43. info.stiltij.nl/publiek/meditatie/soetras2/dhammapada_byrom.pdf. Retrieved March 25, 2014.

Murcott, Susan. *First Buddhist Women, Poems and Stories of Awakening*. Berkeley, CA: Parallax Press, 2006:163.

Wilber, Ken. *Grace and Grit: Spirituality and Healing in the Life and Death of Treya Killam Wilber*. Boston: Shambhala, 1991:99.

Goleman, Daniel. "New Focus on Multiple Personality." May 21, 1985. www.nytimes.com/1985/05/21/science/new-focus-on-multiple-personality.html. Retrieved March 25, 2014.

Tolle, Eckhart. *The Power of Now: A Guide to Spiritual Enlightenment*. Novato, CA: New World Library, 2004:209.

Affirmations: Great Expectations

Müller, Max, and Max Fausböll. *Sacred Books of the East, Vol. 10: The Dhammapada and Sutta Nipata*. Oxford, England: Clarendon Press, 1881:1.2. www.sacred-texts.com/bud/sbe10/sbe1003.htm. Retrieved March 25, 2014.

Hay, Louise. *You Can Heal Your Life Paperback*. Carlsbad, CA: Hay House, 1984:43.

Yogananda, Paramahansa. *Scientific Healing Affirmations: Theory and Practice of Concentration*. Los Angeles: Self-Realization Fellowship, 2007:40.

Anxiety Pills

Berenson, David, and Sheryl Cohen. *A Guide to the Map of Emotions*©, 2011:2-12.

Be Self-full

Siegel, Bernie S. *Love, Medicine, & Miracles: Lessons Learned About Self-healing from a Surgeon's Experience with Exceptional Patients*. New York: Harper & Row, 1986:66, 124.

Woodward, F.L., trans. "The Hidden Treasure." *Some Sayings of the Buddha According to the Pali Canon*. Oxford, England: Oxford University Press, 1945:43.

Blame Games

www.kenwilber.com/Writings/PDF/hi_folks.pdf. Retrieved March 25, 2014.

Mafi, Maryam, and Azima Melita Kolin, trans. *Rūmī: Gardens of the Beloved*. London: Element, 2003:167.

Bucket List: As You Like It

Woodward, F.L., trans. "After Death." i. 279, "Anguttara Nikaya." *Some Sayings of the Buddha According to the Pali Canon*. Oxford, England: Oxford University Press, 1945:43.

Cause of Cancer: Check-mate

Wilber, Ken. *Grace and Grit: Spirituality and Healing in the Life and Death of Treya Killam Wilber*. Boston: Shambhala, 1991:220 (Treya), 261-262 (Ken).

Ornish, Dean. *Love and Survival: The Scientific Basis for the Healing Power of Intimacy*. New York: HarperCollins, 1998:303.

Disease is Evil: A Farewell to Harms

Shoghi Effendi, trans., Baha'u'llah, "CXLVI." *Prayers and Meditations*. Wilmette, IL: Baha'i Publishing Trust, 1996:235.

Yogananda, Paramahansa. *God Talks with Arjuna: The Bhagavad Gita, Royal Science of God-Realization*. Los Angeles: Self-Realization Fellowship, 2001:552-553.

Hagin, Kenneth. *God's Word on Divine Healing*. Tulsa, OK: Faith Library Publications, 2003.

Romans 5:20. King James Bible, Cambridge Ed., 11.

Exercising the Will: How to Tame Your Dragon

Davids, T.W. Rhys, trans. "The Book of that Great Decease." 2:28-30, *Buddhist Suttas*. Oxford: Clarendon Press, 1881. www.sacred-texts.com/bud/sbe11/sbe1103.htm. Retrieved March 26, 2014.

Siegel, Bernie S. *Love, Medicine, & Miracles: Lessons Learned About Self-healing from a Surgeon's Experience with Exceptional Patients*. New York: Harper & Row, 1986:184-5.

Family Patterns: Repetition Compulsion

Villoldo, Alberto. *Shaman, Healer, Sage: How to Heal Yourself and Others with the Energy Medicine of the Americas*. New York: Harmony Books, 2000:59.

Forgiveness: Stairway to Heaven

Jane, Padgett, trans. Jain salutation. "Ahimsa: A Jaina Way of Personal Discipline." 21.

Berenson, David, and Sheryl Cohen. *A Guide to the Map of Emotions*©, 2011.

Gift Nobody Wants

Effendi, Shoghi, trans. Baha'u'llah, *"The Kitab-i-iqan" (The Book of Certitude)*. Wilmette, IL: Bahá'í Pub. Trust, 1983:219.

I Will Survive

Goddard, Dwight. *Tao Teh King*. New York: Brentano's Publishers, 1919:30. www.sacred-texts.com/tao/ltw/tao33.htm. Retrieved March 25, 2014.

Moorjani, Anita. *Dying To Be Me: My Journey from Cancer, to Near Death, to True Healing*. Carlsbad, CA: Hay House, 2012:75.

Image Cycling: The Bengston Technique

www.soundstrue.com/shop/Hands-On-Healing/2656.productdetails. Retrieved March 25, 2014.

Leaving the Land of Confusion

Berenson, David, and Sheryl Cohen. *A Guide to the Map of Emotions*©, 2011:6.

Lucky or Unlucky? God only Knows

Suzuki, D.T., and Paul Carus, trans. *The Canon of Reason and Virtue (Lao-tze's Tao Teh King)*. La Salle, IL: Open Court, 1913:58.

Making Decisions: An Answer is Blowing in the Wind

www.pbs.org/wgbh/nova/ancient/history-pearls.html. Retrieved March 19, 2014.

Questioning Faith

There's a nice summary of the Book of Job at www.sparknotes.com/lit/oldtestament/section11.rhtml. Retrieved March 19, 2014.

1 John 4:8, Christian Bible, New International Version.

Jeremiah 31:2, Jewish Bible.

Qur'an 20:39.

Re-member

Ornish, Dean. *Love and Survival: The Scientific Basis for the Healing Power of Intimacy*. New York: HarperCollins, 1998: Jon Kabat-Zinn, 312.

Resentment: Raging Bull

Hay, Louise. *You Can Heal Your Life*. Carlsbad, CA: Hay House, 1999:180, 185.

Self-Acceptance

Tzu, Lao. *Tao Te Ching*. Lexington, KY: Pacific Publishing Studio, 2010:46.

Songs Bubble Up

Lesko, Barbara S. "Song of praise for the Egyptian Goddess Hathor." *The Great Goddesses of Egypt*. Norman, OK: University of Oklahoma Press, 1999:125.

Petra, "Clean," in "Beat the System." 1990.

Johnny Nash, "I Can See Clearly Now," in "I Can See Clearly Now." 1972.

Using Cancer: Don't Waste Your Sorrows

Woodward, F.L. trans. "It is Time for Me to Go." ii. 120, "Digha Nikaya." *Some Sayings of the Buddha According to the Pali Canon*. Oxford, England: Oxford University Press, 1945:226.

Wilber, Ken. *Grace and Grit: Spirituality and Healing in the Life and Death of Treya Killam Wilber*. Boston: Shambhala, 1991:52.

"The Curious Case of Benjamin Button." Paramount, 2008.

E. Introduction to It Takes a Village: Sharing the Moment...Sharing Life

Ornish, Dean. *Love and Survival: The Scientific Basis for the Healing Power of Intimacy*. New York: HarperCollins, 1998:400.

Dances with Women

Bolen, Jean Shinoda. "The Myth of Amaterasu." *Goddesses in Older Women: Archetypes in Women over Fifty*. New York: HarperCollins Publishers Inc., 2001:104.

Mafi, Maryam, and Azima Melita Kolin, trans. *Rūmī: Gardens of the Beloved*. London: Element, 2003:52.

Erdos, Richard. *Crying for a Dream: The World through Native American Eyes*. Rochester, VT: Bear & Company, 2001:16.

Death and Rebirth Ceremonies

Surinder Deol and Daler Deol, "Meditation 13." *Japji: The Path of Devotional Meditation*. Washington, DC: Mount Meru Books, 1998:36.

Drucker, Karen. "The Heart of Healing." CD.

Gratitude's Gifts

Rūmī, Jalāl ad-Dīn. Barks, Coleman, and John Moyne, trans. *The Essential Rūmī*. New York: HarperOne, 2004:109.

Voskamp, Ann. *One Thousand Gifts: A Dare to Live Fully Right Where You Are*. Grand Rapids, MI: Zondervan, 2011.

Laughter: Have a Joke and a Smile

Bolen, Jean Shinoda. *Goddesses in Older Women: Archetypes in Women over Fifty*. New York: HarperCollins Publishers, 2001:101.

Lubell, Winifred Milius. *The Metamorphosis of Baubo: Myths of Women's Sexual Energy*. Nashville, TN: Vanderbilt University Press, 1994:34.

Siegel, Bernie S. *Love, Medicine, & Miracles: Lessons Learned About Self-healing from a Surgeon's Experience with Exceptional Patients*. New York: Harper & Row, 1986:144.

Integrative Medicine Clinic notebook. The University of Texas MD Anderson Cancer Center Patient Education Office, 2006:1.

F. Soaring with Spirit

Acceptance of Death: Jephthah's Daughter

Thoresen, Lasse. 'Abdu'l-Baha, "Divine Art of Living." *Unlocking the Gate of the Heart*. Oxford, England: George Ronald, 1998:65.

Yogananda, Paramahansa. *God Talks with Arjuna: The Bhagavad Gita, Royal Science of God-Realization*. Los Angeles: Self-Realization Fellowship, 2001:xiv.

Markova, Dawna. *I Will Not Die an Unlived Life: Reclaiming Purpose and Passion*. San Francisco: Conari Press, 2000:99, 107, 115, 127.

Allowing: Loving the Questions

Tzu, Lao. *Tao Te Ching*. Lexington, KY: Pacific Publishing Studio, 2010.

McTaggart, Lynne. *The Field: The Quest for the Secret Force of the Universe*. New York: HarperCollins, 2002:193.

Rilke, Rainer Maria. Herter Norton, trans. "Letter Four," 16 July 1903. *Letters to a Young Poet*. New York: W.W. Norton & Company Inc., 1934:34-35.

Big Dharma

www.wisdomquotes.com/authors/kahlil-gibran/. Retrieved March 19, 2014.

buddhism.about.com/od/theeightfoldpath/a/The-Four-Foundations-Of-Mindfulness.htm. Retrieved March 19, 2014.

Dark Night: Abduction into the Depths

Carlson, Kathie. "Myth of Persephone." *Life's Daughter/Death's Bride: Inner Transformations Through the Goddess Demeter/Persephone*. Boston: Shambhala, 1997:20.

Directed Prayer

Yogananda, Paramahansa. *Whispers from Eternity: A Book of Answered Prayers*. Los Angeles: Self-Realization Publishing House, 1929:8, 14, 16.

Yogananda, Paramahansa. *Scientific Healing Affirmations*. Los Angeles: Self-Realization Publishing House, 1981:52.

Embody the Divine: Transformers

Tsu, Lao. Feng, Gia-Fu, and Jane English, trans. *Tao Te Ching*. New York: Vintage Books, 1972:14.

Sharma, Hari, James G. Meade, Rama K. Mishra, *The Answer to Cancer: Is Never Giving It a Chance to Start*. New York: SelectBooks, Inc., 2002:160-1.

"The Moses Code." Hay House, 2008.

Enlightenment: Knockin' on Heaven's Gate

Brach, Tara. *Radical Acceptance: Embracing Your Life With the Heart of a Buddha*. New York: Bantam Books, 2003:72.

Faith and Trust

"Peter Lundy and the Medicine Hat Stallion." GoodTimes Entertainment, 2006.

Field of Dreams

Erdos, Richard. *Crying for a Dream: The World through Native American Eyes*. Rochester, VT: Bear & Company, 2001:28.

Von Franz, Marie Louise. *The Feminine in Fairy Tales*, rev. ed. Boston: Shambhala, 1993:158.

Intuition: Let Your Heart be Your Guide

Surinder Deol and Daler Deol, "The Japji." 4, *Japji: The Path of Devotional Meditation* (Washington, DC: Mount Meru Books, 1998:31.

Mafi, Maryam, and Azima Melita Kolin, trans. *Rūmī: Gardens of the Beloved*. London: Element, 2003:38.

Qur'an 47:17

Kübler-Ross, Elizabeth, quote in Siegel, Bernie S. *Love, Medicine, & Miracles: Lessons Learned About Self-healing from a Surgeon's Experience with Exceptional Patients*. New York: Harper & Row, 1986:215.

Mindfulness Meditation: Lose Yourself

Sangharakshita, trans. *The Dhammapada: The Way of Truth*. Birmingham, England: Windhorse Publications, 2008:3:37.

www.meditationexpert.com/health-relaxation/h_meditation_methods_to_help_fight_cancer.htm. Retrieved March 24, 2010.

Servan-Schreiber, David. *Anticancer: A New Way of Life*. New York: Viking Penguin, 2008:163.

Mothership: Feminine Transformative Substance

Yogananda, Paramahansa. *The Second Coming of Christ: The Resurrection of the Christ Within You*. Los Angeles: Self-Realization Fellowship, 2008:219, 220.

Not Suffering

Yogananda, Paramahansa. *God Talks with Arjuna: The Bhagavad Gita, Royal Science of God-Realization*. Los Angeles: Self-Realization Fellowship, 2001:201.

Remission: Sustainable Hope

Siegel, Bernie S. *Love, Medicine, & Miracles: Lessons Learned About Self-healing from a Surgeon's Experience with Exceptional Patients*. New York: Harper & Row, 1986:29.

Dossey, Larry. *Healing Words: The Power of Prayer and the Practice of Medicine*. San Francisco: Harper San Francisco, 1993:241-242.

www.meditationexpert.com/health-relaxation/h_meditation_methods_to_help_fight_cancer.htm. Retrieved
March 24, 2010.

Sin Big

Mitchell, Stephen, trans. *Tao Te Ching: A New English Version*. New York: HarperCollins Publishers, 2000:2.

Daly, Mary. "SIN BIG." *The New Yorker*, February 26, 1996.

Surrendering: Offering no Resistance to the Divine

Rodwell, JM. The Koran. London: B. Quaritch, 1876. www.sacred-texts.com/isl/pick/003.htm. Retrieved April 25,
2014.

Yogananda, Paramahansa. *The Second Coming of Christ: The Resurrection of the Christ Within You*. Los Angeles:
Self-Realization Fellowship, 2008:1446.

The Present Moment: It's Now or Never

Deol, Surinder, and Daler Deol. "Meditation 28." *Japji: The Path of Devotional Meditation.* Washington, DC:
Mount Meru Books, 1998:119.

Browning, Elizabeth B. *Aurora Leigh (Oxford World's Classics)*. New York: Oxford University Press, USA,
2008:246.

Undirected Prayer: Help, Thanks

Dossey, Larry. *Healing Words: The Power of Prayer and the Practice of Medicine*. San Francisco: Harper San Francisco, 1993.

Murray, Michael. *How to Prevent and Treat Cancer with Natural Medicine*. New York: Riverhead Books, 2002:192.

www.newbeginningsprayer.org/mertonreflections.html. Retrieved March 20, 2014.

Merton, Thomas. *New Seeds of Contemplation*. New York: New Directions; Reprint Edition, 2007:221.

Upside-down Trees

Villoldo, Alberto. *Shaman, Healer, Sage: How to Heal Yourself and Others with the Energy Medicine of the Americas*. New York: Harmony Books, 2000:52.

Visualizations: Just Imagine

Wilber, Ken. *Grace and Grit: Spirituality and Healing in the Life and Death of Treya Killam Wilber*. Boston: Shambhala, 1991: Ken, 263.

Siegel, Bernie S. *Love, Medicine, & Miracles: Lessons Learned About Self-healing from a Surgeon's Experience with
Exceptional Patients*. New York: Harper & Row, 1986:69, 152, 155, 156.

Murray, Michael. *How to Prevent and Treat Cancer with Natural Medicine*. New York: Riverhead Books, 2002:193.

Servan-Schreiber, David. *Anticancer: A New Way of Life*. New York: Viking Penguin, 2008:31.

Walking the Labyrinth: 'Round 'n' 'Round We Go

Davids, T.W. Rhys, trans. "The Book of the Great Decease." *Buddhist Suttas*. New York: Dover Publications, Inc.,
1969, 2:4.

Sharma, Hari, James G. Meade, Rama K. Mishra. *The Answer to Cancer: Is Never Giving It a Chance to Start*. New
York: SelectBooks, Inc., 2002:138, 139.

labyrinthlocator.com/locate-a-labyrinth. Retrieved March 20, 2014.

G. GPS: Guides Providing and Sustaining, even a Donkey

Asclepius: Lucky Strikes

www.vegetarian-nutrition.info/herbs/cinnamon.php. Retrieved March 20, 2014.

Andrews, Ted. *Animal Speak: The Spiritual & Magical Powers of Creatures Great & Small*. St. Paul, MN: Llewellyn
Publications, 1993:362.

Amma: Are You My Mother?

Canan, Janine. *Messages from Amma: In the Language of the Heart*. Berkeley, CA: Celestial Arts, 2004:71.

Black Panther and Feminine Energy: Bringing Light into Darkness

Sams, Jamie. *Medicine Cards: The Discovery of Power Through the Ways of Animals*. New York: St. Martin's Press,
1999:243.

Andrews, Ted. *Animal Speak: The Spiritual & Magical Powers of Creatures Great & Small*. St. Paul, MN: Llewellyn
Publications, 1993:297, 299.

egyptian-gods.org/egyptian-gods-mafdet/. Retrieved March 20, 2014.

www.wisdomlib.org/definition/mafdet/index.html. Retrieved March 20, 2014.

Black Panther and Masculine Energy: Night Stalker

www.reshafim.org.il/ad/egypt/religion/mafdet.htm. Retrieved March 20, 2014.

Faulkner, R.O. *The Ancient Egyptian Pyramid Texts*. Oxford, England: Oxford University Press, 1998:Utterance 295.

Bruno Gröning: Access the Divine Healing Stream

Haüsler, Grete. *An Introduction to the Teachings of Bruno Gröning*. Hennef/Sieg, Germany: Kreis für geistige Lebenshilfe, 2006:7, 8.

www.bruno-Gröning.org/English/. Retrieved March 20, 2014.

Butterflies are Free to Fly

Tzu, Chuang. C. W. Chan, trans. "The Butterfly Dream," *The Philosopher, Volume LXXXIII No.2*. www.the-philosopher.co.uk/butter.htm. Retrieved April 25, 2014.

www.ehow.com/how-does_4565708_caterpillar-change-butterfly.html#ixzz29JVyvLKG. Retrieved March 20, 2014.

www.differencebetween.com/difference-between-cocoon-and-vs-chrysalis/#ixzz29JcDHEBo. Retrieved March 20, 2014.

Glinda: You have Always had the Power

Williamson, Marianne. *A Return to Love: Reflections on the Principles of "A Course in Miracles."* New York: HarperOne, 1996:190.

Jesus: Wounded Healer

Luke 22:44

John 19:1-2

Luke 24:26

Martha: Subduer of Dragons

Moltmann-Wendel, Elisabeth, and Jurgen Moltmann, *Humanity in God*. Cleveland, OH: Pilgrim Press, 1993:17-34.

Other Guides: The Seen and the Unseen

www.newadvent.org/cathen/01203c.htm. Retrieved March 20, 2014.

www.romancatholicidentity.com/2010/02/st-agatha-patron-saint-of-breast-cancer.html. Retrieved March 20, 2014.

Owl: It's all Inside Me

www.animal-symbols.com/owl-symbol.html. Retrieved March 20, 2014.

Paramahansa Yogananda: God's Boatman

Yogananda, Paramahansa. *Whispers from Eternity, 1929 edition*. Los Angeles: Self-Realization Fellowship, 1929:202-203.

Yogananda, Paramahansa. *Whispers from Eternity*. Los Angeles: Self-Realization Fellowship, 2008:111.

Yogananda, Paramahansa. "God's Boatman," *Songs of the Soul*. Los Angeles: Self-Realization Fellowship, 1983:174-175.

Other Resources

*T*hese are some sample resources not cited in the Sources section; many others are available. Inclusion in this list does not imply endorsement. (All websites retrieved March 23, 2014.)

Organizations

American Association of Naturopathic Physicians members use nutrition and lifestyle changes to assist one's body with healing. (866) 538-2267. www.naturopathic.org.

American Cancer Society, a voluntary national organization, works to eliminate cancer. (800) 227-2345. www.cancer.org.

American Herbalists Guild includes registered herbalists who use plant-based remedies to promote health and well-being. (857) 350-3128. www.americanherbalistsguild.com/

American Osteopathic Association (AOA) provides a guide for finding a doctor of osteopathic medicine. Treatments might include a combination of conventional and complementary therapies, such as manipulation of the joints and muscles. (800) 621-1773. www.osteopathic.org/osteopathic-health/Pages/default.aspx.

CancerCare provides counseling, support groups, education, publications, and financial and co-payment assistance, all free. (800) 813-HOPE (4673). www.cancercare.org/.

Cancer Survivors' Network, hosted by the American Cancer Society, offers peer support and its site contents are contributed by its members. csn.cancer.org/csnhome.

Cleaning for a Reason provides house cleanings for women who are in cancer treatment. www.cleaningforareason.org/

Corporate Angel Network arranges *free* air transportation for *cancer* patients traveling to *treatment* by using the empty seats on corporate jets. www.corpangelnetwork.org.

Livestrong Foundation provides resources for cancer patients. www.livestrong.org/. Among them are "cancer hacks"—tips and tricks from other survivors. cancerhacks.livestrong.org/.

Organic Trade Association represents the organic industry in North America. www.ota.com

Sarcoma Alliance serves those with sarcomas. (415) 381-7236. sarcomaalliance.org/.

Books

Boehmer, Tami. *From Incurable to Incredible: Cancer survivors who beat the odds.* CreateSpace Independent Publishing Platform, 2010.

Bradshaw, John. *Healing the Shame the Binds You.* Deerfield Beach, FL: Health Communications Inc., 2005.

Kerastas, John. *Chief Complaint: Brain Tumor.* Santa Fe, NM: Sunstone Press, 2012.

Lipsenthal, Lee. *Enjoy Every Sandwich: Living Each Day as If It Were Your Last.* New York: Harmony, 2011.

Miller, D. Patrick. *A Little Book of Forgiveness: Challenges and Meditations for Anyone with Something to Forgive.* Berkeley, CA: Fearless Books, 1999.

Moss, Ralph W. *Customized Cancer Treatment: How a Powerful Lab Test Predicts Which Drugs Will Work for You—and Which to Avoid.* Brooklyn, NY: Equinox Press, 2010.

Quillin, Patrick, with Noreen Quillin. *Beating Cancer with Nutrition.* Carlsbad, CA: Nutrition Times Press, Inc. 2005.

Websites
(Active at the time of publication of this book.)

Acupuncture points: Find an atlas at www.chiro.org/acupuncture/ABSTRACTS/Acupuncture%20Points.pdf.

Environmental Working Group: Posted a table showing pesticide residue in produce. www.ewg.org.

Healthy-Steps/Lebed Method: A therapy and movement program done to music and designed to assist with moving lymph through the body. www.gohealthysteps.com/.

Honey: Find sources of local honey through www.honey.com.

Imago Relationship Therapy: Developed by Harville Hendrix, PhD. www.imagorelationships.org/.

Lotsa Helping Hands: Enables groups of people to organize services, such as meals, for cancer patients. www.lotsahelpinghands.com.

National Organic Program: Regulates the federal government's organic program. www.ams.usda.gov/nop.

National Center for Homeopathy: (703) 548-7790. www.nationalcenterforhomeopathy.org

Consumer's Union: Publishes *Consumer Reports* magazine. Click on the food tab. www.consumersunion.org.

National Cancer Institute: The federal government's principal agency for cancer research and training. (800) 422-6237. www.cancer.gov.

NCCAM: A collaborative site between the National Center for Complementary and Alternative Medicine and the National Cancer Institute provides an overview of complementary approaches, including what the science says and any concerns about their safety. nccam.nih.gov/health/cancer/camcancer.htm.

PubMed: National Center for Biotechnology Information, U.S. National Library of Medicine, offers research study results. www.ncbi.nlm.nih.gov/pubmed.